Identifying and Estimating the Genetic Impact of Chemical Mutagens

Committee on Chemical Environmental Mutagens

Board on Toxicology and Environmental
Health Hazards

Commission on Life Sciences

National Research Council

NATIONAL ACADEMY PRESS
Washington, D.C. 1983

   The National Research Council was established by the
National Academy of Sciences in 1916 to associate the broad
community of science and technology with the Academy's
purposes of furthering knowledge and of advising the federal
government. The Council operates in accordance with general
policies determined by the Academy under the authority of
its congressional charter of 1863, which establishes the
Academy as a private, nonprofit, self-governing membership
corporation. The Council has become the principal operating
agency of both the National Academy of Sciences and the
National Academy of Engineering in the conduct of their
services to the government, the public, and the scientific
and engineering communities. It is administered jointly by
both Academies and the Institute of Medicine. The National
Academy of Engineering and the Institute of Medicine were
established in 1964 and 1970, respectively, under the
charter of the National Academy of Sciences.

   The evaluation described in this report has been funded
by the United States Environmental Protection Agency
through Contract Number 68-01-5873; however, the report
has not been subjected to Agency review and, therefore,
may not necessarily reflect the views of the Agency.

Library of Congress Catalog Card Number 82-63011
International Standard Book Number 0-309-03345-4

Available from

NATIONAL ACADEMY PRESS
2101 Constitution Avenue, N.W.
Washington, D.C. 20418

Printed in the United States of America

COMMITTEE ON CHEMICAL ENVIRONMENTAL MUTAGENS

James F. Crow, University of Wisconsin, Madison, Chairman
Seymour Abrahamson, University of Wisconsin, Madison,
 Vice-Chairman
Carter Denniston, University of Wisconsin, Madison
David G. Hoel, National Institute of Environmental Health
 Sciences
Eliezer Huberman, Argonne National Laboratory
Peter N. Magee, Fels Research Institute
Daniel W. Nebert, National Institutes of Health
Thomas Roderick, The Jackson Laboratory
Margery W. Shaw, University of Texas Health Science Center,
 Houston
Fred Sherman, University of Rochester
Vincent F. Simmon, Genex Corporation
H. Eldon Sutton, University of Texas, Austin
Sheldon Wolff, University of California, San Francisco

BOTEHH Liaison Representative

John W. Drake, National Institute of Environmental Health
 Sciences

Consultants

George R. Hoffmann, Holy Cross College (Project Director
 from 1/15/79 to 8/4/81)
Michael D. Hogan, National Institute of Environmental
 Health Sciences
Paul B. Selby, Oak Ridge National Laboratory

Staff

John Delehanty, Project Director
Norman Grossblatt, Editor
Shirley Ash, Administrative Secretary

PREFACE

This volume presents the findings of a study started in the fall of 1979. The study was conducted by the Committee on Chemical Environmental Mutagens of the National Research Council's Board on Toxicology and Environmental Health Hazards. It was supported by a contract between the National Academy of Sciences and the Environmental Protection Agency.

The Committee's main conclusions and recommendations are discussed in Chapters 6 and 9 and summarized in Chapter 1. Research recommendations are in Chapter 10. The other chapters provide background and further details.

From the outset the Committee has been plagued by three uncertainties.

First: The impact of mutation on human health and welfare is enormously diverse--as diverse as the range of genetically influenced traits. The effects are spread over many generations with no certainty about when a particular trait will be expressed. The Committee knows of no reliable way to estimate the total genetic impact of an increased mutation rate. We have to be content with estimating the earlier and more tangible part of the effect, that caused by dominant gene mutations and chromosomal aberrations.

Second: There is no way to detect and measure the rate of occurrence of human germinal mutations. We must rely on information from experimental organisms and cell-culture test systems and on the belief that these tests mimic what happens in human germ cells.

Third: There has been spectacular progress in developing short-term tests that use microorganisms and mammalian cell cultures. These tests are sensitive, efficient, reproducible, and inexpensive, but their relevance for humans is uncertain. Germinal tests on laboratory mice are presumably more relevant, but are less sensitive and more expensive. Do we assign more weight to the consensus of several short-term tests or to a mammalian test? Every group that deals with this situation confronts the same dilemma. Our recommendation is to use short-term tests for initial screening of a large number of compounds and reserve the more expensive mouse tests for the small minority of crucial decisions for which information from a variety of sources is important.

We recognize that the state of knowledge is such that no system can provide complete protection against mutagens. We also recognize that it is possible to be too careful and to be so preoccupied with one kind of risk that other, more important ones are neglected. We believe that the system proposed here provides a practical set of tests that can be applied to a large number of chemicals without inordinate expense and that it provides as adequate protection for the population as is feasible in the present state of knowledge. We emphasize, and urge manufacturers and regulators to recognize, that better information is sure to be forthcoming and that any system must be revised periodically.

The writing of this report was a group effort and used each person's special knowledge. Everyone--members, consultants, project directors--contributed language. The report was considered in detail in Committee meetings and represents the collective judgment of the group.

The Committee members are appreciative of the technical help provided by our consultants, Paul B. Selby and Michael D. Hogan. We were fortunate in having George R. Hoffmann and John Delehanty as scientifically knowledgeable and conscientious project directors and Shirley Ash as an efficient administrative secretary. Norman Grossblatt edited the manuscript. We profited by useful suggestions from Robert Tardiff and Alvin Lazen. We also appreciate the speed and thoroughness with which John Wassom and Elizabeth von Halle at the Environmental Mutagen Information Center provided essential data compilation. Finally, we should like to thank the reviewers of the manuscript; the final product is much better as a result of their detailed, thoughtful, and critical comments.

                              James F. Crow
                              Chairman

CONTENTS

1

SUMMARY AND CONCLUSIONS

There are now some 70,000 synthetic chemicals in commerce, of which more than 25,000 are in common use. In addition, thousands of chemicals occur naturally. Many chemicals are essential for life, and others are of great social and economic benefit. Some chemicals adversely affect the health of humans or the ecosystem. Since the turn of the century, scientists have sought reliable, rapid, and inexpensive ways to test chemicals for deleterious effects.

The concern of the Committee on Chemical Environmental Mutagens is chemicals that cause heritable mutations. In recent years, a number of laboratory tests have been developed to detect mutagenic chemicals. They use various methods and living systems, including bacteria, fungi, mammalian-cell cultures, and insects. Among the approximately 50 such tests described in this report are several that are inexpensive, quick, sensitive, and validated. The development and wide application of such tests contribute to human health and well-being by identifying (before large-scale production) chemicals that can affect germ cells and produce genetic damage that can be passed on to future generations. Mutagenicity tests also may predict a chemical's carcinogenic potential, because there is a strong correlation between carcinogenicity and mutagenicity.

Efficient mutagenicity tests that use experimental organisms and in vitro systems are a product of great advances in basic knowledge and of a substantial research effort. The principal task of the Committee is to study how the results of such tests can be used to assess the risk to future human populations. There are no reliable data from direct human experience, so it is necessary to rely on experimental test systems. Some tests are exquisitely sensitive to chemical mutagens, but use microorganisms or mammalian-cell cultures of uncertain relevance to human

1

germ cell damage. Although there has been great progress
in the development of test systems, it is still not possible
to predict fully the human impact of a mutagen with confidence. There are two reasons for this: first, in the
absence of human data, it is not possible to validate the
test systems, and second, one must assume that they predict
human effects. Even if the damage to human germ cells
could be measured precisely, we lack the knowledge to
translate the measurements into a total impact on the
health and welfare of future generations--this situation is
not likely to change soon.

In view of those problems, the task of this Committee
is to answer two questions:

1. How can data from diverse test systems best be used
to identify possible chemical mutagens and to assess their
potential damage to human germ cells?

2. How can information on mutational damage produced
by chemicals be used to estimate their possible impact on
human welfare in future generations?

In answer to the first question, the Committee suggests
a two-tier system of inexpensive, short-term, sensitive
mutagenicity tests that could be widely applied to identify
substances that may represent a mutagenic hazard. The
first tier uses one microbial test and two mammalian cell-
culture tests. If the results of this tier are inconclusive,
a Drosophila test (the second tier) is used. If the
results are still insufficient for a manufacturing or
control decision, further tests are available, including
those using mice. The test scheme is presented later in
this summary and in more detail in Chapter 9.

To answer the second charge of the Committee, mouse
tests are included. Of the organisms for which germinal
tests have been developed, the mouse is closest to man.
From mouse data, perhaps combined with information from
other tests, the effects in the first half-dozen human
generations can be estimated, although with great uncertainty.
The Committee does not think it feasible to estimate the
total genetic impact, which may spread over hundreds of
generations with very little impact on any single generation.
This opinion is discussed in Chapter 7.

BACKGROUND

The first demonstration that environmental agents could
influence the mutation rate came in the late 1920s. H. J.
Muller, working with Drosophila, and L. J. Stadler, working

with cereals, showed that x rays are mutagenic. During
World War II, Charlotte Auerbach demonstrated chemical
mutagenesis by showing that mustard gas produces mutation
in Drosophila. The early chemical mutagens were all
highly toxic substances, and it was not expected that
there would be any nonaccidental human exposure. In the
early 1960s, this sanguine attitude changed drastically,
when it was discovered that some seemingly harmless,
nontoxic substances were highly mutagenic. It has since
been accepted that mutagenicity testing should be an
integral part of routine testing of chemicals to which
humans are likely to be exposed; excellent short-term
tests have been developed, and a register of mutagenic
chemicals is being kept.

SOME BASIC PRINCIPLES OF GENETICS AND MUTAGENESIS

The unit of heredity is the gene, defined as a stretch
of DNA with a specific function; usually this function is
to produce a protein or protein component. The unit
structure of DNA is the nucleotide, and a gene typically
includes a few thousand nucleotides. Hundreds of genes
are strung together, with large amounts of additional DNA
whose function is generally unknown, to make up a very
long DNA thread. This thread, with adhering proteins, is
a chromosome. A human body cell has 23 pairs of chromosomes.
The total length of DNA in all the chromosomes is more
than 5 billion nucleotides.

Cellular organisms are divided into two broad categories.
Eukaryotes have a distinct cell nucleus, and their chromosomes go through a regular process of mitosis in cell
division. Prokaryotes have no distinct nucleus, and their
chromosomes have a simpler structure. The distinction may
be important because, although all these organisms have
DNA as the basic genetic material, the differences in
chromosomal and cell structure may cause mutagens to act
differently. Bacteria and some primitive algae are
prokaryotes; all higher plants and all animals are eukaryotes.

The classical definition of "mutation" is an abrupt and
heritable genetic change. At the cellular level, "mutation"
means any change in the genetic material of the cell that
is transmitted to descendant cells. A mutation may affect
a single nucleotide of the DNA, several nucleotides in a
gene, several genes, large segments of one or more chromosomes,
or entire chromosomes. In this report, we use the word
"mutation" in its broadest sense and adopt the following
terms:

- Gene <u>mutation</u> affects a single gene.
- <u>Chromosomal</u> <u>mutation</u> affects blocks of genes in one or more chromosomes.
- <u>Genomic</u> <u>mutation</u> affects the number of chromosomes, but does not alter the chromosomal structure itself.

Mutations can occur in any nucleated cell, and some of these may be important in such processes as carcinogenesis and aging. However, the assignment of this Committee is to consider mutations that are transmitted to future generations. Hence our concern is with mutations in germ cells--sperm and egg cells and their precursors.

Chromosomes occur in pairs; of each pair, one member is contributed by the mother and one by the father. Therefore, genes also occur in pairs. A gene that produces its characteristic effect (its phenotype) when only one of its type is present is dominant. If two are required, the gene is recessive. If a mutant gene is recessive, hundreds of generations may pass before it chances to encounter a partner like itself, which permits its effect to be expressed. In contrast, a dominant mutation may be expressed in the generation immediately after it occurs.

Genomic mutations lead to abnormal chromosome numbers. A surplus or a shortage of any chromosome produces an abnormality, usually with a highly deleterious effect. More than one-third of spontaneous abortions are caused by chromosomal and genomic mutations. Chromosomal mutations produce their effect mainly by predisposing the organism to transmit unbalanced combinations of chromosomes.

The spectrum of mutational effects runs the gamut of bodily processes. Genes affect all structures and functions, and so do mutations. The impact ranges from trivial to tragic. Depending on the dominance and severity of a mutation, its effect may be immediate or spread over an enormous period. It is therefore impossible to describe in detail or to quantify all the consequences of an increase in the mutation rate. One generalization is apt, however: the net effect of an increase in mutation rate is harmful, because almost all mutants with any detectable effect are deleterious.

Severe dominant mutations exert their main effects in the first few generations, in contrast with recessive mutations, which are spread out over enormous periods (as are genes with very mild effects). Thus, it is much more feasible to estimate the consequences of dominant mutations than of those whose effects are greatly diluted by time and by space (because of migration, a mutation may be expressed in a different part of the world from that in which it occurred).

Because the chemistry of DNA and some mutagenic mechanisms are so well understood, one might expect it to be possible to predict the mutagenicity of a substance from its chemical properties. That is not now possible, and only rough guesses can be made on the basis of chemical information alone. The final assessment of the mutagenicity of a chemical depends on biologic tests.

It is not yet possible to study the induction of germinal mutations in humans. In fact, there is no direct human evidence of induction of germinal gene mutations in man by an environmental agent--even radiation. Although the consistency of results from a wide range of experimental organisms leaves no doubt that humans are also susceptible to the mutagenic effects of chemicals, we must rely on experimental organisms for most of the information about ourselves. Most of our knowledge of the molecular mechanisms of mutation and of chemical mutagenesis has come from the study of organisms distantly related to man. The most sensitive systems for detecting environmental mutagens involve microorganisms, cell cultures, and insects. It is natural, therefore, to question how much of this information, especially quantitative information, can be applied to man.

Further details of genetic principles and mutagenesis are given in Chapter 3.

METABOLISM OF MUTAGENS AND PROMUTAGENS

Until the 1960s, it was assumed that most mutagenic chemicals acted in the cell in the same form in which they entered the body. There were known to be enzymes that inactivated or detoxified drugs, and some mutagens were thought to be rendered innocuous this way. Now it is understood that, although some chemicals are active in their original form, most are inactive until they are metabolized. Toxification and detoxification go on simultaneously in the same cell, and the causative enzymes are themselves controlled by genes.

The recognition that many innocuous substances become mutagenic because of activating enzymes in the body has led to an entirely different view of mutagen detection. It is no longer sufficient to assume that a chemical is harmless on the grounds that it is nonmutagenic in a simple system. Many chemicals are not mutagenic themselves, but are converted into mutagens in the body, usually in the liver. Reactions with chemicals of external origin lead to a complicated and delicate balance of toxification and detoxification. Intermediate products are often

highly active and can interact with DNA in ways that lead
to mutation. It remains unclear why so many harmless
chemicals are converted into mutagens, but the fact is not
in doubt.

Therefore, test systems must be designed to mimic the
metabolism of the human body. Extracts from rat liver
have proved to be highly effective, and many substances
have been found to be mutagenic in bacteria and cultured
human cells only when such activating systems are included.
Mutation tests are run both with and without activation,
to detect chemicals that are already mutagenic and might
be inactivated, as well as those which require activation
to become mutagenic.

One of the findings of such studies is that different
mammals and even different strains of a given mammal can
differ greatly in their metabolism of particular chemicals.
This makes extrapolation from studies of mice, particularly
of a specific strain of mouse, less certain than was once
thought. Also, results from in vitro tests that require
metabolic activation may differ among species, tissues,
and subcellular fractions. With radiation, one can be
reasonably confident of the dose to the germ cells; with
chemicals, the uncertainties are much greater.

Another consequence of the genetic control of activating
systems is that people can be expected to differ in their
constellations of enzymes, and therefore in their susceptibility to mutagens. Some examples are known, but this
field is in its infancy. It would be desirable to take
account of the fact that some chemicals that are nonmutagenic
for most people may be highly mutagenic for a few. It is
not yet possible to gauge this sensitivity, but it is very
likely to be an important part of the mutation protection
of the future.

A fuller discussion of the metabolism of mutagens and
promutagens appears in Chapter 4.

MUTAGEN TESTING SYSTEMS

The last 15 yr have seen enormous progress in the
development of simple, inexpensive, quick, sensitive,
reproducible tests for mutagenicity. This progress has
resulted not only from the great interest in chemical
mutagens since the 1960s, but also from the great increase
in fundamental understanding of genetics and molecular
biology. The available mutagenicity tests include not
only inexpensive bacterial tests that can be completed in
a few days, but expensive mouse tests that require many
months.

The most sensitive and most widely applied test uses the bacterium Salmonella. The system selects histidine-independent mutants and permits their classification into different kinds of changes at the DNA level. Strains that are specifically susceptible to different kinds of mutation events, especially permeable to external chemicals, and deficient in DNA repair are used. The addition of a mammalian metabolic activation system greatly increases the ability of the test to detect potential human mutagens. The test can be completed in a few days. Similar tests have been and are being developed in other bacteria and in fungi.

Mammalian-cell strains have been developed that strongly select for the tiny fraction of cells that are mutants. One system uses mouse lymphoma cells and detects mutations that cause deficiency of thymidine kinase (TK). Another uses Chinese hamster cells and detects mutations in the gene that produces hypoxanthine-guanine phosphoribosyl transferase (HGPRT). Both tests are efficient, are widely applied, and can be completed in a few weeks. Although not as simple, rapid, and efficient as the Salmonella tests, they have the advantage of being done in a eukaryote. Mammalian-cell cultures are also used to test for chromosomal mutation.

The classical mutation tests in Drosophila use special strains that detect recessive lethal mutations on the X chromosome. They have the advantage that mutations at all lethal-producing loci on the chromosome, and not just those at a few selected loci, are detected. Various germ cell stages can be tested in both sexes. There are also tests for chromosomal breakage and rearrangement. These Drosophila tests require a few weeks.

The organism most closely related to man for which any germinal-mutation rates have been measured is the mouse. The specific-locus test detects recessive gene mutations and small deletions at seven specific gene loci; some of these have dominant effects on vital characters. Because of the small number of loci sampled and the small number of mutations per locus, this test requires a very large number of mice and is therefore unsuitable for routine screening of chemicals. However, it has been very useful in studying the kinetics of radiation and chemical mutagenesis in mammalian germ cells. Another mouse test uses dominant mutations that affect the skeleton, many of which mimic serious human disabilities. A similar, but less sensitive, test looks for cataracts. Also, there are direct tests for chromosomal mutations, based either on direct microscopic observation of germ cells or on partial sterility of the progeny of treated parents.

Another widely used mouse test is the dominant-lethal test. It measures prenatal deaths, which are thought to be caused mainly by chromosomal damage. Relative to other mouse tests, it is inexpensive and easy to carry out. The difficulties are that there is a high background level of spontaneous embryonic death; there is no genetic followup; there may be other, nongenetic causes; and it is less useful for testing females, because of possible maternal effects of the chemical. For risk estimation, there is the further difficulty that the embryonic deaths may be so early as to be of little human consequence. However, this test can be useful in monitoring mammalian germinal chromosomal mutations.

The greatest difficulty with test systems today is that the tests that are most economical and sensitive use cell cultures, or, if they use whole animals, animals that are phylogenetically distant from man. In contrast, tests that use the mouse in ways that are directly comparable with the presumed human experience are too expensive to use for more than a small number of chemicals. Thus, in the tiered screening system detailed in Chapter 9, the Committee recommends that mouse tests be used only when the simpler tests have not provided enough information for a decision or when the chemical in question is so important or widespread in its use that further information is deemed crucial.

The most widely used test systems, as well as some that are still being developed, are described and evaluated in Chapter 5.

STRATEGIES FOR RISK ANALYSIS

There is no universally accepted definition of "risk assessment." Some define it narrowly to mean only the identification of a hazardous substance. Others interpret it to mean the full range of activities, including the risk-benefit analysis and the economic considerations used to make a regulatory decision.

In this report, we visualize five steps in the identification of mutagenic hazards and the estimation of genetic risks:

1. Hazard identification. The determination of whether a substance is mutagenic. For this purpose, inexpensive, quick, sensitive tests are needed.

2. Hazard characterization. A semiquantitative evaluation. Mutagens have vastly different strengths and, even though accurate quantitative evaluation may not be possible, can

be ranked or classified into groups according to relative strength.

3. <u>Risk estimation</u>. The estimation of effect per unit of exposure. There are two components: estimation of mutagenic effects on germ cells (damage) and estimation of effects on health and welfare of future generations (impact).

4. <u>Risk assessment</u>. An assessment of the overall risk to humans from the anticipated use. This involves measurement of the potential effect, not only on the basis of the potency of the mutagen, but also on the basis of the expected extent of human exposure.

5. <u>Risk-benefit analysis</u>. An attempt to weigh the expected risks against the anticipated benefits.

Only the first three items are within the scope of this Committee and this report.

The Committee recommends that hazard evaluation be based chiefly on short-term tests. In most cases, control or decisions in government and industry can be made on the basis of these screening tests. Chemicals that must be characterized more extensively can be tested further in mice.

Although there are many uncertainties in the estimation of human DNA damage on the basis of data on experimental organisms, the estimation of the impact on future generations is even more diffcult. The range of mutational effects is so wide and the future distribution of these effects so unpredictable in time and severity that it is impossible to make any convincing quantitative judgment of total impact. However, the impact can be separated into two components, not entirely distinct, but sufficiently so to make the classification useful: dominant gene mutations and chromosomal mutations whose manifestation is confined mainly to the first half-dozen generations after occurrence of mutation; and mutations with very mild individual effects (such as those which cause a small increase in blood pressure) and recessive mutations whose effects are greatly diluted by time and whose effects on a single generation are much too small to measure. Techniques have been developed for the measurement of the mutational component of human disabilities in which the inheritance is determined by epidemiologic studies and correlations between relatives. However, these have not been tested and applied widely enough for discussion here.

The strategy adopted by this Committee, as well as by United Nations committees and other National Research Council committees in connection with radiation effects, is to concentrate on risk estimation for genetic effects that can be expected within the first half-dozen generations.

Strategies for risk estimation are discussed further in Chapters 6 and 7.

TESTING AND MONITORING HUMAN POPULATIONS

There is always a possibility, despite an efficient testing system, that a mutagen--natural or man-made--will escape detection and that people will be exposed to it. It is important to develop methods for identifying those who have been exposed to a mutagen and for locating the source of such exposure. There are a number of potentially useful tests, but none is well-enough developed to be recommended for wide use.

There are tests for DNA alkylation and repair, for chromosomal aberrations, and for gene mutations in somatic cells. Sister chromatid exchange is a particularly sensitive indicator and, because of its simplicity and low cost, could be widely applied. It is possible to examine body fluids, especially urine, for mutagenic substances. Finally, one can monitor the incidence of specific dominant phenotypes in newborns; an increase might indicate an increase in the mutation rate. Sperm abnormalities might also indicate mutational changes.

Three promising direct tests are the study of peripheral lymphocytes for chromosomal changes, analysis of body fluids for mutagenic substances (as identified in microbial systems), and in vitro and in vivo sister chromatid exchange. Although large-scale population monitoring seems premature, these could be used in more localized circumstances, as in populations of workers in chemical factories. Such a population might consist of a number of persons in one location exposed to the same chemical, possibly at relatively high concentrations. These tests could become a routine part of good industrial hygiene.

Inasmuch as carcinogenicity is highly correlated with mutagenicity, it may be possible to monitor human populations through the extensive existing registries of cancer incidence and mortality. Populations with a high incidence of cancer may have been exposed to a chemical mutagen.

People who are particularly sensitive to environmental agents might be identified by such systems as are mentioned above. Research aimed at better methods of monitoring and identifying mutagen-sensitive people could be of great value.

Population monitoring is discussed more fully in Chapter 8.

A MUTAGEN ASSESSMENT PROGRAM

One of the two major tasks of the Committee is to determine how data from diverse test systems can best be used to assess mutagenic damage to human germ cells. Chapter 9 details a program for this purpose, but it is summarized here. The proposed program has five levels:

1. Screening of many chemicals with short-term tests. To the extent feasible, this should include all chemicals to which humans are routinely exposed. New chemicals should be tested before they are put into large-scale production. In most cases, the outcomes of such tests will be sufficient to support industrial or governmental control.

2. Classification of chemicals by mutagenic potency in individual test systems. It is not feasible to be fully quantitative, because there are inconsistencies among tests, but a rough classification based on relative potency is useful for decision-making when a simple, all-or-none classification (i.e., mutagenic or nonmutagenic) is insufficient.

3. Consideration of available carcinogenicity data. Although some compounds that increase cancer rates have not been shown to be mutagens, the correlation between mutagenicity and carcinogenicity is so high that the finding of one property strongly suggests the presence of the other. Furthermore, a decision to modify the use of a chemical may be made on the basis of carcinogenicity, in which case limited resources for mammalian mutagenicity testing may be conserved for other chemicals.

4. Testing in rodents. Especially important chemicals are further classified by rodent tests. So far only the mouse is used, but it would be good to broaden the basis for extrapolation to man by developing tests that use other small mammals.

5. Estimation of risk. This is based on mouse data perhaps supplemented with ancillary information from other sources, to be used by those who have to make risk-benefit analyses.

Figure 9-1 is a flow chart for a mutagen assessment system; the suggested decision function for short-term tests is shown in Table 9-2.

For the short-term tests, we recommend a two-tier system. Tier I consists of a microbial gene-mutation test (Salmonella/microsome test), a mammalian cell-culture gene-mutation test (HGPRT or TK), and a mammalian cell-culture chromosomal-breakage test. All these are to be done both with and without metabolic activation. If the outcomes or all three tests are negative, the chemical is classified as a presumed mammalian nonmutagen. If two or more tests have positive results, the chemical is a presumed mammalian mutagen. If one test is positive, testing moves to Tier II, which is a Drosophila X-linked lethal test. If this is positive, the chemical is classified as a presumed mammalian mutagen; if negative, the chemical is a presumed mammalian nonmutagen. An examination of 36 mutagenic chemicals in which several of these tests had been done showed that at least 31 would have been identified by Tier I tests alone. This suggests that the more expensive Drosophila tests would not be needed for most chemicals. We caution, however, that many of the data come from strong mutagens; when more tests for weaker mutagens are carried out, the Tier I results may not be decisive so often.

If a simple yes-no result at Level 1 (screening) is insufficient for a decision, we recommend that the program move to Level 2. Risk-benefit decisions may require information about relative potencies of mutagens. We suggest that chemicals be assigned class numbers. For example, in Class 0 are chemicals with no statistically significant mutagenic effect. Class 1 contains the weakest mutagenic chemicals, and each unit increase in class number indicates a 10-fold increase in mutagenic potency.

At Level 3 of the program, one introduces information, when available, from carcinogenicity tests to help in judging the mutagenic hazard.

If a decision still cannot be reached reliably in Level 3, a mammalian test (Level 4) is recommended. If the expected effect is chromosomal, a dominant-lethal test is appropriate. If the expected effect is genic, then the specific-locus test is appropriate. A positive result in either test is sufficient to classify a chemical as a mammalian mutagen, regardless of the results of short-term tests. However, the dominant-lethal test may sometimes detect effects that are nongenetic.

A combination of a negative test in the mouse with positive results in the screening system creates a dilemma. One possibility is that the number of mice used in the test was insufficient to demonstrate a small effect. There are other possibilities: the material did not reach the germ cells; the chemical was inactivated in the mouse body; the DNA damage was almost completely repaired by a mouse repair system; the cell stages treated were insensitive; cell death eliminated the mutagenized cells. If humans respond in the same way as mice, it is arguable that human germ cells will be similarly unaffected. However, the human system may not be the same as that of the mouse, and substances that do not produce a detectable increase in the mouse rate could be important human mutagens. In some cases, it may be possible to decide between these two possibilities by investigating such things as metabolic paths in the two species, but such information will usually not be available. The Committee is unwilling to assume that negative mouse data necessarily outweigh the consensus of a variety of short-term tests. There is no uniform rule, and the decision will have to be made in uncertainty. All the evidence needs to be taken into account, and the decision based on the weight of the evidence in each case.

Finally, the best currently available method for risk estimation is the use of skeletal mutations and cataracts in mice for dominant gene mutations and heritable trans-locations for chromosomal mutations. These provide an estimate of the first-generation effect. We suggest that this estimate of first-generation effect be multiplied by 4 to give the total effect. It should be recognized that this estimate does not include the effects of recessive mutations and the minor effects of gene mutations; those effects would be much more dilute and not measurable by any present methods. It should also be recognized that in the absence of human data there is no way that these estimates can be validated. One can only make the reasonable assumption that the organism closest to man provides the most relevant information.

There are a number of other good short-term systems, some of which have been extensively tested. If the tier tests lead to inconsistent, ambiguous, or doubtful results, it may be desirable to use other short-term tests; these may resolve the doubts without the necessity for mouse tests. Another reason for using supplementary tests is that the primary tests may be inappropriate for a particular chemical; for example, one may not want to test insecticides in Drosophila.

Further details about the suggested testing scheme, with relevant data, are given in Chapter 9.

CONCLUSIONS

1. Although genetic disease has a large impact on human health and welfare, the contribution of recurrent mutation to this burden is not known.

2. It is not possible now to assess the total impact of an increased mutation rate on future generations, nor is this likely to be possible with any confidence in the near future.

3. The best present basis for a <u>partial</u> assessment of the impact is dominant gene and chromosomal mutations, which constitute the major mutational impact in the next half-dozen generations. It is within the time span of only a few human generations that the preponderance of mutation impact will occur.

4. The number of chemicals to be screened is so great that it is important to have several rapid, sensitive, inexpensive tests available. Some tests involving microorganisms and cell cultures have been developed.

5. The most sensitive and inexpensive tests involve microorganisms and cell cultures, whereas the tests most closely related to the human situation are the relatively insensitive germinal tests in the mouse.

6. A battery of short-term tests can be used to identify presumed mammalian mutagens. Several of these have been used widely in different laboratories with reasonably consistent results. The tests have been devised to measure a variety of mutational end points. It is neither necessary nor feasible to use mammals for initial screening.

7. There is as yet no validated short-term test for genomic mutations (aneuploidy and polyploidy).

8. For most chemicals, short-term tests are sufficient for a regulatory or manufacturing decision. For the most crucial decisions, direct information from mammalian germ cell tests may be desirable. Two tests are available for mammalian germinal screening: the specific-locus test detects gene mutations and small deletions; the dominant-lethal test detects prenatal deaths, thought to be caused mainly by chromosomal mutations.

9. If the short-term tests and mammalian tests are both negative, the chemical is regarded as a mammalian nonmutagen and is presumed to be safe for man. If any mouse test is positive, the substance is regarded as a mammalian mutagen, regardless of the outcome of the short-term tests. If the short-term tests are positive and the mouse test negative, the decision must be made case by case with all relevant evidence taken into account. The Committee feels that it is prudent to regard the chemical as a potential human mutagen unless there is specific evidence that the mouse is a good human surrogate for this chemical.

10. For risk estimation, other mouse tests are appropriate. Dominant phenotypes (skeletal effects, possibly supplemented by cataracts) in mice provide the only current basis for assessing the early-generation phenotypic effects in man. These estimates must be regarded as very uncertain until there have been more comparative studies in mice and

other species and in various germ cell stages. Germinal
cytogenetic tests in the mouse can be used to predict
human damage from chromosomal mutations.

11. Research in better mutation-detection systems and
in molecular dosimetry is progressing rapidly, and it is
likely that better procedures for mutagen detection and
risk assessment will be forthcoming. This means that some
of our recommended testing procedures are likely to be
superseded in a few years.

12. The technology for monitoring mutation in the
human population is not yet sufficiently developed for
wide application. However, there are systems that could
be applied to selected populations, such as workers in a
chemical factory.

RECOMMENDATIONS

1. Our recommended mutagen assessment program has five
levels (outlined in Figure 9-1):

Level 1. Screening of a large number of chemicals in
      short-term tests.
Level 2. Classification of chemicals by mutagenic
      potency in individual test systems.
Level 3. Consideration of available animal carcinogenicity
      data.
Level 4. Further testing in mice of chemicals of crucial
      importance.
Level 5. Risk estimation.

At any level, a regulatory or manufacturing decision can
be made, or one can proceed to a higher level.

2. The recommended screening system consists of two
tiers. Tier I consists of (1) the Salmonella/microsome
gene-mutation test, (2) a mammalian-cell gene-mutation
test, and (3) a mammalian-cell chromosomal-breakage test.
Tier II consists of a Drosophila X-linked lethal-mutation
test. A positive finding in any two of the three Tier I
tests classifies the chemical as a presumed mammalian
mutagen. If all three are negative, it is a presumed
mammalian nonmutagen. If only one test is positive, the
Tier II test is used. If this is positive, the chemical
is a presumed mammalian mutagen; if negative, it is a
presumed mammalian nonmutagen. (This scheme is presented
in decision-function form in Table 9-2.)

3. If the decision requires an estimation of relative
potency, we recommend that the results in a particular
test be placed in groups of equal width on a geometric

scale of potencies. Each group corresponds to one decade (power of 10).

4. Many chemicals will also be tested for carcinogenicity. We recommend that, in cases where Levels 1 and 2 have not led to a decision, carcinogenicity data be considered in arriving at an overall decision.

5. For further screening of the most crucial chemicals, a mouse test may be necessary. To test whether a chemical is mutagenic in mammalian germ cells, a specific-locus test is appropriate. If the effect is primarily chromosomal mutations, a dominant-lethal test is appropriate. If the short-term tests are positive and the mouse test negative, we recommend that the decision be made on the basis of all the relevant information.

6. For risk estimation based on information most closely related to the expected human impact, the mouse test for dominant skeletal abnormalities (possibly supple-mented by a cataract test) is appropriate. Because these tests have not been validated by comparisons in different laboratories, different species, and different cell stages in both sexes, and because the similarity of humans to mice remains uncertain, we recommend that the risk aspect of any risk-benefit decision be based on all relevant mutational and toxicologic information.

7. We recommend that systematic, centralized recording of data on chemical mutagens be maintained and specifically recommend that there be a regular system for recording negative data and making them available.

8. Recommendations for research are presented in Chapter 10.

2

INTRODUCTION

Besides the large number of biologically active compounds
that occur naturally, there are about 70,000 synthetic
chemicals in commerce, of which more than 25,000 are
produced in large quantities.[122] [170] Chemical Abstracts
lists over 5.3 million chemicals. Over 1,000 chemicals
are newly synthesized each year. Many of these chemicals
are beneficial and contribute substantially to our society's
high standard of living. However, among them are chemicals
that are mutagenic in experimental test systems or that
have metabolic derivatives that are mutagenic. Because
effects of induced mutations are generally detrimental, it
is important to identify potential mutagens and to assess
their possible impact on future human health. To compare
the benefits and risks of particular chemicals requires
some estimate of the risks.

Mutagens can exert their detrimental effects in somatic
cells or germ cells. Genetic damage to somatic cells is
transmitted only to descendant somatic cells and is therefore
restricted to the individual exposed. Such damage is
usually unimportant, but not always; somatic cell damage
may lead to cancer and possibly atherosclerosis.[28] Genetic
damage to germ cells (sperm and egg cells and their
precursors) can be transmitted to offspring and by them to
future generations. It is with transmitted genetic
damage that this report is concerned.

The development of efficient mutagenicity tests with
experimental organisms and in vitro systems is the product
of a substantial research effort. The principal task of
the Committee on Chemical Environmental Mutagens is to
study how the results of such tests can be used to assess
the risk to human populations of the future. It must be
recognized that there are very few data from direct human
experience, so it is necessary to rely on experimental

17

test systems. Some test systems are exquisitely sensitive
to chemical mutagens, but they use microorganisms or
specific end points in mammalian cell systems with uncertain
relevance to human germ cell damage. It is necessary to
recognize at the outset that, although there has been
great progress in development of test systems, it is still
not possible to predict with confidence the total human
impact of exposure to a chemical. There are two reasons
for this. One is that, in the absence of direct human
data, it is not possible to calibrate the test systems;
one must simply assume that the test systems predict the
human effect. The second reason is that, even if the
damage to human germ cells could be measured precisely, we
lack the knowledge to translate the measurements into a
total impact on the health and welfare of future generations,
nor is this situation likely to change in the near future.
(We shall continue to use the words "damage" and "impact"
with this distinction in meaning.) We must do the best we
can with information that is indirect and uncertain.

   In view of these two major problems, it is convenient
to describe the first task of the Committee by asking two
questions:

   • How can data from diverse test systems best be used to
estimate mutagenic damage to human germ cells?
   • How can information on mutational damage to human
germ cells yield information on the impact on human welfare
in future generations?

   The Committee's second task is a feasibility study of
the predictive value of short-term mutagenicity tests for
carcinogenicity. This report is concerned with only the
first task.

HISTORY OF RADIATION PROTECTION

   The first unequivocal demonstration that environmental
agents could produce mutations came with the work of H. J.
Muller[293] that showed that x rays are mutagenic in Drosophila.
L. J. Stadler[431] independently discovered x-ray mutagenesis
in barley. In his earliest writings on this subject,
Muller called attention to the risk to future generations
from exposure of the germ cells to ionizing radiation.
But genetic risks to the population did not become a major
consideration in determining acceptable radiation doses
until after World War II. Before then, exposure standards

for radiation, as for chemicals, had been based on prevention of harmful effects in the exposed persons themselves.*

In the mid-1950s, there was great public concern about possible long-range effects of nuclear radiation, especially from aboveground nuclear explosions. The National Research Council Committee on the Biological Effects of Atomic Radiation (BEAR) issued its first report in 1956 and recommended that man-made radiation be so restricted that the average person would not be exposed to more than 10 roentgens (10 R) before the mean age of reproduction, which was taken to be 30 yr.

At the same time, a committee appointed by the British Medical Research Council suggested that, in planning for radiation-producing facilities, the average radiation dose to the population from these sources be kept no greater than approximately the normal background, which at that time was estimated at about 5 R in a 30-yr period. Specifically, the report said that "those responsible for authorizing the development and use of sources of ionizing radiation should be advised that the upper limit, which future knowledge may set to the total dose of extra radiation which may be received by the population as a whole, is not likely to be more than twice the dose which is already received from the natural background. The recommended figure may indeed be appreciably less than this."

The 10-R exposure recommended by BEAR included an estimated 5 R from medical radiation, with the remainder derived from all other radiation. The National Council on Radiation Protection and Measurements (NCRP) immediately accepted this recommendation in its report, issued in January 1957. It stated that the population dose "shall not exceed 14 million man-rems per million of population over the period from conception up to age 30 and one-third that amount in each decade thereafter." The age of 30 yr is the approximate average age of reproduction. Background radiation was assumed to be about 4 million rems per million persons and medical radiation about 5 million

---

*"Exposure" refers to material ingested, inhaled, injected, or simply found in the environment; it is expressed in appropriate units, such as milligrams per kilogram (mg/kg) or parts per million (ppm). "Dose" refers to the amount of material reaching the target; it is measured in such units as adducts per nucleotide. Because, by this definition, dose can hardly ever be measured, we use "dose" as a synonym for "exposure" when the meaning is clear from the context.

rems, leaving 5 million rems for occupational and general exposures. It was estimated that nonmedical man-made sources accounted for considerably less than 1 million rems, leaving a cushion of 4 million rems per million persons for future needs. It also was recommended that radiation-producing facilities be designed to make it improbable that any person in the general population would receive a dose of more than 0.5 rem in any year.

In 1958, the International Commission on Radiological Protection (ICRP) recommended that the genetic dose to the general population, excluding natural background radiation, not exceed 5 rems plus the lowest practicable contribution from medical exposure in a 30-yr period, or 170 mrems/yr. The NCRP calculated the same value.

Founded over 50 yr ago, the ICRP and NCRP have been concerned continuously with potential harmful effects of ionizing radiation. The history of concern about radiation protection has been summarized by Taylor.[456]

Three more National Research Council committees (the first, second, and third Committees on the Biological Effects of Ionizing Radiations--BEIR I, II, and III) issued reports in 1972, 1977, and 1980.[301-303] They emphasized risk estimation, rather than recommendation of standards. There also has been discussion of carcinogenicity as a low-dose, delayed effect. The United Nations, through its Scientific Committee on the Effects of Atomic Radiation, has continued to produce periodic encyclopedic reviews of the literature.[468-473]

CONCERN ABOUT CHEMICAL MUTAGENS

Although there were scattered reports of chemical mutagenesis in the 1930s and early 1940s, none was sufficiently impressive to convince a largely skeptical community of geneticists. The first definitive studies were performed in Britain during World War II by Charlotte Auerbach.[19] After the observation that injuries from war gases resembled x-ray burns, Auerbach demonstrated unequivocally that mustard gas induced sex-linked recessive lethal mutations in Drosophila. At about the same time, I. A. Rapoport[361] independently reported that several other chemicals induced gene mutations and chromosomal aberrations. Their work ushered in the era of chemical studies of mutation, and within a few years a large number of chemical mutagens had been identified.

There was some discussion that chemicals might constitute a genetic hazard as great as, if not greater than, radiation (e.g., Lederberg[234]), but at the time radiation was regarded as a more serious threat. Most of the chemicals that had been discovered to be mutagenic were highly toxic, and substantial human exposure was not expected. This situation changed abruptly in the early 1960s, with the discovery of compounds that were highly mutagenic at concentrations that produced no toxic effects or decrease in fertility. Among the early examples were ethyl methanesulfonate and N-methyl-N'-nitro-N-nitrosoguanidine, both potent mutagens in a variety of experimental organisms.

At the instigation of Matthew Meselson, the Genetics Study Section of the Division of Research Grants, National Institutes of Health, sponsored a small conference at the Jackson Laboratory on September 14, 1966. A report of the conference[77] contained four recommendations:

• That an up-to-date register of mutagenic chemicals be kept and the information be made generally available.
• That tests for mutagenicity be a routine part of the testing of chemicals that are used in food or drugs or to which large numbers of persons may be exposed.
• That research to develop more sensitive and less expensive assays of mutagenicity and chromosomal breakage or assays based on organisms more closely related to man be encouraged and supported.
• That the feasibility of genetic monitoring of the human population for chromosomal breakage and increased genetic disease be explored.

The first three recommendations were quickly put into effect by the concerted action of a number of groups, and the fourth has been continuously under consideration ever since (see Chapter 8).

E. M. Mrak[291] chaired a committee formed in response to a request from the Secretary of the Department of Health, Education, and Welfare to study toxic properties of pesticides, including mutagenicity. The Food and Drug Administration also sponsored several conferences and studies related to mutagenicity. Various recommendations were made as to how mutagenicity, teratogenicity, and carcinogenicity could be detected and controlled. The concern was international, with groups active in Japan, Canada, and various European nations, as well as in the United States.

Largely through the efforts of Alexander Hollaender and Frederick de Serres, the Environmental Mutagen Society (EMS) was formed in the United States in 1969 to encourage work on mutagenesis and its relationship to public health. Among the early accomplishments of the EMS was the facilitation of information exchange in environmental mutagenesis through meetings, publications, and the establishment of the Environmental Mutagen Information Center (EMIC). Since 1969, environmental mutagen societies have been formed in Europe, Japan, and other parts of the world.

EMIC was organized in the fall of 1969, and its growth has paralleled the growth of the field of chemical mutagenesis. Operated by a staff of geneticists, biochemists, linguists, and information specialists, EMIC provides easy access to a collection of over 36,000 publications. The activities of EMIC in literature searching, indexing, query response, publication, and providing access to collected literature have contributed substantially to progress in genetic toxicology.

The literature on chemical mutagenesis reflects the concern about potential health hazards posed by chemical mutagens. The journal Mutation Research was founded in 1964. During the last 8 yr, sections of Mutation Research entitled "Environmental Mutagenesis and Related Subjects," "Reviews in Genetic Toxicology," "Genetic Toxicology Testing," and "Mutation Research Letters" have been established. Other journals on chemical mutagenesis have also been established, including Environmental Mutagenesis, Mutagenesis, Teratogenesis and Carcinogenesis, and Mutagens and Toxicology (Japan).

In 1975, the report of Committee 17 of the Environmental Mutagen Society, chaired by J. W. Drake,[98] considered in detail several important issues in environmental mutagenesis. It described criteria for good test systems and discussed which systems were feasible. It also considered pharmacologic problems of dosage and of persistence and distribution of chemicals within the body. It suggested how risk analysis might be made and gave specific examples of calculations. Finally, it considered some regulatory principles and issues. That report was a milestone in environmental mutagenesis and risk assessment for chemical mutagens, and the present report is in some ways a followup to it.

The International Commission for Protection against Environmental Mutagens and Carcinogens (ICPEMC) was founded in 1977 under the sponsorship of the Institut de la Vie. The Commission has an international membership drawn from universities, research institutions, industry, and national health organizations. Its objectives are "to identify and promote scientific principles in the fields of environmental mutagenesis, carcinogenesis, and genetic toxicology"[182,256] and "to prevent and minimize the deleterious effects resulting from the interaction of chemicals with the genetic material of man."[425] To pursue these objectives, ICPEMC prepares documents that evaluate current knowledge and that can serve as a basis for guidelines and regulations or establish priorities for research. The Commission has established committees and task groups devoted to short-term mutagenicity test systems, the correlation between carcinogenesis and mutagenesis, regulations and legislation related to mutagenesis, risk estimation procedures and exposure limits, epidemiologic studies on populations exposed to mutagens, and the evaluation of risks posed by specific chemicals.

In the decades since the discovery of chemical mutagenesis, data from more than 100 systems for mutagenicity assay of chemicals have been published.[486] The data, however, are uneven in quality, and the assay systems vary widely in stage of development, use, validation, and effectiveness. As mutagen testing becomes accepted as a part of the toxicologic evaluation of chemicals, regulatory-agency personnel are faced with the difficult problem of interpreting data that were collected from diverse organisms and assay systems under a vast range of experimental conditions. Their task is complicated by studies in which the experimental design and procedures and the interpretation of results were inadequate.

To simplify the task of interpreting existing mutagenicity studies and to assist in designing future studies, the U. S. Environmental Protection Agency (EPA) initiated a program entitled "Evaluation of Current Status of Bioassays in Genetic Toxicology." The objective of this program, which has come to be called the "GENE-TOX Program," is to evaluate selected genetic-toxicology assay systems on the basis of published literature.[486] To accomplish this goal, 23 work groups have been formed.[475] Each work group is devoted to a particular assay and is composed of scientists who are knowledgeable in its use.

The GENE-TOX Program will soon enter a phase of summary evaluation and assessment, when the task of the work groups is completed. This phase will include establishment of a computer file of genetic-toxicology data, assimilation of the work groups' reports for the purpose of proposing testing strategies, and publication of the results of the entire GENE-TOX Program in the scientific literature.[486]

The work of the GENE-TOX Program is related to the task of the Committee on Chemical Environmental Mutagens. The principal distinction between the two is that the GENE-TOX Program is concerned primarily with the evaluation and comparison of test systems, whereas this Committee emphasizes issues pertaining to the use of test results in identifying and assessing genetic risks to human health.

3

A PRIMER ON GENETICS, MUTATION, MUTAGENS,
AND THE IMPLICATIONS OF MUTAGENESIS

This chapter presents an elementary account of the
principles of genetics and mutagenesis that are required
to understand problems in mutagenicity testing and to
assess the effects of an increased mutation rate on human
welfare. The assessment relies heavily on data from
experimental organisms and from in vitro systems, because
direct assessment of human germinal mutation is largely
beyond present methods. Therefore, much of the discussion
will concern experimental organisms.

CELLS, CHROMOSOMES, AND GENES

All higher organisms are composed of cells of many
kinds, such as blood, skin, liver, and nerve cells. The
many trillions of cells in a human body arise by successive
divisions starting from a single cell. Whatever is transmitted genetically must be carried by the egg and sperm,
which fuse to form the fertilized egg, or zygote, from
which an organism develops. Events that happen in most
body cells are not transmitted to future generations.
Only damage that occurs in the sperm and egg cells or in
cells ancestral to them (collectively designated germ
cells*) has any chance of being transmitted to future
generations. Consequently, if chemicals are to produce
any heritable effects, they must reach and act on the germ
cells, which (except in very early embryos) are in the
testis or ovary.

"Genetic effect" is used in two ways. Some regard any

---

*Asterisk denotes that the term is defined in the Glossary.

24

change in the DNA in any kind of cell as genetic, because DNA is the genetic material. However, in this report, "genetic effect" refers to genetic changes that occur in germ cells and therefore may be transmitted to future generations. A change induced in any germ cell may be transmitted to descendant cells and finally to a sperm or egg, possibly many cell generations later.

Within the cell nucleus are the chromosomes*--thread-like or rod-shaped bodies that, with proper treatment and staining, can be seen through a microscope. Every species has a characteristic number of chromosomes--46 in the typical human somatic cell*. The process of cell division is organized so that the chromosome number is constant; each chromosome replicates itself, and one of the two copies goes to each of the two daughter cells as the cell divides. This process of precise assortment of the chromosomes during cell division is called mitosis*. The process ensures that, except for errors and for some special tissues, each cell in the body has the same number of chromosomes as the zygote* from which the organism arose.

The regular exception to this process occurs during meiosis*, the process creating sperm and eggs (collectively called gametes*). Meiosis consists of two nuclear divisions after but a single chromosomal replication. It thus results in a halving of the number of chromosomes. The halving is not random: chromosomes occur in pairs, and the meiotic process ensures that each gamete gets one and only one representative of each pair. Thus, a human sperm or egg has 23 chromosomes. When fertilization takes place, the original number, 46 (or 23 pairs), is restored.

Because the two members of a pair came from two parents, each gamete produced by a person contains one member of each chromosome pair from each parent. In addition, during meiosis the paternal and maternal chromosomes pair up and exchange parts (called crossing-over*). The result is that each gamete contains a mixture of paternal and maternal chromosomal segments. There is a thorough scrambling of chromosomal material, so a child has a random sample from each of its parents, or from four grandparents.

A cell whose chromosomes are in pairs, like most cells in the human body, is diploid*. A cell with a single set of chromosomes, such as a gamete, is called haploid*. Most higher animals and plants are diploid. Some of the most important experimental species, such as the bacterium Escherichia coli, are haploid. Still others, such as yeasts, may be either haploid or diploid.

Most hereditary traits are transmitted from parent to child via the chromosomes, but some extranuclear cell organelles, such as mitochondria*, are exceptional in that they code for many functions related to their replication. This leads to a small additional amount of inheritance, which is mainly, if not entirely, through the egg, because the sperm transmits very little nonnuclear material. The extrachromosomal inheritance is such a small part of the total inheritance that, for purposes of this report, it will be neglected.

A chromosome has a surprisingly simple structure. Essentially, it is a very long thread of deoxyribonucleic acid (DNA). DNA can be an extremely long molecule; the DNA of an average human chromosome would be about an inch long if it were uncoiled. DNA is surrounded by protein material, but the genetic message is carried by the DNA alone, and the protein plays a role only in determining chromosomal structure and regulating the expression of the genetic message.

Because the cell nucleus is only about 0.001 mm in diameter, the DNA thread must be very tightly packed; this is done by coiling and supercoiling. How the DNA thread can replicate itself and separate without becoming hopelessly tangled is only partially understood.

The DNA molecule is composed of two parts. One is a repeating sequence of a 5-carbon sugar (deoxyribose) and phosphate that makes up the backbone of the molecule. The second part is one of four bases associated with each repeat unit in the backbone: two purines, adenine* (A) and guanine* (G), and two pyrimidines, cytosine* (C) and thymine* (T). DNA consists of two vertical backbones bonded horizontally by a purine-pyrimidine pair at each sugar-phosphate unit. A purine or pyrimidine with its associated sugar and phosphate is called a nucleotide*.

The purine-pyrimidine bridge is held together by chemical bonds (hydrogen bonds) that are much weaker than the bonds holding the rest of the molecule together. The structure of these bases is such that only two pairs fit together well--A with T and G with C. Thus, there are four kinds of bridges: A:T, T:A, G:C, and C:G. When the DNA molecule replicates, it splits apart at the hydrogen bonds. Each half then acts as a template for synthesizing a complementary strand identical with its former partner. The replication process proceeds zipper-like along the chromosome. In this way, two new double structures are produced, each consisting of one new and one old strand. These processes are catalyzed by highly specific enzymes, each with its own role.

The sugar-phosphate backbone of the DNA molecule is completely repetitious and therefore cannot carry any message. Consequently, the genetic information must be encoded in the sequences of the four bases, which can

occur in the molecule in any order. The order determines
the difference between genes; the genetic information is
spelled out with the four-letter alphabet, A, T, C, and G.

Proteins perform most biologic functions--e.g., as
hemoglobin, tubules, antibodies, and enzymes. The primary
function of the genes is to carry the message for synthesis
of proteins. One way to define "gene" is to say that it
is a region of DNA that carries a single message. A
typical gene is a stretch of DNA 1,000-10,000 nucleotides
long and carries the coded information to produce a chain
of amino acids* that makes up a single polypeptide*. A
protein consists of one or more polypeptides folded into a
characteristic three-dimensional structure responsible for
its special properties. The information carried in the
sequence of nucleotides of the DNA is transcribed onto a
corresponding sequence in another, similar nucleic acid--
ribonucleic acid (RNA). This messenger RNA moves to the
cytoplasm of the cell, where it is translated into a
sequence of amino acids on cellular particles called
ribosomes. Thus, the linear sequence of nucleotides in
the DNA is translated into a specific sequence of amino
acids in the protein, and this sequence in turn determines
the structure and biologic properties of the protein. A
sequence of three nucleotides specifies one amino acid.
The gene also includes DNA that is not translated directly
into the amino acids of the protein, but is responsible
for starting and stopping the process, for regulating the
rate of protein synthesis, and for other cellular functions.
Doubtless, many such functions remain to be discovered.

The number of genes in Escherichia coli is about 3,000.
The number in the fruit fly Drosophila melanogaster is
about 6,000 per gamete, or 12,000 in a diploid cell. The
number of human genes is not known, but the haploid number
is probably at least 10,000.

Only a small part of the DNA is required for known gene
functions. The haploid chromosomes of a human cell contain
about 3×10^9 base pairs. If there are 10,000 genes, each
with 3,000 base pairs, this is about 1% of the DNA; if the
gene number is 10 times as large, this is still only 10%.
Some DNA at either end of the translated region is used to
regulate the transcription and translation of the gene
message. Furthermore, one of the biggest recent surprises
was the discovery of regions of DNA within the gene,
called intervening sequences, or "introns," that are not
translated into protein. These regions are cut out of the
RNA (processed) before translation. One inherited form of
thalassemia (a kind of anemia) is caused by a defect in
the RNA processing. The function of most of the extra DNA
both within and between genes is not understood.

The picture of the chromosome that emerges from this description is of a very long thread of DNA with associated proteins. Interspersed along this thread are regions of DNA that carry specific messages. We designate these regions as genes. Long before their molecular basis was understood, genes were recognized by their effects, and most genes are still identified this way. For example, there is a gene in humans that is responsible for red hair. Another is responsible for early baldness. Others have effects that are not recognized externally, but are detected by laboratory procedures--e.g., blood groups and histocompatibility types, which are important factors in a blood transfusion or organ transplant. Recent molecular studies have shown that the so-called normal (or, in experimental organisms, "wild-type") genes may exist in two or more types that cannot be distinguished by any superficial criterion and have little or no detectable difference in function. Yet they may differ in one or more nucleotides, and that difference can lead to the presence of a different amino acid at some position. Most proteins can function with some amino acids changed, although there may be subtle differences. Other amino acids are crucial and cannot be changed without impairment of protein function.

The concern here is not with normal gene-determined variability, but rather with genetic changes that are harmful. The range of gene-determined deleterious effects is enormous. Some abnormal genes cause only very mild disease or abnormality; others are lethal. Every part of the body and every known function are genetically determined. Normal development is a process of coordinated action of many genes. The failure of any one of these is likely to result in some impairment, disease, or, in extreme cases, death--the effect depends on the importance of the particular gene and the extent to which normal and abnormal genes differ in their capacity to carry out an assigned function. Many differences are within the range that is regarded as normal; but of course there is a continuous gradation, and no sharp distinction exists between normal and abnormal.

RULES OF INHERITANCE

The rules of inheritance can be deduced from the rules of chromosomal behavior. Because chromosomes occur in pairs, so do individual genes. A person receives one member of each gene pair from the mother and the other from the father. The gene is the unit of inheritance.

The position of a gene along the chromosome is its

locus*. Two corresponding (homologous) genes that differ in some way from each other are alleles*. If a person carries a gene for red hair and one for nonred, the person's child will inherit one of these alleles, but not both.

Alleles are classified by how they interact with each other. The red-hair allele is recessive*--i.e., one such gene on each member of the chromosome pair is required for the trait to be manifest. The nonred-hair allele, in contrast, is dominant*--i.e., a person with either one or two of these genes has nonred hair. It is customary to designate dominant alleles with capital letters and recessive alleles with lower-case letters. If r stands for the red-hair gene and R for its alternative, rr persons will have red hair, and Rr and RR will not.

The genetic makeup of a person (or other organism) is the genotype*. If two alleles are alike (RR or rr), the person is homozygous* for the trait in question. If they are different (Rr), the person is heterozygous*. The manifestation of the trait itself, in this case hair color, is the phenotype*. Two persons, one with Rr and the other with RR, have different genotypes, but the same phenotype.

Sometimes both members of a pair of alleles express their phenotypes. In such cases, the alleles are codominant*. An example is found in blood groups: a person with both A and B genes has both A and B antigens and has blood type AB. Dominance is often incomplete, the heterozygote being somewhere between the two homozygotes in its phenotype. This is discussed later.

The rules of chromosomal behavior in meiosis ensure that the two alleles at a locus segregate, that is, they separate and go to different gametes. Furthermore, the exchange of parts between homologous chromosomes and the independent behavior of different chromosomal pairs ensure that the paternally and maternally derived genes are scrambled thoroughly. These two rules--the segregation of alleles at the same locus and the independent assortment of genes at different loci--were first deduced from pea-breeding experiments by Gregor Mendel and published in 1865. It has since been shown that genes that are close together on a chromosome are not inherited independently, but tend to be linked. In other words, there is not a complete scramble with every sexual generation. However, there is a process (crossing-over*) by which homologous chromosomes exchange corresponding parts. As in card-shuffling, in which neighboring cards may stay together through a few shuffles, but eventually are all randomized, genes that are on the same chromosome may remain linked for several generations, but eventually are separated.

Many human diseases are caused by abnormal genes. For example, phenylketonuria, cystic fibrosis, sickle-cell anemia, and Tay-Sachs disease are caused by recessive genes; achondroplasia, polydactyly, and Huntington's disease are caused by dominant genes. In human genetics, it is often true that the heterozygous state of an abnormal gene produces a disease, whereas the homozygous state is unknown, very rare, or lethal. Such abnormal genes are conventionally considered dominant, even if the heterozygous and homozygous states do not have the same phenotype.

One pair of chromosomes are the sex chromosomes. The two members of this pair, called the X and Y chromosomes, are not identical in size and shape; the Y is much smaller. A human female has two X chromosomes, and a male has an X and a Y chromosome. In the human, the Y chromosome is almost without genes, but the X chromosome has an average number. Because the X and Y chromosomes determine sex, traits caused by genes on the X chromosome will be associated with gender, although the traits themselves (e.g., color-blindness) have nothing to do with sex. In particular, because the male has only one X chromosome, even an unpaired recessive gene is expressed in the absence of a dominant allele to mask it. A consequence is that X-linked recessive diseases are much more common in males than in females. Some familiar examples of X-linked recessive conditions are color-blindness, hemophilia, and two forms of muscular dystrophy.

The latest compendium[279] of human traits that are inherited as single-gene differences listed 736 dominant (plus 753 more that are less well established), 521 recessive (plus 596 less certain), and 107 X-linked (plus 98), for totals of 1,364 well-established Mendelian traits and an additional 1,447 traits that are provisionally Mendelian, or 2,811 all together. Today, more than 3,000 are known. Almost all these are pathologic, ranging from mildly to lethally. The list continues to grow by about 100 new genes per year as discoveries are made, so the stated total is clearly a minimum. That is especially true of recessive diseases, inasmuch as they are not likely to be found in relatives of affected persons (except siblings) and hence are less likely to be recognized as genetic.

It is important to emphasize that much genetic variability in the population is not caused by genes with conspicuous individual effects. Many genes, such as those determining height, have effects that are covert, mild, or cumulative. Height is influenced mainly by a large number of genes that cause small increases or decreases in size; a person's height is determined by the relative numbers of height-

increasing and height-decreasing genes. It is also typical
that traits determined by the cumulative action of many
genes are also influenced by the environment. It is often
as hard to distinguish between genetic and environmental
influences as it is to sort out the contributions of
individual genes.

THE ANATOMY OF MUTATION

Mutagenesis comprises the array of ways in which the
highly evolved and finely tuned fidelity of DNA function
can go awry. We begin by listing the major categories of
mutation and then describe mechanisms and their genetic
determinants. For more detailed discussion, see Drake,[99]
Hollaender,[164-167] Hollaender and de Serres,[168] Auerbach,[18]
Drake and Baltz,[100] and Drake and Koch.[76]

"Mutation" can be defined at the phenotypic and the
molecular level. The classical definition of mutation is
"an abrupt and heritable phenotypic change," it being
implicit in this definition that modes of mutation expression
and heritability depend on the chromosomal mechanics
characteristic of the particular organism. From the early
1950s, it became fashionable to use the more molecular
definition, "a change in nucleotide sequence," which,
although more precise, is less readily amenable to
experimental verification. Both definitions exclude
changes that are due only to crossing-over.

We use the word "mutation" to refer to either the
mutation process or the resulting DNA alteration, whereas
"mutant"* refers to the individual organism that harbors
the mutation. One also speaks of a "mutant gene," to
distinguish it from the normal allele.

Mutation may change a normal gene into a mutant gene or
vice versa (forward mutation* and reverse mutation*,
respectively). "Normal" is a somewhat arbitrary designation,
however, in that "wild" populations comprise many genetically
distinct but functionally normal individuals. Because
most newly arisen and readily recognized mutations are
deleterious, "forward mutation" usually (but not always)
connotes a gene-damaging alteration. Reverse mutation may
either restore the original DNA sequence or compensate for
the damage by mutations at other sites (suppressor mutation).
The analysis of the complexities of specific pathways of
forward and reverse mutation is crucial to the understanding
of mutagenic mechanisms, but it is only infrequently a
conceptual or operational component of mutagen screening.

Mutation may be recessive, dominant, partially dominant,
or codominant, as was mentioned earlier. Most "recessive"

deleterious mutations are partially dominant, in that the heterozygous phenotype is influenced by both alleles. The evidence for this is strongest for Drosophila,[79][421] but there is good reason to think that the rule holds also for mammals.

A particularly important difference between forward- and reverse-mutation screening systems is target size. A forward-mutation system that detects events that occur at any of the hundreds to thousands of DNA base pairs in a gene usually exhibits much greater absolute frequencies of mutation than does a reverse-mutation system that detects only the few specific base-pair changes that are capable of reversing the original error. High mutation rates themselves are rarely as important for mutagen detection as are large increases over the spontaneous-mutation frequency, because the latter determines the quantitative sensitivity of the system. A mutagen that induces only particular types of mutation may produce only a small factor of increase in a forward-mutation system, because other noninduced spontaneous mutations may contribute heavily to the background frequency; conversely, the same mutagen may produce a very large increase in a reverse-mutation system that responds well to the particular type of mutation induced by that mutagen. To gain a qualitative response comparable with that of a forward-mutation system, therefore, reverse-mutation screening typically uses several strains in parallel, each responding to a different class of mutational events. An important exception to this pattern of differential modes of response of forward- and reverse-mutation systems is seen in some (but not all) drug-resistance screening systems. Forward mutation to drug resistance often requires very specific nucleotide-sequence changes and thus resembles reverse mutation in its small and qualitatively restricted targets.

We consider next the specific molecular or chromosomal classes of mutation. The nomenclature that describes these lesions is by no means universal, even among geneticists. However, we adopt the following scheme: Gene mutation* affects but a single gene, often inactivating it, but sometimes changing its expression. Chromosomal mutation* affects blocks of genes, either within or between chromosomes. Genomic mutation* changes the number of chromosomes in the genome (the haploid set of all chromosomes), but does not alter genes or gene arrangements within chromosomes. There is a practical reason for so classifying genetic changes. Agents that produce aneuploidy* or polyploidy* (genomic mutation) are often different from those which produce chromosomal or gene mutation. Gain or loss of whole chromosomes usually is caused by failure of the

chromosomes to separate normally during cell division.
The effect may not be on DNA at all. For example, a
chemical may poison the spindle fibers that are responsible
for chromosomal movement during cell division. However,
gene mutation and chromosomal mutation are produced typically
by direct effects on the DNA. Some agents, such as ionizing
radiation, are very effective at breaking chromosomes and
thus leading to chromosomal rearrangement, but are less
effective at producing changes in individual nucleotides.
Some chemicals produce gene mutation by affecting the
purines and pyrimidines directly, but are less effective
at breaking chromosomes.

Although this scheme is simple, the specific sizes and
shapes of mutational lesions are very complex. Gene
mutation, for instance, includes both point mutation*
(involving only one or a few DNA base pairs) and larger
but still wholly intragenic changes (such as small deletions)
that probably correspond on a smaller scale to multigenic
chromosomal mutations. Gene mutation and point mutation
frequently are confused; operationally, mutation that
affects a specific gene is first termed "gene mutation"
and should be termed "point mutation" only when further
analysis reveals its appropriately small dimensions;
however, reverse mutation selected in a well-characterized
system usually can be safely assumed to be point mutation.

Point mutation consists of base-pair substitution*
(such as adenine:thymine to guanine:cytosine) and frameshift
mutation* (deletion or addition of a small number of base
pairs). Base-pair substitution, in turn, consists of
transition* (in which the purine:pyrimidine base-pair
orientation is preserved, as in the above example of
A:T → G:C) and transversion* (in which the orientation is
reversed, as in A:T → T:A). Frameshift mutation takes its
name from the codon reading frame defined by the correspondence of three bases to one amino acid in the genetic
code. Addition or deletion of one or a few bases (in
messenger RNA) or base pairs (in DNA) makes nonsense of
the rest of the message. (Note that addition or deletion
of multiples of three base pairs between sets of triplet
nucleotides that code for amino acids fails to shift the
reading frame. However, it does result in the addition or
removal of amino acids from the protein, which is very apt
to be deleterious. Thus, amino acid substitution can
occur by base-pair substitution or by replacement of a set
of three nucleotides in the proper reading frame.) Base-
pair substitution and frameshift mutation have character-
istically different impacts on organisms.

Chromosomal mutation consists of deletion* or deficiency*
(loss of long rows of base pairs), duplication* (tandem or

reverse-tandem repeat of long rows of base pairs), inversion*
(simple reversal of segments of DNA within a single
chromosome), transposition* (relocation of a long DNA
sequence within a single chromosome), and translocation*
(relocation of nonhomologous segments, usually terminal
fractions of arms, from one chromosome to another or,
often, reciprocally). Deletions and duplications are most
important in the first generation of children. In addition,
insertion sequences* (additions of long foreign DNA sequences
that are innately able to change chromosomal locations)
are known to occur in bacteria and in eukaryotes--such as
yeasts, Drosophila, and maize--and recently have been
found to occur in mammals. The larger chromosomal mutations
usually are detected by cytogenetic examination, by altered
gene linkage patterns, or by their extremely deleterious
effects. The smaller chromosomal mutations usually are
detected first as gene mutations; involving small segments
of DNA, they may not be recognized as chromosomal mutations
without fine-scale mapping tests. The often severe and
dominant effects of a considerable proportion of large
chromosomal mutations arise from three causes: gene imbalances
in first-generation heterozygotes (one or three copies of
many genes, rather than two); distorted meiotic segregation
patterns that produce abnormal gametes with unbalanced
chromosomes, decreased fertility, or abnormal offspring;
and possibly altered gene activity due to relocation of
genes to relatively inactive regions of chromosomes (the
"position effect" known to be important in Drosophila, but
of uncertain generality).

The first class of chromosomal mutation, deletion, is
of great importance, because it occurs frequently and
because the loss of several genes almost always causes
some deleterious effect. Rearrangements of chromosomal
segments usually have no effect unless a break is inside
or near a gene; this is generally not the case in humans,
because so much of the DNA is not genic. But chromosomal
rearrangements invite complications at meiosis, which lead
to gametes with genic imbalance.

Genomic mutation is caused by an aberration of chromosomal
segregation, often as a result of nondisjunction (failure
of a chromosome pair to separate and migrate to opposite
daughter cells) or anaphase lag (failure of a single
chromosome to migrate to its pole). The result is monosomy
or trisomy (one or three copies of a chromosome, rather
than two). Sometimes, asynchrony between chromosomal and
cellular divisions leads to gains or losses of entire sets
of chromosomes and produces haploidy (one chromosome set,
rather than two), triploidy (three sets), and, in somatic

cells, tetraploidy and above. The gene imbalance resulting
from monosomy and trisomy usually leads to death, often by
early abortion or drastic deformity; the expression of
deleterious recessive mutations in monosomy and haploidy
also has drastic consequences. The higher ploidies in
germ cells are also lethal in mammals, although often
viable in plants and insects.

A final class of mutation affects cytoplasmic, rather
than nuclear, DNA. For reasons mentioned before, this is
believed to be of less consequence than nuclear mutation.

THE INDUCERS OF MUTATION

Mutation is induced mainly by radiation and chemicals.
The former includes ionizing radiation (x rays, gamma
rays, and other kinds), ultraviolet light, and sometimes
visible light (when it excites a chemical that transfers
this energy to DNA). With the possible exception of
effects due to heating or shearing, radiation of longer
wavelength than visible radiation is probably an ineffective
mutagen.

Although the number of radiation mutagens is quite
small, the number of chemical mutagens, and even classes
of chemical mutagens, is large. For instance, a recent
list of chemical mutagens and carcinogens[370] grouped them
into about 40 chemical classes, a number that represents
a minimum. The responses of the chemicals in a given
class are diverse even in a single test system, and the
probability of scoring a carcinogen as a mutagen also
varies considerably among chemical classes.

The literature is replete with interesting studies of
structure-function comparisons in closely related families
of chemicals, but they rarely provide a reliable basis for
predicting mutagenicity in an untested chemical. However,
structure-function correlations do provide an important
basis for ranking previously uncharacterized chemicals for
mutagenicity testing; untested chemicals from classes
richly populated with mutagens are indeed likely to be
mutagens--e.g., nitroso compounds, aromatic amines, nitro-
aromatics, haloaliphatics, mustards, and hydrazines. The
extension of structure-function extrapolations from
qualitative measures to predictors of either quantitative
responses or classes of mutation (chromosomal mutation,
base-pair substitution, frameshift mutation, etc.) is not
now feasible. A goal of research in this field is some
combination of pharmacologic and genetic measurement that
eventually will achieve such predictive power.

THE MECHANICS OF MUTATION

During the course of evolution, a complex set of enzymatic mechanisms developed to maintain the fidelity of DNA before and during its replication. Any damage to this apparatus, including the structure of DNA itself, may result in mutation.

The contemporary theory of frameshift mutagenesis comfortably encompasses the available experimental data, but is by no means fully established. The mutagenic process begins with a DNA strand interruption, as might occur during DNA replication, crossing-over, or excision repair. At ordinary temperatures, the strand terminus will rapidly and repeatedly melt back by one or a few bases and then reanneal. Occasionally, however, reannealing occurs out of register, especially if the strand terminus is at or near a region of local sequence redundancy (...AAAAA..., for instance). If this misalignment happens to be sealed into DNA strand continuity by normal replicative or repair synthesis before being reversed by a later melt, a mutation is created. Several classes of chemicals are adept in the induction of frameshift mutation: large aromatic planar structures that can adhere to the flat surfaces of the bases, agents that directly break DNA strands, and agents that induce strand breakage as a result of excision repair.

Recently, a quite different model has been proposed that accounts for the appearance of many kinds of mutations, including base pair substitutions, additions and deletions, and small chromosomal mutations of the type that would usually be classified as gene mutations. The model accounts for frequent palindromic sequences (more exactly, imperfect palindromes or quasipalindromes) in DNA that can predispose to alternative DNA structures (e.g., clover leaves) that differ from the usual double helix. The alternative or "secondary" structures can then be acted on by any of a variety of DNA-processing enzymes in ways that may ultimately lead to mutations. The details of these processes are only now becoming manifest, but the general model clearly explains many hitherto mysterious mutational phenomena.[371]

Two general models are available to describe base-pair substitution mutagenesis. Again, although each satisfies numerous experimental results, neither is fully established, particularly in the case of mammalian cells. In the first model, base mispairing occurs during DNA synthesis because the parental or the progeny base assumes an altered configuration that specifically favors this mispairing. The change may occur spontaneously (by internal proton migration, for instance) or as the result of reaction with an attacking species (a classical example is the deamination of cytosine by nitrous acid to generate uracil, which pairs the way thymine does). In the second model, template bases are so grossly altered that they exhibit virtually no pairing potential, and progeny bases may be inserted opposite them virtually at random.

Chromosomal mutagenesis generally is attributed either to chromosomal breakage and attachment of broken ends in new ways or to aberrations of normal recombination.[471] Break-rejoin schemes are attractive, because some mutagens, such as ionizing radiation, both break chromosomes and generate chromosomal mutations efficiently and because higher eukaryotic chromosomes contain reiterated DNA sequences scattered throughout the genome; the latter provides a conceptual basis for ready misjoining by means of limited DNA sequence homologies. The recombinational model also assumes that the rejoining of fragments occurs through regions of DNA sequence homology, but primarily as a consequence of otherwise normal meiotic processes, rather than chemically induced chromosomal breakage.

Genomic mutagenesis generally is attributed to abnormalities of chromosomal segregation at anaphase--an event that may be triggered by chemical damage to proteins, rather than to DNA. For instance, some agents that interfere with spindle-fiber formation, but appear not to affect DNA directly, are effective inducers of numerical changes, such as aneuploidy and polyploidy.

Some mutational processes are considered to be fairly direct, others indirect. Frameshift mutagenesis, directly induced base mispairing, and chromosomal and genomic mutation are relatively direct processes, albeit representing escapes from a variety of avoidance mechanisms to be mentioned below. The more indirect processes are those in which the chemically altered DNA bases are unable to specify any progeny base at all; in which the primary target of chemical damage is an enzyme of DNA metabolism, rather than DNA itself; or in which a major component of the mutational target is a portion of DNA different from the ultimately mutated sequence.

Evidence is accumulating that the cell's mutational response to many mutagens may require gene regulation, transcription, and translation.[498] Indeed, the mutagenicity of many agents can be abolished by mutations that block this response--usually at the cost of increased cellular sensitivity to the killing effects that typically accompany mutagen action. Often, the inducing signal appears to be DNA damage itself, although not necessarily at the ultimately mutated sites. The frequently simultaneous induction of capacities for mutagenesis and DNA repair has generated

much jargon for these processes, despite a somewhat
scanty experimental base: "error-prone repair," "misrepair,"
and "mutagenic repair." The underlying mechanisms are
virtually unknown.

An elegant and extremely sophisticated set of mutation-
avoidance mechanisms operates within cells; so effective
are these that only once in 10^3-10^8 possibilities is a
potentially mutagenic lesion not circumvented. These
mechanisms operate at three distinct times during the cell
cycle: before, during, and shortly after DNA replication.
The first mechanism operates to remove DNA damage, whereupon
the missing genetic information is resynthesized chemically
according to instructions received from the complementary
strand (e.g., excision repair or direct reversal of damage,
as by photoreactivation and dealkylation). The second
mechanism acts as a part of, or in close association with,
DNA polymerase. In an energetic sense, the event consists
of well-informed prior base selection (better informed
than base pairing itself) and base rejection after
polymerization (e.g., by 3'-exonuclease action). The
third mechanism is rather diverse. First, mispair correction
recognizes base mispairing and, being informed as to which
is the progeny and which the template strand, achieves
highly effective excision repair. Second, recombinational
repair operates on progeny-strand gaps (induced, for
instance, by an inability to insert any base at all),
correcting this deficiency by a series of DNA strand
exchanges designed to relocate nonpairing lesions opposite
intact strands. Third, mutagenic repair occurs. It
should be noted, however, that these mechanisms generally
have been characterized in microorganisms, and the extent
(if any) to which they operate in humans is unknown.

In addition to the primary mutagenic mechanisms described
above, two other general mechanisms contribute crucially.
The first comprises metabolic processing of otherwise
genetically innocuous chemicals to mutationally active
products, a process that is imperfectly countered by the
degradation of the mutagens to genotoxic inertness. This
is apt to be a species-, organ-, and individual-specific
process and can confound the species-to-species extrapolation
of mutational-response profiles. The second process,
probably of little consequence for mutation risk assessment,
comprises events that promote the expression of recessive
mutations. The full expression of a recessive mutation
usually is delayed for many sexual generations, until
homozygosity can occur. Somatic cell expression may be
more prompt if the mutation is rendered homozygous by
special cellular events. One such event is loss of the

wild-type allele by chromosomal mutation (a deletion, for
instance) or genomic mutation (monosomy, for instance).
Although such gross changes usually would be lethal if
borne by every cell in the body, single cells and many of
their descendants may survive as islands surrounded by
supportive normal cells. Another event is mitotic
recombination, an exchange between homologous chromosomes
followed by a segregation pattern that sometimes renders
the mutant gene homozygous. Mitotic recombination has not
yet been demonstrated in vivo in humans. But it is readily
induced in numerous nonhuman systems and in human cell
cultures by the same sorts of chemicals that induce mutations.

It should be clear from the above that the mutation
process may be described (although very imperfectly) in
specific physicochemical terms. Thus, the same fundamental
restraints apply to mutation rates as to rates of other
complex chemical reactions. Specifically, although mutation
rates in principle can be reduced by the application of
ever more numerous and sophisticated avoidance systems,
they can neither be reduced to zero nor be reduced in
contemporary practice by any known means of human intervention
other than the obvious one of restricting exposure to
mutagens.

THE GENETICS OF MUTATION

Mutation rates depend on the particular target gene, on
the individual and the species, and on germ cell stage and
sex. The role of germ cell stage is particularly important
in the evaluation of human hazard.

It will often be necessary to extrapolate from test
systems to humans; therefore, we need to understand the
degree to which underlying mutagenic mechanisms are similar.
Our understanding of mammalian mechanisms of mutation is
very primitive; few genetic probes possess the resolving
power available for prokaryotic and eukaryotic microorganisms.
What follows, although partly speculative, may nevertheless
indicate likely general directions for future research.

It is clear that rates of spontaneous and induced
mutation themselves have evolved. Many of the genes that
determine these rates have been identified in model microbial
systems, although very few are characterized in higher
eukaryotes. Rates of spontaneous mutation per gene per
generation tend to decrease as genome size increases, but
this tendency has been measured only among viruses, bacteria,
and fungi; the rate of spontaneous mutation per gene per
generation is approximately inversely proportional to the

size of the genome, so that the total rate per genome remains nearly invariant. Among animals, however, the average mutation rate per gene per generation is roughly the same in Drosophila, mouse, and man, despite large differences in the amount of DNA.

Approximate constancy of mutation per gene per generation is not equivalent to constancy per gene per year. For example, the Drosophila life cycle is completed in about one-thousandth the time of the human cycle. Therefore, the Drosophila mutation rate is about 1,000 times as great (measured in absolute time units). Mutation rates correspond to the generation length in such a way that the number of mutations per gene per generation is approximately constant.

There are many ways in which mutation rates might be heritably increased, and individually inherited sensitivities are already known in Drosophila, mice, and humans. In view of the large number of enzymatic steps involved in mutation avoidance and in the metabolic pathways that affect the processing of xenobiotics*, it is to be expected that individual humans will differ substantially in sensitivity to particular chemical mutagens. Indeed, it is estimated that a few percent of humans are heterozygous for genes that determine sensitivity to radiation and chemical damage to DNA by defects in repair capacities,[348] [449] [454] [455] and some of the heterozygotes may be at increased risk of cancer. It has been suggested that as much as 5% of all cancer patients may be heterozygotes for ataxia telangiectasia.[450] By analogy with some microbial systems, it is possible that a majority of deleterious mutations that enter the human gene pool may originate in such heterozygotes. Thought needs to be given to ways to identify such susceptible persons.

Even within a genetically homogeneous population, individual genes vary greatly in rates of spontaneous and induced mutation. Only a part of this variation is attributable to gene-size differences; greater contributions probably come from differences in the intrinsic mutability of particular sites within the gene--the "mutational hot spots" that so heavily dominate the mutational responses of individual genes. These differences will have to be taken into account in extrapolating from one or a few test genes to entire genomes; they are largely irrelevant, however, when large banks of genes are screened simultaneously, as in the Drosophila recessive-lethal systems.

Known differences in mutational response between sexes and between germ cell stages are still limited largely to spontaneous mutation and that induced by ionizing radiation.[299] [386] [472] [473] On the one hand, there are indications of

increasing frequencies of germinal gene mutation with age
in human males--a result consistent with the ongoing
process of spermatogenesis. On the other hand, genomic
mutation resulting from meiotic nondisjunction appears to
increase with maternal age, the most notable example being
in Down's syndrome.

Environmental effects on mutation rates (other than
those attributable to mutagens themselves) have yet to be
documented in mammals, although they probably exist.
Examples expected to emerge are drug effects on mutagen
activation or DNA repair.

TRANSPOSABLE GENETIC ELEMENTS

Until recently, the mechanisms for increasing the
overall mutation rate were thought to involve DNA-copying
enzymes or the process of DNA repair. However, high
mutation rate is now known to be caused by another genetic
mechanism--transposable genetic elements.

Transposons* are small pieces of DNA that are capable
of inserting themselves into chromosomal DNA. If a transposon
inserts into a region where no gene exists, there is
little effect; but, if the insertion occurs in a gene's
coding or regulatory sequences, function may be impaired
or destroyed. Under some circumstances, the frequency
with which transposable elements move about and generate
mutations becomes very large, and they may even contribute
a majority of phenotypically expressed spontaneous mutations.

Mutation schemes of this kind have been known in maize
for many years, but the basic mechanism of action has only
recently become understood. Most information is derived
from bacteria and yeast, but examples are also well known
in Drosophila, and there is evidence of transposons in
mammals. The fraction of mutations that occur by this
mechanism is unknown, but transposition probably accounts
for the high mutability that is seen in various species
from time to time.

If transposons cause human mutation in significant
numbers, this will necessitate some revision in mutagenicity
testing. The mechanisms of transposition may be more akin
to those of crossing-over. It is quite likely that many
chemicals that induce base substitutions or chromosomal
breaks may have little influence on transposon-induced
mutation, whereas other chemicals may affect transposons
specifically. In this regard, it is interesting that some
transposons act exclusively in germ cells, but not in
somatic cells.

THE IMPACT OF MUTATION

The health consequence of deleterious mutation in populations is poorly understood, despite the large effort that has been expended in the study of mutation. Spontaneous-mutation rates are known only roughly, the forces that maintain or alter gene frequencies in populations are not well understood, and the relative impacts of different types of mutations are obscure.

Rates of human spontaneous mutation per gene per generation have been estimated to range from less than 10^{-6} to as high as 10^{-4}, and the numbers of genes at risk from 10^4 to 10^5. These ranges are likely to narrow considerably as improved gene- and mutation-detection technologies are applied in the next decade. However, of greater importance in assessing the impact of mutations is the unknown fraction of the human load of deleterious mutations that is maintained by balanced selective forces, compared with the fraction maintained by selection pressures, such as heterozygote advantage and the existence of genes favorable in one environment or in one genotype but not in others.

Another problem is the impact of "mild" mutations--those which produce only small effects, which arise at relatively high rates, and which are inefficiently selected out of populations. Although it is currently virtually impossible to detect such effects clinically in humans, it is clear that they contribute markedly to the total mutational load in Drosophila, where they outnumber "severe" (recessive lethal and semilethal) mutations by a factor of at least 10 and significantly reduce the health of the typical wild fly. The same is true for mutations induced by ethyl methanesulfonate, but other chemicals have not been tested. The human situation is not understood, but it is possible that, for every severe mutation detected by laboratory test systems, 20 or more mildly deleterious mutations also occur.

An assessment of the impact of mutations also must take into account the severities of different types of mutations. Chromosomal and genomic mutations, for instance, are apt to produce severe dominant effects--so much so that zygotic death occurs early in embryonic development and zygotes that survive may be seriously burdened.[471-473] The severity of point mutations depends on the specific nature of the lesion.[421 497] Base-addition and -deletion mutations often generate null mutations (e.g., no gene product whatsoever, the functional equivalent of a gene-sized deletion), and their severity therefore is apt to reflect the consequences of altered amount of gene product in the heterozygote. Base-pair substitutions may generate amino

acid substitutions that in many cases lead to the presence
of a defective gene product, because the consequences of
defective gene products are in some cases greater than
those of no gene product. Such mutations may be less
fully recessive and have a greater social impact than will
base additions and deletions. Eventually, differences
like these will have to be taken into account if the
mutational impact of environmental chemicals on humans is
to be estimated adequately.

IS AN INCREASED MUTATION RATE NECESSARILY DETRIMENTAL?

It is commonly believed that mutations are almost
invariably harmful, whether they are genic, chromosomal,
or genomic. Some mutations have effects so minute as to
be undetectable. Whether these are neutral or only nearly
so is a matter of considerable discussion and experimentation.
Nevertheless, we can say confidently that the overwhelming
majority of mutations that have any overt effect at all
are harmful. A geneticist has to search to find examples
of mutations that are clearly beneficial to the organism.
Usually, these are found when the environment has been
drastically altered. One example is DDT resistance in
insects, but here it is worth noting that, in the absence
of DDT, the resistance genes are usually mildly harmful.[421]
There are also a number of examples of benefit from the
human viewpoint, but hardly from that of the animal in its
wild state--for example, hornless cattle or nonbrooding
hens.

All organisms are the products of a long evolutionary
history during which favorable genes have been preserved
and deleterious genes eliminated by natural selection.
Beneficial mutations of the past are part of the present
population. A random change is much more likely to make
things worse than better. In the framework of genetic
possibility, a mutation is essentially a random change.
Thus, the general harmfulness of mutation is both an
empirical fact and an expectation based on evolutionary
reasoning.

Of course, some mutations must be beneficial, or we
would not have evolved at all. There may be some mutant
genes that are beneficial in some combinations or in some
circumstances. Nevertheless, it is clear that the aggregate
effect of all mutation is deleterious.

It is sometimes said that, were it not for mutations,
we would run out of genetic variability and thus cut off
any possibility of future human evolution. Such statements
do not take account of the extremely low rate at which

genetic variability decays. If the human mutation rate
were to drop to zero, we probably would observe no effect
except the disappearance of some of our most severe genetic
diseases. According to the prevailing neo-Darwinian view,
the variability on which future evolution depends involves
mainly inconspicuous genes, often with quantitative rather
than sharply qualitative effects. Mendelian inheritance
is very effective in conserving variability. The rate of
decrease of genetic variance is 1/2N per generation, where
N is the effective population number,[506] which is roughly
the number of reproducing adults. Thus, any loss of
genetic variability because of the failure of new mutations
to occur would be extremely slow. In our view, even the
current rate of "spontaneous" mutation is not optimal for
human welfare; our descendants for the next few centuries,
and probably beyond, would be better off if we could find
a way to reduce the rate of spontaneous mutation.

THE RARITY OF COMPLETELY RECESSIVE MUTANT GENES

It is generally recognized that the frequency of recessive
lethal mutation in the Drosophila population is less than
would be expected from the known mutation rate. The
explanation is that the typical "recessive" lethal mutation
is not completely recessive, but is slightly deleterious
in the heterozygous condition. Calculations based on the
observed frequency of recessive lethal mutants in natural
populations of D. melanogaster and the spontaneous-
mutation rates measured in many laboratory experiments
show that the mutant heterozygotes have viability and
fertility about 2% lower than normal homozygotes.[79] This
has been confirmed by direct viability and fertility
studies in the laboratory. Because the mutants that are
found in a natural population are a selected sample weighted
in favor of those with the mildest effects (these being
the ones that would persist longest in nature), we should
expect a group of newly occurring lethal mutations to have
a greater heterozygous effect. That is found to be true,
and the value is about twice that found in natural,
equilibrium populations.

The evidence in the human population is not as strong,
but is consistent. If most recessive mutations were
completely recessive, they should accumulate to such an
extent that almost every cousin marriage would lead to
offspring that die early or have gross abnormalities.
Thus, the human data are qualitatively consistent with the
Drosophila data, although there is no way yet to determine
the quantitative consistency.

An example of the many partially recessive genes in the human population is the autosomal gene causing Type II hyper-β-lipoproteinemia.[126] Both homozygotes and heterozygotes have high concentrations of low-density lipoproteins, but the concentration is much higher in homozygotes. As a result, homozygotes manifest the disease early and more severely; such people rarely live past adolescence. Heterozygotes have much milder symptoms, and vascular disease does not start until middle age.

A completely recessive autosomal mutation is almost never expressed immediately. The recessive trait will appear only if the mutant gene becomes homozygous, which can occur if the recessive gene happens to combine in the same individual with a gene like itself. Because such mutant genes are very rare in the population, this kind of combination is very unlikely, and a typical recessive mutant gene in a large, non-inbred human population might wait for 100 or more generations for this to happen. Another way for the mutant gene to become homozygous is through the mating of two descendants of the person in whom the mutation occurred. Consanguineous marriages are rare in most parts of the developed world, so homozygosity of a mutant gene by this process is also infrequent. Because a recessive mutation so rarely becomes homozygous, it is eliminated by natural selection primarily because of its deleterious heterozygous effects. This can occur even if the heterozygous effect reduces survival and fertility by only 2-5%.

In contrast with rare, lethal recessive mutation, extensive studies in Drosophila have shown that the most frequent mutations are those with only mild effects. In Drosophila, these are detected as a small reduction in the probability of surviving to adulthood or a small decrease in fertility. Such mutations also are not completely recessive. Therefore, they, like their more drastic recessive counterparts, are eliminated from the population in the heterozygous state.

We have very little idea what the human counterparts of these mildly deleterious Drosophila mutations are. Presumably, they are heterogeneous functional impairments that are individually mild, but collectively can add up to a substantial genetic load. Such a mild mutation can remain in the population for many generations, weakening each individual slightly until it tips the balance between survival and premature death or sterility and is eliminated from the population. This kind of condition is not likely to be the clear-cut genetic disease for which biochemistry, cytogenetics, and molecular biology seek cures. Such mutation may have a significant cumulative impact on distant future generations. However, they may have non-specific effects that are ameliorated by improvements in living standards and health care. This is the most uncertain part of genetic risk assessment.

THE TIME DISTRIBUTION OF EFFECTS OF MUTATIONS

If a sudden increase in the mutation rate occurred, perhaps because of the temporary widespread presence of a chemical mutagen, it would add new mutant genes in the population. The greatest impact of these new mutations would be on the next generation, and the effect would diminish over time as the mutations were eliminated. Mutations that have a severe heterozygous effect do a great deal of harm in the early generations, but are eliminated relatively rapidly. However, if they are mild, the mutations will cause little harm in any one generation, but will persist longer. This is illustrated in Figure 3-1.

The effect of a mutation-induced impairment on human well-being is not necessarily the same as its effect on survival and fertility (Darwinian fitness). A mutant gene or altered chromosome may cause great pain or anguish without any great effect on survival and fertility. A mutation that causes early embryonic death is severe from the standpoint of Darwinian fitness, but with little social impact; it is eliminated quickly from the population. Despite these exceptions and reservations, there is

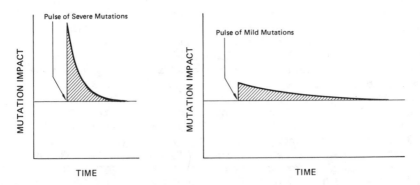

FIGURE 3-1 Distribution of the impact of a single-generation pulse of mutations. Shaded area shows the total impact. Left, distribution of impact for a mutation with severe effect; right, more dilute effect of milder mutations.

an overall positive association between the severity of a
mutation from the humanitarian standpoint and its effect
on survival and fertility. If we adopt a system of mutation
cost-accounting that equates a small amount of harm to a
large number of people with a great amount of harm to a
small number of people, mild mutations can have as great
consequences as severe ones, or greater. For this reason,
the two curves in Figure 3-1 have been drawn to have
approximately the same total hatched area. (The shape of
the true curve is complex. For any one kind of mutant
gene, the approach to equilibrium is exponential, the rate
depending on its dominance and its effect on fitness--the
more severe the effect, the more rapid the approach to
equilibrium. Considering all mutations, the approach is a
family of exponentials; and, of course, there are changing
conditions and random fluctuations.)

The graphs in Figure 3-1 are based on the assumption
that the dominant heterozygous effects of the mutations
are the most important. Severe recessive diseases also
occur, but their impact would be spread over hundreds or
thousands of generations, and the effect on any one generation
would be very small indeed. As emphasized above, if we
can generalize from Drosophila data, most recessive mutations
are eliminated from the population through their heterozygous
effects before they ever become homozygous. Their impact
is through a general nonspecific weakening. It is very
hard to predict the effect of future environmental changes
on the impact of such mutations.

Figure 3-1 assumes that, after the induced mutant genes
are eliminated, the mutation impact will return to its
previous level. If the environment remains constant for a
long time, there will eventually be an equilibrium between
the spontaneous occurrence of new mutations and their
elimination by natural selection. In recent decades,
however, there have been enormous improvements in sanitation,
living standards, nutrition, and medical care. One
consequence is that a mutant gene that formerly had a
severe effect may now have a milder one. The population
is now out of equilibrium: mutations are accumulating
faster, but each mutation has a milder effect than it used
to, so the overall impact is smaller. Therefore, Figure
3-1 would be more accurate if the horizontal line were
sloping downward. Nevertheless, the total shaded area
would be roughly the same.

Figure 3-2 shows the combined effects of mutation
increase and environmental improvement. If there is an
increase in the mutation rate and no change in environment,
the number of mutants in the population will increase
gradually until a new equilibrium is approached. Figure

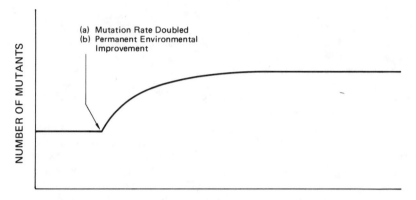

FIGURE 3-2 Change in number of mutants in a population
after (a) doubling of the mutation rate or (b) environmental improvement that causes halving of the effect of
the mutations on preadult mortality and sterility.

3-2 also shows the effect of an improved environment. If
there is a new environment in which each mutant gene
causes only half its previous reduction in fitness, the
number of mutants in the population will double. The
curve will be essentially the same as that caused by an
overall doubling of the mutation rate. From this viewpoint,
an increased mutation rate and an environmental improvement
have the same effect--an increased number of mutant genes
and chromosomes.
     One should not conclude from this analysis that, from
the standpoint of human welfare, environmental improvement
can be equated to an increased mutation rate. The difference
is brought out in Figure 3-3, which, instead of showing
the number of mutant genes, shows their total impact. A
doubling of the mutation rate, with no change in the
environment, eventually will lead to a doubling of the
personal and social burden of mutation. An improvement in
economic standards, health care, and other aspects of the
environment will lessen the impact of the mutations. If
there is no additional improvement in the environment, the
impact gradually will increase to its former value as the
mutant-gene frequencies approach twice their previous
equilibrium frequencies. Whether the final frequency is
the same as that before the environmental improvement
depends on the complex relationship between the human
impact of the mutations and their effect on survival and

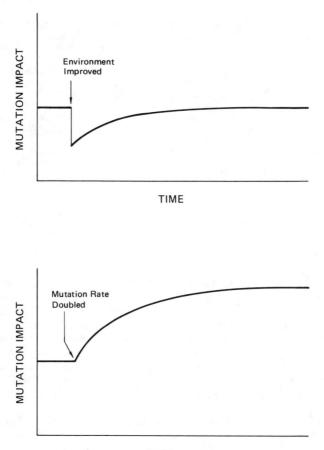

FIGURE 3-3 Effect of (top) environmental improvement on mutation impact and (bottom) increased mutation rate.

fertility. The proportion of homozygote recessives would remain small, however.

Figure 3-4 shows the effect of a series of environmental improvements, each occurring before there has been time for a new mutational equilibrium to be reached. The actual situation in the last 200 yr is probably much like this, except that the environmental improvements have been gradual, rather than abrupt, and what has been observed could probably be shown simply as a decreasing curve of total mutation impact.

Predicting environmental trends is very uncertain. Optimistically, we might expect technologic advances and

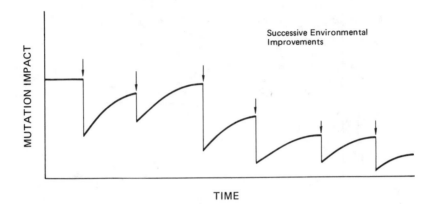

FIGURE 3-4 Effect of a series of environmental improvements.

the ability to ameliorate the effect of mutant genes to continue. To the extent that that expectation is borne out, the population can neutralize the accumulation of mutations as it is doing now. However, epidemic, nuclear war, or overpopulation may force a return to the kind of environment that our ancestors lived in. The population then would suffer a mutation impact comparable with that of the past plus the impact of mutations that have accumulated during the recent period of relaxed natural selection. This is illustrated in Figure 3-5.

Thus, environmental improvement has its price: the obligation to keep improving the environment. The alternative (these are not necessarily mutually exclusive) is some sort of genetic intervention, perhaps with the aid of new techniques that will be revealed by cell and molecular biology of the future.

We need to consider the possibility that there will be a pulse of mutations induced by some environmental agent. If the cause were discovered and removed, the result would be as shown in Figure 3-6. There is a large effect in the immediately ensuing generations, then a rapid decrease and a long tail after the more severe mutants are eliminated. In a stable environment, the total effect of mild mutations on viability and fertility will probably be greater than that of the more severe ones. In a changing environment, the long-range impact of minor mutations depends very much on long-term environmental trends. The effect on a single generation would be minute. This suggests a strategy of concentrating on severe mutations and cytogenetic effects for risk estimation, in the expectation that future knowledge

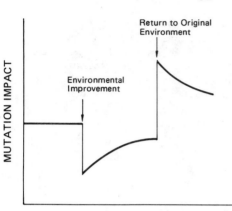

FIGURE 3-5 Effect of an environmental improvement
followed by a return to the original environment.

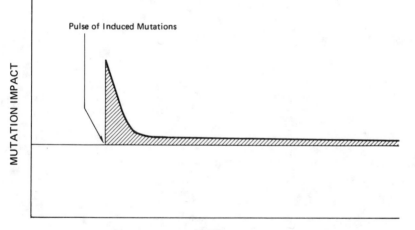

FIGURE 3-6 Distribution of the impact of heterogeneous
group of mutations, as might be expected after a sudden
increase in the mutation rate. Mutations with the most
severe effects produce their damage soon and are eliminated
in a few generations, whereas the effects of milder mutations
are spread out over a very long time.

will reveal more about mild effects. Because the impact
of a one-generation pulse of recessive or mild dominant
mutations on a single generation is extremely small, it
may be wiser not to try now to obtain risk estimates,
except for severe, dominant effects. That is the policy
followed in the BEIR[303] and UNSCEAR[472] reports on estimation
of radiation risks.

4

METABOLISM AND PHARMACOLOGIC DISPOSITION OF MUTAGENS AND PROMUTAGENS

GENERAL INTRODUCTION TO MUTAGEN METABOLISM

Less than 30 years ago, it was generally believed that all drugs and other environmental chemicals were pharmacologically active, toxic, carcinogenic, or mutagenic in their parent (nonmetabolized) form. The function of drug-metabolizing enzymes was therefore regarded as detoxification, i.e., "inactivation" of the active parent drug. Now it is evident that, although some chemicals are indeed active in their nonmetabolized form, most are inactive until they are metabolized;[141][284] this process is called "toxification." Detoxification and metabolic activation enzymes coexist in the same cell, in some instances architecturally next to one another in the same membrane. Furthermore, any given enzyme may be involved in detoxifying one chemical while toxifying a second chemical. Examples are given later in this chapter. Each enzyme is controlled by one or more genes. Each enzyme is likely to differ from one tissue, organ, strain, or species to another and to differ between cells in culture and an intact animal. Such factors as age, hormonal and nutritional variations, diurnal and seasonal rhythms, pH at the enzyme active site, and substrate concentrations (saturating vs. nonsaturating) also contribute to the function of each of these enzymes. Thus, there is a delicate and very complicated balance between detoxification and toxification.

Most drugs and other environmental pollutants are so fat-soluble that they would remain in the body indefinitely were it not for metabolism to more water-soluble derivatives. These enzyme systems--which are principally in the liver, but probably also present to some degree in virtually all tissues of the body--are usually divided into two groups: Phase I and Phase II. During Phase I metabolism, one or

more water-soluble groups (such as hydroxyl) are introduced
into the fat-soluble parent molecule, thus allowing a
"handle," or a position, for the Phase II conjugating
enzymes to attack. Many Phase I products, but especially
the conjugated Phase II products, are sufficiently water-
soluble for these chemicals to be readily excreted from
the body.[141]

Table 4-1 lists a large number of potentially relevant
metabolic reactions that may be important in detoxification
or toxification of mutagens or promutagens. Basically,
whenever a chemical bond is cleaved or electrons are
passed one at a time, there is a possibility of unwanted
reactions of metabolic intermediates with nucleic acid or
protein. The reactions can be complicated by various
factors, including the degree of stability of short-lived
chemical intermediates, the redox state, movement of
unpaired electrons from one molecule (free radical) to
another, and lipid peroxidation. Reactions involving DNA
are believed to be most important for mutagenesis (and
probably for carcinogenesis). It is certainly possible
for mutagens to interact with nucleic acid polymerases,
endonucleases, processing enzymes, or other important
proteins and thus lead to heritable changes in gene expression.

Most Phase I oxidations are performed by cytochrome P-
450. "Cytochrome," derived from Greek, literally means
"colored substance in the cell." The color is derived
from the properties of the outer electrons of the transition
element iron. "P-450" denotes a reddish pigment with the
unusual property of having its major optical absorption
peak (Soret maximum) at about 450 nm, when it has been
reduced and combined with carbon monoxide.[330] Although
the name "P-450" was intended to be temporary (until more
was known about the substance), the terminology has persisted
for 18 yr because of the increasing complexity of this
enzyme system and because of the lack of agreement on new
nomenclature.

Cytochrome P-450 is a multigene family of hemoproteins
with catalytic activity toward thousands of substrates.
This collection of enzymes is known to metabolize almost
all drugs and laboratory reagents; small chemicals, such
as benzene, thiocyanate, and ethanol; polycyclic aromatic
hydrocarbons, such as benzo[a]pyrene (ubiquitous in city
smog and present in cigarette smoke and charcoal-cooked
foods) and biphenyl; halogenated hydrocarbons, such as
polychlorinated and polybrominated biphenyls, herbicides,
insecticides, and ingredients of soaps and deodorants;
some fungal toxins and antibiotics; many of the chemicals
used to treat human cancer; strong mutagens, such as N-
methyl-N'-nitro-N-nitrosoguanidine and alkyl nitrosamines;

TABLE 4-1 Metabolic Reactions That May Be Important
in Environmental Mutagenesis

A. Phase I metabolism: oxidation

    1. Aromatic or aliphatic C-oxygenation (epoxidation,
       hydroxylation)
    2. N-, O-, or S-dealkylation
    3. N-oxidation or N-hydroxylation
    4. S-oxidation
    5. Deamination
    6. Dehalogenation
    7. Metalloalkane dealkylation
    8. Desulfuration
    9. Alcohol or aldehyde dehydrogenation
   10. Xanthine (or other purine) oxidation
   11. Tyrosine hydroxylation
   12. Monoamine (including catecholamine) oxidation

B. Phase I metabolism: reduction

    1. Azo reduction
    2. Nitro reduction
    3. Arene oxide reduction
    4. N-hydroxyl reduction
    5. Quinone reduction
    6. Carbonyl sulfide reduction by carbonic anhydrase
    7. Reduction of transition-metal ion salt

C. Phase I metabolism: hydrolysis

    1. Hydrolysis of ester
    2. Hydrolysis of amide
    3. Hydrolysis of peptide

D. Phase II metabolism: conjugation

    1. Glucuronidation
    2. Sulfate conjugation
    3. Glutathione conjugation
    4. Acetylation
    5. Glycine conjugation
    6. Serine conjugation
    7. N-, O-, or S-methylation
    8. Ribonucleoside or ribonucleotide formation
    9. Glycoside conjugation
   10. Water conjugation

E. Beyond phase II metabolism

    1. C-oxygenation
    2. Glucuronidation
    3. Glycosidation
    4. Deacetylation

F. Direct chemical reaction

    1. Oxidation/reduction

aminoazo dyes and diazo compounds; many chemicals found in
cosmetics and perfumes; numerous aromatic amines, such as
those found in hair dyes, nitro aromatics, and heterocyclics;
N-acetylarylamines and nitrofurans; wood terpenes; epoxides;
carbamates; alkyl halides; safrole derivatives; antioxidants,
other food additives, and many ingredients of foodstuffs,
fermentative alcoholic beverages, and spices; both endogenous
and synthetic steroids; prostaglandins; and other endogenous
compounds, such as biogenic amines, indoles, thyroxine,
and fatty acids.

The consensus among most laboratories[149 259 307 389] has
been that there are a substantial but limited number of P-
450s and that overlapping substrate specificity accounts
for the diversity seen when thousands of different chemicals
are metabolized. The number of forms might be considerably
larger than 20.

A monooxygenase is an enzyme that inserts one atom of
atmospheric oxygen into its substrate. The various forms
of P-450 constitute a large subset of all monooxygenases.
In monooxygenation, the P-450 hemoprotein receives two
electrons from cofactor NADPH or NADH, or both; these
electrons are received one at a time, usually via reductases
(flavoproteins). In most organisms, the electron chain is
deeply embedded principally in the endoplasmic reticulum
(and to some degree in the inner mitochondrial membrane
and nuclear envelope). After sheering of the membrane
during homogenization, the endoplasmic reticulum is centri-
fuged at 100,000 g for an hour, and the product is called
the "microsomal pellet." The microsomal electron chain
contains reductase and P-450.

P-450-mediated monooxygenase activities are found in
virtually all living things--some kinds of bacteria and
presumably all plants and animals.[149 204] For example,
types of bacteria are being developed to destroy oil
spilled in the ocean; this catalytic activity represents
Phase I metabolism and the P-450-mediated monooxygenase
system.

P-450-mediated monooxygenase activities (Table 4-1)
include aromatic and aliphatic hydroxylations of carbon
atoms; N-, O-, and S-dealkylations; N-oxidations and N-
hydroxylations; S-oxidations, deaminations; dehalogenations;
metalloalkane dealkylations; desulfurations; some purine
and monoamine oxidations; azo and nitro reductions; and
some arene oxide and N-hydroxyl reductions. Removal of
methyl or ethyl groups from substrates (dealkylation) can
result in the covalent binding of reactive intermediates
(alkylation) to nucleic acid or protein--a potentially
important mechanism for mutagenesis, tumorigenesis, or
drug toxicity. Tetraethyl lead in gasoline, for example,

is metabolized by P-450 in this manner to a reactive
intermediate that is toxic to the central nervous system.[141]
Chromate is one of a number of inorganic chemical carcinogens.
P-450 has been reported[192] to reduce in vitro some metals,
such as Cr(VI) to Cr(III); this may be an important
detoxification pathway for chromate.

Human liver alcohol dehydrogenase (Table 4-1) catalyzes
the oxidation of digitoxigenin and derivatives. This is a
potentially important detoxification pathway. Liver
alcohol dehydrogenase may also toxify chemicals, metabolizing
several xylyl alcohols to aldehydes that are toxic to lung
and allyl alcohol to the extremely neurotoxic acrolein.
Alcohol dehydrogenase is therefore an excellent example of
the dual nature of an enzyme designed to metabolize endogenous
substrates: the enzyme can detoxify one foreign chemical
and toxify another.

Quinone reduction by DT diaphorase[251] has been postulated
to be an important step leading to a substrate for glucuronide
conjugation (Table 4-1). Quinone-derived free radicals
might also be generated by this catalytic activity or by
some similar activity other than DT diaphorase. Carbonyl
sulfide has recently been shown to be metabolized to
hydrogen sulfide by carbonic anhydrase; hydrogen sulfide
is responsible for carbonyl sulfide toxicity.[61] Carbonic
anhydrase therefore is involved in a metabolic pathway
leading to toxification.

Drugs and other foreign chemicals are most commonly
conjugated with glucuronide, sulfate, or glutathione
(Table 4-1). Characterization of the sulfotransferases
has only begun.[262] Glutathione transferases act on a
large number of chemicals--including arene oxides, epoxides,
chlorodinitrobenzene, bromosulfophthalein (for testing
liver function), and bilirubin; at least six glutathione
transferases have been characterized so far.[191] Sulfotransferases and glutathione transferases are isozymes,
are cytosolic, and have overlapping substrate specificities.
Epoxide hydrolase adds water to arene oxides or epoxides
to form dihydrodiols; this "water conjugation" occurs, for
example, during the metabolism of carcinogenic polycyclic
hydrocarbons. Epoxide hydrolase is nuclear, cytosolic,
and microsomal; it activates polycyclic aromatic hydrocarbons
and inactivates aflatoxin B_1 epoxide.

Although dihydrodiols are, in general, readily excreted,
it is now clear[284] that diol-epoxides are formed and that
these highly reactive intermediates may be important in
mutagenicity, tumorigenesis, toxicity, and birth defects.[284,418]
Diols can therefore undergo further C-oxygenations (Table
4-1).

The general belief has been that, once a conjugate is

formed, the substance is excreted. The glucuronide of 3-hydroxybenzo[a]pyrene treated with β-glucuronidase, however, forms reactive intermediates capable of binding covalently with nucleic acid and protein.[208] β-Glucuronidase activity is extremely high in kidney and bladder. By a similar mechanism, glycosides react with various glycosidases, and the reaction results in reactive intermediates capable of binding covalently with nucleic acid and protein. After conjugation with acetyl CoA, many drugs can be deacetylated (Table 4-1) to form reactive intermediates.

Some chemicals, by their molecular properties, have a high redox potential. o-Aminophenol, for example, can oxidize ferrohemoglobin to ferrihemoglobin. Nitrates also cause methemoglobinemia. Such one-electron chemical reactions may play a role in mutagenesis.

In conclusion, perhaps only a few enzymes in the body take care of only foreign chemicals. Apparently, many enzymes that react with normal-body substrates, however, can interact with most mutagens and promutagens. The result is a complicated and delicate balance of detoxification and toxification.

INTRACELLULAR LOCALIZATION OF DRUG-METABOLIZING ENZYMES

Of the reactions listed in Table 4-1, more than 98% is in the cytoplasm--endoplasmic reticulum (microsomes) and soluble (cytosolic) fractions. Mitochondrial enzymes performing some of these reactions generally appear to account for much less than 5% and enzymes of the nuclear envelope less than 1% of the total cellular metabolic activity. Many recent reports have described "nuclear-membrane P-450" and other enzymes capable of forming reactive mutagens-carcinogens. If a short-lived intermediate is formed in the proximity of nuclear DNA, this might be far more important than reactive-intermediate formation farther from DNA on the other side of the nuclear membrane in the cytoplasm. Although this hypothesis remains attractive, most studies have relied on light microscopy to determine the "degree of purity" of nuclear membranes. Minuscule contamination of nuclear fractions with 100 or 1,000 times more metabolically active microsomal fragments would cause artifactual data. Studies of nuclear-membrane "drug-metabolizing enzyme activity" will require verification to show that there is not microsomal contamination of the isolated nuclear-membrane fraction.

Benzo[a]pyrene 7,8-diol-9,10-epoxide, for example, is considered to be highly reactive and extremely short-lived. Yet, given intraperitoneally to newborn mice, this chemical causes tumors in distant tissues and organs.[47] Short-lived intermediates apparently can be stabilized by proteins and lipids in solution. It remains to be proved, therefore, whether nuclear-membrane P-450 is any more important than cytoplasmic P-450 in forming this highly reactive potent mutagen-carcinogen. It must be emphasized that the possible role of nuclear drug-metabolizing capacity in mutagenesis should be examined further.

INTERACTIONS OF REACTIVE ELECTROPHILES WITH DNA

Benzo[a]pyrene trans-7,8-diol-9,10-epoxide binds covalently predominantly to guanine and lies in the minor groove of DNA, although one-tenth or one-hundredth of this amount of covalent binding between the diol-epoxide and both adenine and cytosine has also been found. This good fit with DNA[488] leads to decreases in RNA polymerase transcription and to relatively slow recognition by the DNA polymerase system;[241] these aberrations may be important in making this particular diol-epoxide such a potent mutagen-carcinogen. Benzo[a]pyrene cis-7,8-diol-epoxide and benzo[a]pyrene 4,5-oxide appear not to fit very well in the minor DNA groove. Other potentially important well-characterized adducts include N-hydroxy-2-acetylamino-fluorene and aflatoxin B_1 2,3-oxide binding to guanine. How these "specific binding sites" for metabolites in the DNA are related to mutagenesis, cancer, or toxicity, however, remains to be determined. One recent hypothesis[48 489] is that covalently bound reactive metabolites cause the movement of transposable elements to new locations in genomic DNA and that this process represents carcinogenic "initiation."

EVOLUTION AND THE METABOLISM OF FOREIGN CHEMICALS

Some types of bacteria (such as Pseudomonas, Aerobacter, and Klebsiella) utilize camphor, toluene, and other hydrocarbons as energy sources; the induced enzymes are soluble forms of P-450, and in some instances the induction process appears to be controlled by plasmid genes.[58] Simple eukaryotic cells, such as fungi,[57 250] as well as simple and more highly evolved plants and animals,[204 389] have detectable P-450-mediated monooxygenase activities that can be induced by chemicals under the proper conditions. At some undetermined point in evolution, the function of these induced enzymes apparently changed from efficient utilization of an energy source to detoxification. In organisms with fatty tissues, most hydrophobic drugs and other environmental pollutants would remain indefinitely in these fatty depots--to the point of interruption of normal cell processes--were it not for metabolism of the inert parent chemicals to more polar, excretable intermediates and products. The resistance of insects to various insecticides, for example, is a recently understood phenomenon with world-wide implications for agriculture and economy:[352] exposed to a chemical requiring toxification, insects lacking particular P-450s become resistant; exposed to a toxic parent chemical, insects with high concentrations of particular P-450s are resistant because of increased detoxification.

Toxification pathways account for well over 90% of the formation of active mutagens. Such pathways appear to be self-destructive to the organism, and it is not clear why toxification pathways should ever have evolved. It is also not completely understood how bacteria, plants, or animals "sense" and "respond" to the presence of an inducer of drug-metabolizing enzymes and use this inducing chemical as an energy source, for toxification, or for detoxification. One sensor system is known to involve a specific cytosolic receptor: the Ah locus.[309] [312] In the Ah system, the receptor appears to bind avidly only to particular planar foreign chemicals commonly found in combustion processes. Whether the Ah receptor has a naturally occurring normal-body compound as its most specific ligand is not known. Whether other drug-metabolizing enzyme induction processes use specific receptors remains to be determined. Additional studies[317] [465] involving the cloning of P-450 genes should provide valuable insight into the mechanism of drug-metabolizing enzyme induction and the evolution of this interesting, phylogenetically very old, life process.

All organisms have a number of genetically regulated mechanisms with which to cope with rapid adverse changes in the environment. If the regulation of P-450 induction (and induction of many other drug-metabolizing enzymes) resembles in any way the other methods by which prokaryotes and eukaryotes cope genetically with numerous forms of environmental adversity, mammalian tissues may have the capacity to produce a large number of distinct inducible forms of these drug-metabolizing enzyme systems. Extrapolation of mutagenesis data on laboratory animals or in vitro test systems to individual (and unique) human beings therefore might be extremely difficult.

Many forms of control of P-450 and other enzymes responsible for the reactions listed in Table 4-1 must have evolved for metabolizing important endogenous substrates. These enzymes are not induced by foreign chemicals. In some

instances, induction of specific P-450 forms by peptide
hormone--adrenocorticotropic hormone (ACTH), luteinizing
hormone (LH), and gastrin--is known to occur.[346]

GENETIC DIFFERENCES IN THE METABOLISM
OF MUTAGENS AND PROMUTAGENS

SPECIES AND STRAIN DIFFERENCES

Thousands of reports have described species and strain
differences in drug-metabolizing enzymes.[141 149 259 307 389]
The data are totally empirical. Whereas one enzyme may be
undetectable in the hamster, high in the dog, and very
high in the rat, a second may be just the reverse. Many
of these activities tend to be much higher in the adult
male than in the adult female rat; many are higher in the
mature female than in the mature male mouse. There are
many unexplained cases of striking species differences in
drug toxicity, teratogenesis, and carcinogenesis. Thalidomide,
for example, is highly teratogenic in the rabbit, monkey,
and human, but not in the rat, mouse, or hamster. Strain
differences in drug-metabolizing enzymes--within one
species--are known to occur in the rat, mouse, and other
laboratory animals.[310]

The mutagenesis test systems described in this report
include Drosophila, Neurospora, Tradescantia, yeast,
mouse, Salmonella, and other bacteria in combination with
polychlorinated biphenyl (PCB)-induced rat-liver homogenate
and cell-culture systems. DNA appears to be similar among
all eukaryotes and might be regarded as an infinite,
nonspecific target. Probably none of these test systems
contains all the mutagen-activating enzymes listed in
Table 4-1. Metabolism of mutagens and promutagens in
Neurospora, for example, probably does not approximate
that in the human. Metabolism of several drugs and chemical
carcinogens in Drosophila has been shown to be different
from that in rat liver.[150 151]

INDIVIDUAL DIFFERENCES

Several pharmacogenetic disorders have been described;[305
306 308] these disorders do not represent dissimilarities
of 10% or 40%, but rather differences of a factor of 3, 5,
or more than 20 among individuals in their response to
some drug or other foreign chemical. Marked differences
may occur even between siblings. Hence, even if there are
two or three dozen competing enzymatic reactions for a

foreign chemical, if one relatively important (e.g., rate-limiting) enzyme activity differs genetically by a factor of 20 between two individuals, minor differences (10% or 40%) in each of the other drug-metabolizing enzyme activities are insignificant in the ultimate outcome of mutagenesis, carcinogenesis, or toxicity.

In the 1960s, clinical pharmacologists had hoped to "categorize" all drugs into three, five, or 10 classes. If a patient were to receive an anesthetic from "Class A," it was hoped, clinical pharmacologists could give some test compound from Class A and determine whether the patient was a fast or slow metabolizer and thus how much Class A anesthetic would be required. After hundreds of such studies, however, the conclusion became clear. Each patient appears to be genetically unique, and knowledge of the rate of metabolism of one drug cannot predict the rate of metabolism of other drugs. Drug response has become extremely empirical and anecdotal. Two recent interesting examples may be cited. In some genetically predisposed people, rifampicin appears to induce sufficient enzyme activity that anovulatory drugs are metabolized more rapidly; this has resulted in unplanned pregnancies among some patients taking both rifampicin and birth-control tablets.[324] Isoniazid (an antituberculosis drug), in some genetically susceptible people, apparently induces a form of P-450 that metabolizes enflurane much more rapidly;[368] this has resulted in a requirement of a much larger dose of enflurane for maintenance anesthesia among some patients who are taking isoniazid.

The genetic heterogeneity of the human population may be viewed in two distinct ways: as an underlying predisposition to promutagen and mutagen metabolism by the endogenous enzymes listed in Table 4-1; and as a response to induction of these enzymes by foreign compounds. The number of foreign-chemical inducers of drug-metabolizing enzymes is estimated at hundreds or thousands. Whereas it is recognized that each individual may be unique with respect to metabolism of these promutagens and mutagens, it is far less complicated to focus on the human population as a whole.

GENETIC SPECIFICITY OF METABOLISM OF MUTAGENS AND PROMUTAGENS AND NONSPECIFICITY OF TARGETS FOR REACTIVE MUTAGENS

How does genetics interact with mutagenesis caused by environmental agents? Figure 4-1 is an attempt to include all possibilities of specific sites or enzymes (that are controlled by gene expression), compared with all nonspecific

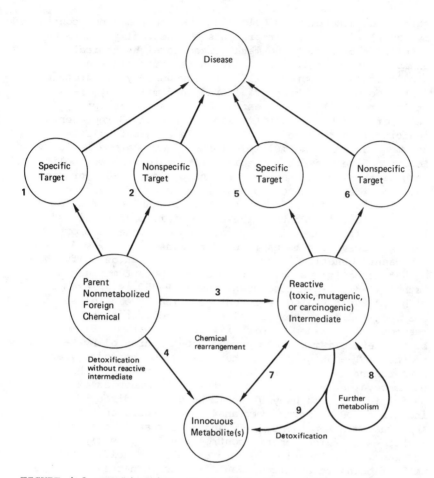

FIGURE 4-1 Combination of possible fates of parent (non-metabolized foreign chemical, whether it is an active mutagen or an inert promutagen that requires metabolism to become active. "Disease" is used here to connote mutation, malignancy, or toxicity. Locations 1 and 5 and pathways 3, 4, 8, and 9 are controlled by enzymes and therefore would be under specific genetic control. Locations 2 and 6 and pathway 7 are nonspecific and would not be affected by genetic differences in drug-metabolizing enzymes. See text for discussion.

sites, targets, or chemical reactions (that are not controlled
by genes). Location 1 represents a genetically determined
specific site for the nonmetabolized foreign chemical;
examples might include the insulin receptor (lacking in
some forms of diabetes mellitus), low-density lipoprotein
(LDL) receptor (lacking or altered in familial hypercholesterolemia),[43] the postulated coumarin "receptor,"[333] the Ah
receptor,[312] and α-1 antitrypsin.[59] Pathway 3 represents
genetically determined differences in drug-metabolizing
enzymes, such as the multiple forms of cytochrome P-450.
Location 5 represents a specific target for the metabolite,
such as the N-2 of guanine for benzopyrene 7,8-dihydrodiol-
9,10-epoxide,[141] the C-8 of guanine for N-hydroxylated 2-
acetylaminofluorene,[183] and the N-7 of guanine for aflatoxin
B_1 2,3-oxide.[114] Whether these "specific binding sites"
for metabolites are directly related to mutagenesis or
cancer, however, remains to be determined. Pathway 4
represents genetically expressed enzymes that detoxify the
parent molecule; detoxification of the potent mutagen N-
methyl-N'-nitro-N-nitrosoguanidine by P-450 is an example.[83]
Pathways 8 and 9 also represent genetically controlled
enzymes leading to toxification and detoxification,
respectively. Examples of toxification (pathway 8) would
be the metabolism of benzopyrene 7,8-dihydrodiol by P-450
to the diol-epoxide[422] and the cleavage of benzo[a]pyrene
glucuronide by β-glucuronidase to an intermediate that
binds covalently to DNA and protein.[208] Examples of
detoxification (pathway 9) would be genetic differences in
inducible UDP glucuronosyltransferase associated with the
Ah locus.[337] Locations 2, 6, and 7 represent nonspecific
reactions in which genetic control would not be expected.
An example for location 2 would be sulfuric acid, which,
without being metabolized, would indiscriminately destroy
nucleic acid and protein, regardless of genetic differences.
Reactive metabolites, as potent electrophiles, presumably
seek out macromolecular nucleophilic sites in a random
fashion; covalent interaction of small reactive metabolities
with DNA is therefore an example of location 6. The
chemical rearrangement of a reactive epoxide to a less
reactive phenol would also occur nonenzymatically; this is
an example of pathway 7.

In summary, genetic differences in drug-metabolizing
enzymes are poorly understood and contribute by far the
most to the problems surrounding heterogeneity of species
and individuals within a species. Generation of mutagens
by metabolism depends on specific genes. The damage
inflicted on nucleic acids and proteins by the mutagens
involves a nonspecific, stochastic process. Emphasis on
genetic differences in these enzymes therefore should be

the most important consideration in the ultimate attempt
to extrapolate mutagenesis test data to human populations.

METABOLIC DIFFERENCES AMONG VARIOUS
EXPERIMENTAL SYSTEMS

SUBCELLULAR FRACTIONS

In addition to species, strain, and individual genetic
differences in the metabolism of mutagens and promutagens,
one must consider differences related to experimental
techniques. Some enzyme activities in the intact cell
differ from those in isolated subcellular fractions.
Among the best examples are the UDP glucuronosyltransferases,
generally regarded as much more important in detoxification
than in toxification. These transferases are active in
the intact cell, but isolation of microsomes or the 9,000
g postmitochondrial supernatant (S-9) fraction inhibits
these activities, for unknown reasons. To study these
microsomal transferase activities in vitro, one generally
adds detergents or organic solvents in low concentrations,
and this mild treatment somehow restores the activity. In
the usual Salmonella/microsome test, however, no such
detergents or other solvents are used; therefore, UDP
glucuronosyltransferase activities can play no role in the
interpretation of data from this assay. The results from
the Salmonella/microsome assay thus reflect only the
aggregate activities of all active (toxifying plus detoxifying)
enzymes in the microsomes and cytosolic fractions.

INTACT CELLS

It has long been known that drug metabolism in fetal
rat primary hepatocytes[337] and in continuous hepatoma-
derived cell lines differs from that in intact liver.[336]
The benzo[a]pyrene metabolite profile changes as a function
of time in culture,[414] and the induction of drug-
metabolizing enzymes by phenobarbital in culture clearly
is not the same as that in the intact animal.[119] In
addition, subcellular fractions differ from intact cells
in the profile of metabolites[86 413] and DNA adducts[32 318]
formed after metabolism of various promutagens, such as
aflatoxin B_1, benzo[a]pyrene, and 7,12-dimethylbenz[a]-
anthracene. These data reflect the rapid loss of many
forms of P-450 and perhaps other drug-metabolizing enzymes
as soon as cells are treated with trypsin and put into
culture.[35] The reason for such a loss is not understood,

but the loss must be considered in any study involving the activation of promutagens to mutagens.

The toxification of benzo[a]pyrene and most other polycyclic aromatic hydrocarbons to mutagenic intermediates by continuous cell lines has been reported dozens of times, whereas toxification of aflatoxin B_1 to mutagenic intermediates in some cell lines does not occur.[225] These data can be explained by the fact that the forms of P-450 necessary for polycyclic-hydrocarbon toxification remain in cultured primary and continuous cell lines, whereas the forms of P-450 responsible for the 2,3-oxide formation of aflatoxin B_1 disappear rapidly in culture, for unknown reasons. Studies involving cultured human tissues may have this same major liability. The choice of cell culture for any particular compound therefore can be important.

One common assay combines Chinese hamster ovary cells (which have markers for determining mutagenic frequency, but little drug-metabolizing capacity) with irradiated secondary cultures of fetal hamster fibroblasts (which have drug-metabolizing capacity, but cannot survive).[177] This test suffers from the absence of some drug-metabolizing enzymes. Another assay combines microsomes or postmito-chondrial supernatant fractions with V79 cells in culture;[222] the hypothesis is that the microsomes or postmitochondrial supernatant fractions would provide the necessary drug-metabolizing capacity. This test would have some of the same shortcomings described in the previous section.

After perfusion of liver (or other organ) with colla-genase, hyaluronidase, and other degradative enzymes, it is possible to isolate freshly prepared intact cells.[30] Liver cells appear to maintain most of their drug-metabolizing capacity for at least some 24 h after isolation. Many forms of P-450, active UDP glucuronosyltransferases, epoxide hydrolase, and other enzyme activities are presumed to exist in these freshly prepared cells, whereas they do not exist to the same degree (and some do not exist at all) in subcellular fractions and cell cultures. Several laboratories have applied this fresh liver-cell system to study drug toxicity.[459] These studies also have been extended to isolated cells from rat small intestine[142] and kidney.[334] The advantage of this system is that all drug-metabolizing enzymes appear to be active and able to excrete mutagenic, carcinogenic, or toxic intermediates into the medium, as well as into neighboring cells. The multiplicity of P-450 forms has not yet been characterized with this system, however, so it is still conceivable that metabolite profiles of some promutagens would differ between these intact cells and the cells in the intact organ. The major disadvantage of this system is that

these cells are no longer in the same architectural
arrangement as in the intact organ. The cells are principally parenchymal cells with the mesenchymal stroma
removed. If the proximity of one "high-metabolizing" cell
to another "target" cell is important within the same
organ--and such hypotheses abound, especially among the
various cell types in the lung[33 68]--the mutagenic data on
freshly prepared cells in vitro may differ from data on
the intact organ.

PERFUSED ORGAN

Studies involving perfused liver,[200] lung,[200 476]
testis,[236] and other organs are increasingly popular.
Concerning metabolism of mutagens and promutagens, perfusion systems obviously approximate what occurs in the
intact animal. Unless a reactive intermediate is extremely
short-lived, therefore, it should be possible to expose
freshly formed mutagens in the perfusate to some cell or
bacterium that has markers for determining mutagenic
frequency. The disadvantage of this system is that
extremely reactive intermediates, perhaps mutagenic in the
cell in which they were formed or to nearby cells, would
no longer be mutagenic in the perfusate. Furthermore, if
a mutagenic intermediate is formed in one tissue and then
travels to another organ or tissue before hitting its
target, one would not be able to assess the possibility
with this test system, unless the perfusate from one
tissue were delivered to a second (perfused) tissue.

INTACT ANIMAL

With regard to metabolic and pharmacologic factors,
whole-animal testing has obvious advantages over any
perfused-organ or in vitro assay. The animal is a combination
of all organs and tissues interconnected by blood and
lymphatic vessels, with the architectural arrangement of
each cell intact in each tissue, and with the inter-
relationship of all subcellular organelles intact in each
cell. The disadvantages of whole-animal mutagenesis
testing include the decision as to which laboratory animal
species most closely approximates the human.
Bacteria have characteristic drug-metabolizing capacities,
and laboratory animals and humans have numerous types of
bacteria, principally in the colon. Bacterial cells, in
fact, account for approximately half of human fecal
solids.[436] The naturally occurring glucoside cycasein

from the ancient gymnospermous plants called "cycads" is
known to undergo toxification by the microbial enzymes of
the gut flora.[226] "Fecalase," a preparation of human
feces, has recently been proposed as a model for studying
the toxification of dietary glycosides to mutagens by
intestinal flora.[452] As mentioned earlier, the formation
of glucuronides and glycosides (Phase II drug metabolism)
does not ensure detoxification and excretion of these
innocuous products. Glucuronidases (especially concen-
trated in the kidney and urinary bladder) and glycosidases
(especially from bacteria in the colon) therefore provide
mechanisms for producing mutagenic intermediates from many
Phase II products. If these intermediates are extremely
short-lived, mutagenesis, carcinogenesis, or toxicity
occurs in the kidney, bladder, or colon epithelium; if the
intermediates are longer-lived (with half-lives measured
in seconds), even distant organs might be targets for such
mutagens. Such a complicated arrangement certainly cannot
be taken into account in studies of perfused organ, studies
of cells in culture, or in vitro mutagenesis assays.

METABOLISM AND PHARMACOKINETICS WITH REGARD
TO GERMINAL TISSUE

It is important to address the question of whether
promutagens and mutagens reach the gonadal tissue. The
mouse specific-locus test, the mouse spot test, the
heritable-translocation test in mice, the dominant-lethal
test, and the sex-chromosome loss and nondisjunction assay
are all based on the fact that chemicals given to the
intact laboratory animal, by whatever route of administration,
produce mutations in germinal tissue. A number of chemicals
have been studied in these various whole-animal assays and
have been found to be mutagenic; therefore, there is no
doubt that mutagens and promutagens are able to reach
germinal tissue. Special concern has been expressed for
mutagenic activity of male antifertility drugs,[435] diethylstilbestrol,[159] and dibromochloropropane[457] in the human.
Chemicals that have caused reproductive toxicity in humans
include alkylating agents, such as cyclophosphamide and
other drugs used for treating neoplastic and nonneoplastic
diseases;[161] chlorcyclizine;[504] p,p'-DDT;[133] halogenated
aromatic compounds;[8] hexachlorobenzene;[178] cadmium;[97]
boron oxides;[97] agents in cigarette smoke;[193] salicylazo-
sulfapyridine;[247] 6-mercaptopurine, the active metabolite
of the widely used immunosuppressive drug azathioprine;[366]
cimetidine;[479] and alcohol.[478] However, it is not possible
to determine in humans whether these have a mutagenic

effect. Male oligospermia, azoospermia, gynecomastia, and infertility and female ovarian failure, infertility, and earlier onset of menopause are the usual clinical effects described. Toxification of all these chemicals in the gonads by the drug-metabolizing enzymes listed in Table 4-1 therefore must be seriously considered.

In germinal tissue itself, there is no doubt that promutagens can undergo toxification, because in vitro metabolism by gonadal subcellular fractions has been examined.[158] Recent supportive studies have used the isolated perfused testis[236] and mouse egg cylinders 3.5-8.5 d after conception[130] that were cultured in a dish free of maternal tissues or placenta. Mutagens can also undergo detoxification in both ovary and testis.[235] [292] Repair mechanisms for DNA damage in the gonad,[244] in the oocyte before and after fertilization,[349] in the developing spermatozoon,[96] and in sperm DNA after fertilization[138] have been described. With respect to its drug-metabolizing enzyme capabilities in handling promutagens and mutagens, as well as the likelihood of receiving via the bloodstream mutagens that have been converted to their active form elsewhere in the body, therefore, germinal tissue should be recognized as very similar to liver or virtually any other tissue in the body. Hence, toxification, detoxification, and repair of mutagenic lesions all are known to occur in the gonad.

PHARMACOKINETICS OF MUTAGENS AND PROMUTAGENS: IMPORTANCE OF THE ROUTE OF ADMINISTRATION

The murine Ah locus controls the induction by numerous polycyclic aromatic compounds of many drug-metabolizing enzyme activities.[309] [312] A cytosolic receptor highly specific for these inducers has been shown to be essential for the induction process.[329] "Ah-responsive" mice have high concentrations of this receptor, and drug-metabolizing enzymes are therefore easily inducible by these polycyclic aromatic compounds. "Ah-nonresponsive" mice, however, lack detectable Ah receptor and thus have drug-metabolizing enzymes that are much more difficult to induce with the same polycyclic compounds.

In studies of various types of tumorigenesis and toxicity, a pattern has emerged in the use of these mice.[306] If the chemical administered to intact mice is an inducer of P-450 forms that are controlled by the Ah receptor, not only are the dose and its timing important, but the route of administration and the site at which the tumor or toxicity occurs--relative to the route of administration--are critical. Hence, polycyclic aromatic compounds applied topically, subcutaneously, or intratracheally are more likely to cause tumors or toxicity in tissues at the site of administration--epidermal carcinoma or ulceration, subcutaneous fibrosarcoma, and various types of pulmonary tumors, respectively--in Ah-responsive mice than in Ah-nonresponsive mice. Administered intraperitoneally, these compounds are more likely to cause hepatic necrosis and ovarian toxicity in Ah-responsive mice; again, liver and ovary are viewed as intraperitoneal organs close to the site of the administered drug.

On the other hand, polycyclic aromatic compounds given orally or subcutaneously are more likely to cause aplastic anemia, leukemia, and lymphatic tumors in Ah-nonresponsive mice. These effects are manifest in tissues distant from the site of drug administration. In the example of oral benzo[a]pyrene, pharmacokinetic studies have shown a 10- and 20-fold higher uptake in the marrow and spleen of Ah-nonresponsive than of Ah-responsive mice; this confirms the phenomenon called "first-pass elimination kinetics." In essence, first-pass elimination kinetics means that, if a chemical administered by any route is metabolized before it reaches a target tissue, it will cause no response in that tissue. Hence, the forms of P-450 induced in the intestine and liver metabolize most of the benzo[a]pyrene given orally to the Ah-responsive mouse; the amount of parent drug or its metabolites reaching the bone marrow is therefore greatly decreased.

In the case of malignancy or toxicity at the site of administration, therefore, the compound induces its own metabolism via particular forms of P-450--much more readily in Ah-responsive than in Ah-nonresponsive mice--and that leads to high concentrations of reactive intermediates that cause the local cancer or toxicity. In the case of malignancy or toxicity in tissues distal to the site of administration, the compound in cells at the site of administration induces its own metabolism much more readily in Ah-responsive mice, but the detoxification pathways also appear to be important. The concentration of non-metabolized parent drug that reaches distal tissues, such as bone marrow and lymph nodes, is therefore much greater in Ah-nonresponsive mice. This higher concentration of chemical somehow causes more toxicity or malignancy in Ah-nonresponsive mice.

If mutagenesis is determined in the Salmonella/microsome test, the degree of positive or negative findings is based on toxification by the postmitochondrial supernatant fraction from the liver of rats previously treated with Aroclor 1254. Likewise, any mutagenicity index for a

given chemical is based solely on which drug-metabolizing
enzyme systems were used for toxification and what the
balance of toxification to detoxification was.[321] If a
chemical painted on mouse skin induces a particular form
of P-450 that enhances the toxification of that chemical,
for example, the tumorigenicity of the chemical need not
be correlated with mutagenicity determined by the Salmonella/-
microsome test if the same form of P-450 is not present in
the rat-liver fraction. In the intact animal, therefore,
drug-drug interactions, chemicals that promote cancer, and
agents that enhance carcinogenesis may likewise act in
concert in a manner not possible to interpret in any in
vitro or culture test system.

SUMMARY

An intact animal is a combination of organs interconnected by blood and lymphatic vessels. There is a
microbial contribution to the metabolism of mutagens and
promutagens in the gut. Many of the aspects discussed
here are summarized in Table 4-2. Pharmacokinetic

TABLE 4-2 Summary of Test Systems with Drug-Metabolizing
Capability and with Markers for Assessing Mutagenesis

Intact Animal, Perfused Organ, Cells, or Subcellular Fraction	Drug-Metabolizing Capability	Presence of Markers for Determining Mutagenic Frequency[a]
V79 Chinese hamster ovary cells	±	Yes
Fetal hamster fibroblast cultures (lethally irradiated feeder layer)	++	No
Human cells, such as HeLa	±	Yes
Rat liver S-9[b]	+++	No
Liver S-9 from rats pretreated with Aroclor 1254	+++++	No
Isolated freshly prepared hepatocytes	+++++++	No
Perfused liver or liver slice from rats treated with Aroclor 1254	+++++++	No
Intact laboratory animal	+++++++++	Yes

a. Markers include ouabain, 8-azaguanine, or thioguanine resistance and
thymidine kinase or hypoxanthine-guanine phosphoribosyltransferase deficiency.
b. "S-9" refers to 9,000-g postmitochondrial supernatant fraction.

phenomena, especially those which occur during chronic administration of chemicals that are inducers of drug-metabolizing enzymes, can never be taken into account in studies of perfused organs or cells in culture or in in vitro mutagenesis assays.

The toxification of promutagens to mutagens and the detoxification of mutagens by freshly prepared intact human cells or perfused healthy organs would most closely approximate human metabolism. The use of biochemical genetic markers in human cells to determine mutagenesis would most closely approximate the target for potential human mutagens. Individual differences in drug metabolism among the human population must be recognized, but cannot be included easily in tests designed to identify potential human mutagens. If fresh human cells or perfused organs cannot be easily obtained for use in such metabolism studies, it is difficult to know which intact laboratory animal most closely approximates the human with respect to drug-metabolizing capability.

5

THE NATURE OF TEST SYSTEMS

EXTRAPOLATION TO MAN

A fundamental issue in genetic toxicology is that
environmental chemicals may cause mutation in human germ
cells and thereby pose a health risk for future generations.
Because of this possibility, there is a major effort to
detect chemicals that induce mutation in man. However,
mutagenesis is not amenable to the collection of data on
human populations, except for effects in somatic cells.

Thus, we must rely on extrapolations from test systems
in nonhuman and often nonmammalian organisms. Although
extrapolating from one species to another poses difficult
problems, there is at least a conceptual basis for extrapolation with respect to mutagenesis: DNA is the hereditary
material in all cellular organisms. A chemical that
interacts with DNA to produce mutation in one species is
likely to do so in others. But there are no easy
generalizations, because species differ in the way exogenous
substances enter the body, in metabolism and pharmacologic
disposition of toxicants, and in capacity to repair genetic
damage. More reliable extrapolation from one species to
another is likely if measurements are made in similar
organisms and on corresponding cells and stages of
development.

The conceptual basis for extrapolating among species
has some experimental support: chemicals that are mutagenic
in one species also are generally mutagenic in other
species.[90][170] There are also semiquantitative consistencies:
chemicals that are strong mutagens in one species tend to
be strong mutagens in others. It is highly unlikely that
a chemical that is mutagenic in all test systems is innocuous
in man. In contrast, a chemical that is nonmutagenic in a

wide variety of sensitive test systems may be presumed to be safe for man.

Studies on carcinogenesis lend some support to the extrapolation of mutagenesis data to man. Despite some uncertainties,[357] carcinogenicity in experimental rodents is regularly assumed to predict carcinogenicity in man.[76] [359] [460] Moreover, most evidence on mechanisms of chemical carcinogenesis indicates the involvement of mutation in the initiation of cancer,[441] and there is a rather strong correlation between the carcinogenicity of an agent in mammals and its mutagenicity in experimental test systems, including submammalian tests.[27] [49] [275] [276] [358] When substances known to be carcinogenic in mammals are tested in short-term tests, the overwhelming majority are mutagenic. The converse is not true: several substances that are active in short-term mutagenicity tests are not known to cause cancer in mammals, although this may simply reflect the greater sensitivity of short-term tests. Brusick[44] has estimated that 88% of animal carcinogens are bacterial mutagens and that about 85% of animal noncarcinogens have no mutagenic activity in bacteria. Thus, there is an experimental link between mutagenicity in experimental systems and health consequences in people--short-term mutagenicity tests can predict carcinogenicity in rodents, and rodent carcinogenicity tests are useful for predicting carcinogenicity in man.

The link to human carcinogenicity and the observation that an agent mutagenic in one species is generally mutagenic in others argue that short-term mutagenicity tests have predictive value not only for carcinogenicity, but also for mutagenicity in man. Because of differences in such characteristics as metabolism and DNA repair, the correlation is imperfect. Several carcinogens that induced mutations in short-term tests (e.g., diethlynitrosamine) yielded negative results in tests for mutations in germs cells of mice.[385] However, ethyl nitrosourea (ENU) is strongly mutagenic in the mouse; such a striking difference would not have been predicted from short-term tests. This argues that pharmacokinetics can markedly influence the quantitative effect. Clearly, an agent that yields a positive result in mutagenicity tests in experimental organisms is more likely to be mutagenic in humans than one that does not. In the absence of germ cell data from whole mammals, the presumption of human mutagenicity is stronger if the positive short-term test result is combined with evidence that the agent in question actually reaches the germinal tissue in whole animals. This could be monitored, for example, by the formation of DNA adducts in germ cells.

Although the use of simple test systems to predict
genetic effects in whole mammals is desirable, comparison
of dosages in submammalian systems with human exposure is
extremely complex. The nature of the exposure, cellular
toxicity, and units of measurement differ markedly from
one type of organism to another. Molecular dosimetry that
measures adducts in DNA is promising,[1-3] [237-239] but the
ability to relate exposures in short-term test systems,
including mammalian cell cultures, to human risks is
primitive. There are much better grounds for qualitative
than for quantitative extrapolation.

EXTRAPOLATION FROM HIGH CONCENTRATIONS
AND DOSAGES: THE THRESHOLD PROBLEM

The early studies of the kinetics of induction of
recessive lethal mutations in Drosophila showed linearity
at low doses and no evidence of a threshold. The contention
that there is no threshold, or "safe" dose, has dominated
genetic thinking on radiation effects and has carried over
to chemicals. However, it was long assumed that carcinogenic
effects of radiation and chemicals had a threshold. It
may be helpful to review some of the recent studies of
carcinogenesis.

Carcinogenicity tests are performed at much higher and
more acute doses than those to which people are normally
exposed. This is necessary because testing at low doses
or low dose rates would require prohibitively large numbers
of experimental animals or prohibitively long times.
Several mathematical models have been proposed for calculating
from high-dose experiment data to predicted low-dose
effects.[72] [82] [110] [124] [274] [303] [395] When only high-dose
data are available, it is usually possible to fit several
different plausible curves to the data, and these may lead
to different predictions of effects of exposure at low
doses.

In particular, high-dose data usually cannot identify a
threshold. A threshold is a dose or exposure below which
there is no effect. It is often assumed that there is no
threshold for an end point, like a gene mutation, that may
involve one molecule of the toxicant and one target molecule;
in such a case, the dose-response relationship would be
linear at low doses. If the observed relationship is
linear over the dose range studied and if the fitted line
is extrapolated to no effect (or the background frequency
of effects) at zero dose, linear kinetics with no threshold
are likely. But data are usually not clear. Even such a
large carcinogenesis study as the ED_{01} study conducted by

the National Center for Toxicological Research[432] was unable to demonstrate a threshold empirically. The ED_{01} study used 24,142 mice to study dose-response relationships in carcinogenesis associated with chronic oral exposures to the carcinogen 2-acetylaminofluorene at relatively low doses. The summary[132] stated: "Compatibility of the data with a threshold model does not constitute proof as non-threshold models also fit the data." The threshold issue is therefore unresolved for cancer. Furthermore, there is evidence that when a chemical is given in small amounts over long time periods, the organism may become adapted to the compound and be less affected by it.

Similar considerations apply to genetic effects of chemicals. But in one respect genetic effects are simpler. Carcinogenesis may involve initiation and promotion, and the two processes often have different kinetics. In particular, promotion is often temporary or reversible. Genetic damage is thought to be simpler, in that the DNA damage, once established, is heritable in this form and not subsequently modified. Therefore, it is less likely that there is a threshold for genetic effects, and in the absence of evidence to the contrary it is usually assumed that even the smallest doses will have some effect. However, depending on the shape of the dose-response curve, the low-dose effect may be very small.

For most chemicals, there are empirical uncertainties and poor theoretical understanding that would determine the form of the dose-response curve. There is, however, one generalization: the deviations from linearity are almost always in the direction of a curve that is accelerating (i.e., has a positive second derivative). It is usually true that linear interpolation between the high-dose data and the spontaneous rate at zero dose will overestimate, rather than underestimate, the low-dose effect. So an assumption of linearity is often justified on the grounds of prudence--on the grounds that being too safe is of less consequence than not being safe enough.

One cannot automatically be sure of this assumption. One possibility is that there is differential susceptibility to both mutation and killing among the cells. If, for example, there are two populations of cells, the high-dose data reflect the mutation rate of the component more resistant to killing. If these cells are also resistant to mutation, the resistance of the total cell population is underestimated. Another possibility is that there is a mutation-repair mechanism that is turned on at high doses. Deviations from either of these causes can usually be detected by the shape and slope of the curve at high doses; for example, linear extrapolation from high-dose data may lead to a zero-dose prediction higher than the known spontaneous rate. Better, of course, is the direct observation of cell-killing and induced repair mechanisms. Similarly, an accelerating curve may show a negative effect from extrapolation to zero dose.

The approach taken by this Committee is that, unless there is evidence to the contrary, it will be assumed that there is no threshold. If it is necessary to extrapolate from high-dose data, the best procedure is to interpolate linearly between the effect at zero dose and the lowest reliable data point(s). The lower the doses studied, the more reliable is this interpolation.

Two earlier National Research Council committees[300][304] accepted this approach. The report of the Committee on Safe Drinking Water stated that, "if an effect can be caused by a single hit, a single molecule, or a single unit of exposure, then the effect in question cannot have a threshold in the dose-response relationship, no matter how unlikely it is that the single hit or event will produce the effect." This statement also reflects the approach of the Environmental Protection Agency in "Mutagenicity Risk Assessment: Proposed Guidelines"[475] and in its water-quality criteria.[474]

VALIDITY, RELIABILITY, AND SENSITIVITY OF TEST SYSTEMS

In traditional statistical testing theory--e.g., as applied in educational testing--the words "reliability" and "validity" have specific meanings.

"Reliability" means the same as "repeatability"; it is a measure of how often a test gives consistent results when applied to different groups and how often tests that purport to measure the same thing agree with each other. It is usually measured by correlating the results of repeat tests.

"Validity" is the extent to which a test measures what it is supposed to measure. A test can have high reliability and low validity if it measures repeatedly the wrong thing.

Neither of these words is used with such precise definitions in mutagen testing. A correlation definition of "reliability" is not usually feasible, because mutation tests are not usually scaled in appropriate numerical units. It is much more troublesome that the end point is human genetic damage (and its impact). Because this cannot now be assessed, there is no way in which proper validation can be done. We have to make do with something less, and "validation" has come to be applied to assessments of nonhuman genetic damage.

"Validation" as used in mutagen testing programs has two components:

• The first component is how well the test is or can be run and how reproducible the results are from one laboratory to another. This component is determined by sending out blind samples to various laboratories on several occasions. The test results are compared with predetermined criteria for consistency. This usually consists of classifying each result as showing no significant mutagenicity, a small amount, or a great amount; if these are concordant among the different laboratories, this is regarded as reasonable validation of the test. This classification is quite proper in a period of rapid test improvement, as we are in now. It is expected that sharper criteria will evolve as test protocols improve.

• The second component cannot achieve its purpose, if its purpose is to validate test results against human response. In the commonly accepted compromise, the test is applied to a considerable number of chemicals, which represent a wide range of classes of chemicals and reactive groups, and the results are inspected for concordance with other widely used tests that purport to detect the same or related end points.

In general, there is a tendency to accept a positive response as more valid than a negative one when comparing tests, because we know more ways in which a test can fail than in which it can give a falsely positive result.

In mutagenicity testing, it is desirable to reduce to a minimum both false positives (nonmutagens classified as mutagenic) and false negatives (mutagens classified as nonmutagenic). "Sensitivity" is defined as the proportion of known mutagens that are positive in the system being evaluated; "specificity" is the proportion of nonmutagens that are negative.

However, because there is no way of measuring human germinal-mutation induction, these terms cannot be used with their proper meanings. Instead, we use "sensitivity" to mean the capacity of the test to detect small increases in the mutation rate. In this usage, "sensitivity" has essentially the same meaning as "statistical power." A sensitive test is one that is capable of detecting a statistically significant increase in mutation with a small increase in concentration of the chemical. The smaller the concentration that can be detected, the more sensitive the test. One way of making a test more sensitive is to increase the number of test organisms, genes scored, or replications. There is always greater than binomial variance, and another way to increase sensitivity is to decrease the nonbinomial component by greater uniformity of test conditions. Because the induced mutations are detected against a background of spontaneous mutants, a system that reduces this background noise increases sensitivity. For this reason, reverse-mutation systems are sometimes preferred.

A REVIEW OF MUTAGEN TEST SYSTEMS

Because mutagenic agents possibly can cause heritable genetic damage or cancer in people, considerable effort has been devoted to developing and validating methods for detecting mutagens.[44 90 92 164-168 170 207 338 358 369 486] A brief overview of major assay systems in genetic toxicology is presented in Table 5-1. The inclusion of particular assays is somewhat subjective. Nevertheless, the table provides ready reference to the major assays, including all those discussed in this report.

Before a discussion of particular tests, which have been categorized by phylogenetic rank of test organism or by genetic end point, it should be emphasized that an exhaustive treatment of mutagenicity tests is not intended. Rather, the most widely used tests, their strengths and weaknesses, and some promising future possibilities are described. The purpose of this review is to provide background information for other parts of the report.

BACTERIAL GENOTOXICITY ASSAYS

It is not by accident that bacteria have been the principal tool of biologic research. As with most fields of genetics and biochemistry, genetic toxicology has derived much of its initial success from experiments with these organisms. Genetic toxicologists are attracted to bacterial tests because they are rapid and relatively inexpensive. In the hands of trained personnel, the tests reproducibly and efficiently detect chemicals that are mutagenic in mammals. As will be discussed, bacterial strains have been constructed that are extremely sensitive to mutagenic chemicals (see Table 5-2 for partial list of strains). Furthermore, to make bacterial systems more compatible with conditions in higher organisms, an exogenous metabolic activation system from mammalian liver has been included in most microbial assays.[12 14] Although the

TABLE 5-1 The Characteristics of the Most Common Genetic Toxicology Tests[a]

Category	Organism and/or Cell Type	System and/or Strain	End Points Measured	Test Duration	Cost[b] Capital	Cost[b] Operation	Data Base[c]	U.S. Testing Capacity, chemicals/yr[d]
Bacteria: Mutation	Salmonella typhimurium	Salmonella/microsome test; histidine reversions	Point mutations; reversion by base-pair substitution or frameshift mutation	<3 wk	L	L	L	H
Mutation	Salmonella typhimurium	Azaguanine-resistant	Gene mutations (forward mutations)	<3 wk	L	L	M	NA
Mutation	Escherichia coli	WP2 tryptophan reversions	Point mutations (base-pair substitutions)	<3 wk	L	L	M	M
Mutation	Escherichia coli	Strain 343/113 (Mohn strain)	Gene mutations (forward mutations and reversions) at several loci	<3 wk	L	L	S	NA
Repair tests	Escherichia coli	polA+ vs polA-	Differential killing (via DNA damage)	<3 wk	L	L	L	H
Repair tests	Bacillus subtilis	rec+ vs rec-	Differential killing (via DNA damage)	<3 wk	L	L	M	NA
Inductest	Escherichia coli	λ-lysogen	Phage or enzyme induction	<3 wk	L	L	M	NA
Fungi: Mutation	Saccharomyces cerevisiae	Reversion of auxotrophic mutations (e.g. ilv in strain D7; several in strain XV185-14C)	Point mutations	<3 wk	L	L	S-M	NA
Mutation	Schizosaccharomyces pombe	White mutants in a red ad-7 strain	Gene mutations (forward mutations at five loci)	<1 mo	L	L-M	S-M	NA
Fungi: Mutation	Neurospora crassa	ad-3 system: red adenine mutants	Gene (forward) mutations and small deletions in ad3A and ad3B	<2 mo	M	M	M	L
Mutation	Neurospora crassa	Reversion of adenine auxotrophy in strains N23 and N24	Gene mutations	<1 mo	L	L	S	NA
Mutation	Aspergillus nidulans	Suppressors of meth-1	Gene (forward) mutations	<1 mo	L	L	S	NA

Mutation	Aspergillus nidulans	XDH conidial color system	Forward mutations and reversions	<1 mo	L	M	S	NA
Mitotic recombination	Saccharomyces cerevisiae	Strain D1	Mitotic crossing-over	<1 mo	L	L	S	NA
Mitotic recombination	Saccharomyces cerevisiae	Strain D3	Mitotic crossing-over	<1 mo	L	L	M	M
Mitotic recombination	Saccharomyces cerevisiae	Strain D4	Mitotic gene conversion	<3 wk	L	L	M	M
Mitotic recombination	Saccharomyces cerevisiae	Strain D5	Mitotic crossing-over	<1 mo	L	L	S-M	NA
Mitotic recombination	Saccharomyces cerevisiae	Strain D7	Mitotic crossing-over and gene conversion	<1 mo	L	L	S-M	NA
Aneuploidy	Neurospora crassa	Multiply marked linkage group I	Meiotic nondisjunction	<1 mo	L	L	S	NA
Aneuploidy	Saccharomyces cerevisiae	Strain D6	Mitotic aneuploidy	<1 mo	L	L	S	NA
Aneuploidy	Saccharomyces cerevisiae	Strain D9	Meiotic nondisjunction	<1 mo	L	L	S	NA
Vascular Plants:								
Mutation	Barley and other species	Chlorophyll mutations	Forward mutations	<3 mo	M	M	M	NA
Mutation	Tradescantia	Stamen hair pigmentation	Gene (forward) mutations	<3 mo	M	M	S	L
Mutation	Zea mays	Waxy locus system; staining of starchy pollen grains	Gene mutations (forward mutations and reversions)	<4 mo	M	M	S-M	L
Cytogenetic damage	Vicia faba and other species	Root-tip cytogenetics	Chromosomal and chromatid aberrations	<1 mo	L	M	M	NA
Cytogenetic damage	Barley and other species	Microsporocyte cytogenetics	Chromosomal aberrations	<3 mo	M	M	S	NA
Insects:								
Mutation	Drosophila melanogaster	Sex-linked recessive lethal test	Gene mutations and small deletions	<3 mo	M	H	L	M
Translocations	Drosophila melanogaster	Chromosome II/III exchanges (i.e., bw/st system)	Reciprocal exchanges	<3 mo	M	H	M	NA

TABLE 5-1 continued

Category	Organism and/or Cell Type	System and/or Strain	End Points Measured	Test Duration	Cost[b] Capital	Operation	Data Base[c]	U.S. Testing Capacity, chemicals/yr[d]
Sex-chromosome loss	Drosophila melanogaster	Sex-chromosome loss	Loss of sex-linked markers; nondisjunction and/or breakage	<2 mo	M	M	M	NA
Mammalian cells:								
Mutation	Mouse lymphoma L5178Y cells	Thymidine kinase (TK) system	Gene (forward) mutations	<2 mo	M	M	M	H
Mutation	Chinese hamster V79 lung cells	HGPRT system	Gene (forward) mutations	<2 mo	M	M	M	H
Mutation	Chinese hamster ovary (CHO) cells	HGPRT system	Gene (forward) mutations	<2 mo	M	M	M	H
Mutation	Human fibroblasts	HGPRT system	Gene (forward) mutations	<2 mo	M	M	S	NA
Mammalian cells:								
Cytogenetic damage	CHO or other cell types	In vitro cytogenetic analysis	Chromosomal aberrations	<3 mo	M	M	M	H
Cytogenetic damage	Human lymphocytes or fibroblasts and other cell types	In vitro cytogenetic analysis	Sister chromatid exchanges	<2 mo	M	M	M	H
DNA repair	Human fibroblasts, rat hepatocytes, or other cell types	Unscheduled DNA synthesis	Repair of DNA damage, detected by [^{3}H]TdR incorporation in DNA	<3 mo	M	M	M	M
Mammals:								
Mutation	Mouse	Specific-locus test	Forward mutations and/or small deletions at 7 loci	<9 mo	H	VH	S	L
Mutation	Mouse	Somatic cell specific-locus test (spot test)	Forward mutations and small deletions at 7 loci	<3 mo	M	H	S	L
Mutation	Mouse	Electrophoretic variants	Forward mutations at 21 loci	<9 mo	H	VH	S	L
Mutation	Mouse	Skeletal mutations	Forward mutations	<9 mo	H	VH	S	L
Mutation	Mouse	Cataracts	Forward mutations	<9 mo	H	VH	S	L
Cytogenetic damage	Mouse or rat bone marrow	In vivo cytogenetic analysis	Chromosomal aberrations	<3 mo	M	H	M	M

Type of damage	Organism	Test	Endpoint	Time	[b]	[c]	[d]
Cytogenetic damage	Mouse (or other species) blood (lymphocytes)	In vivo cytogenetic analysis	Chromosomal aberrations	<2 mo	M	M	H	M
Cytogenetic damage	Mouse spermatocytes	In vivo cytogenetic analysis	Chromosomal rearrangements	<3 mo	M	H	S	NA
Cytogenetic damage	Mouse	Micronucleus test	Chromosomal fragments in erythrocyte stem cells	<1 mo	M	M	M	M
Mammals:							
Cytogenetic damage	Mouse	Heritable-translocation test	Semisterility, confirmed by cytogenetic detection of translocations	<9 mo	M	VH	M	L
Dominant lethals	Mouse or rat	Dominant-lethal test	Chromosomal damage	<3 mo	M	H	M	M
Abnormal sperm	Mouse or other species	Sperm-abnormality test	Morphologically abnormal sperm	<3 mo	M	M	M	M
Host-mediated assays	Mouse or rat	Uses microbial indicator organisms or cell cultures	As in indicator test system	1 mo	M	M	M	NA
Body-fluid analysis	Mouse, rat, man, or others; most commonly uses urine sample concentrates	Uses microbial indicator organisms or cell cultures	As in indicator test system	1 mo	M	M	S	M

a. Data from Brusick;[44] Brusick, personal communication, 1981; Drake;[98] and Hoffmann.[163]

b. L (low) <$1,500; M (moderate) = $1,500-6,000; H (high) = $6,000-24,000; VH (very high) >$24,000.

c. S = small; M = moderate; L = large. Data from Environmental Mutagen Information Center, Oak Ridge, Tennessee, 1980, provided by J.S. Wassom and E.S. von Halle.

d. L (low) <150; M (moderate) = 150-1,000; H (high) >1,000; NA = not applicable because test not in general use for screening.

TABLE 5-2 Bacterial Strains Used in Mutagenicity and Genotoxicity Assays

Strain	Significant Genetic Markers	Plasmid	Use
Salmonella typhimurium TA1535	his uvrB rfa	--	Reverse mutation: base-pair substitution
Salmonella typhimurium TA1537	his uvrB rfa	--	Reverse mutation: frameshift
Salmonella typhimurium TA1538	his uvrB rfa	--	Reverse mutation: frameshift
Salmonella typhimurium TA98	his uvrB rfa	pKM101	Reverse mutation: frameshift
Salmonella typhimurium TA100	his uvrB rfa	pKM101	Reverse mutation: base-pair substitution and some frameshift
Salmonella typhimurium TM35	his⁺	--	Forward mutation: 8-azaguanine resistance
Salmonella typhimurium TM677	his⁺	pKM101	Forward mutation: 8-azaguanine resistance
Escherichia coli WP2	trp uvrA or uvrB	±pKM101	Reverse mutation: base-pair substitution
Escherichia coli K12 343/113(λ)	arg gal nad	--	Reverse mutation: frameshift and base-pair substitution
		--	Forward mutation: 6-MT resistance, loss of ability to ferment galactose
		--	Induction of prophage
Escherichia coli W3110/p3478	polA⁺/polA	--	DNA damage assay
Escherichia coli GY5031	envA uvrB(λ)	--	Prophage induction and forward mutation
Escherichia coli BR513	λ-lac fusion, envA, uvrB	--	β-Galactosidase induction
Bacillus subtilis 168 & derivatives	can be hcr⁻ or rec⁻	--	Forward mutation: sporulation mutants
Bacillus subtilis H17/M45	rec⁺/rec⁻	--	DNA damage assay

enzyme preparation is difficult to standardize,[103] it has greatly increased the fraction of carcinogens that are detected as mutagens.[276]

In general, bacterial mutagenicity assays rely on one of three mutational schemes: reverse mutation, forward mutation, and DNA damage.

REVERSE-MUTATION ASSAYS

Assays that detect reverse mutation are most popular, largely because of the development of the Salmonella/microsome assay by Bruce Ames and his co-workers.[10][13] All five of the strains that are currently recommended[95] contain point mutations that prevent the biosynthesis of histidine. Unless histidine is provided in the growth medium, the bacteria cannot grow. However, if a new mutation occurs at the site of the original mutation and "reverses" its effect, growth without histidine can take place.

Aside from the expression of histidine mutations that are easily detected, other properties have been built into the Salmonella strains by mutation to increase their sensitivity. The strains are defective in DNA excision repair (uvrB). In this case, the increased sensitivity probably is due to the failure to remove some DNA adducts that could lead to mutation. The strains also possess a mutation (rfa) that removes part of the lipopolysaccharide barrier of the bacterial cell wall and thereby makes the cells more permeable to some chemicals. Finally, Salmonella strains TA98 and TA100 contain the R-factor plasmid pkM101,[277] which increases sensitivity probably by increasing the activity of an error-prone DNA-repair system.

Although not as frequently, several strains of Escherichia coli also are used in genotoxicity testing. E. coli WP2 and its derivatives possess a base-pair substitution in a tryptophan gene.[144] Reversion to tryptophan independence can be caused by base-pair substitution mutagens and even some frameshift mutagens. DNA-repair mutations and the pkM101 plasmid have been introduced into WP2 strains to increase sensitivity.

E. coli K12 343/113 contains three markers that are detected by reverse mutation: reversion to arginine independence, reversion to nicotinic acid independence, and reversion to the ability to ferment galactose.[289] The arg site seems to be more sensitive to chemicals that cause base-pair substitution mutation, whereas the gal and nad sites appear to be more sensitive to chemicals that cause frameshift mutation.

Investigators using reverse-mutation assays can distinguish between mutagens that primarily cause base-pair substitution and mutagens that primarily cause frameshift mutation by observing which strains are most sensitive to the mutagen. However, the discrimination in many cases is relative, rather than absolute. For example, N-methyl-N'-nitro-N-nitrosoguanidine (a base-pair substitution mutagen) and 2-aminoanthracene (a frameshift mutagen) are detected as mutagens in the five Salmonella strains.

Microbial tests based on reverse mutation are specific, because a unique mutation must undergo precise reversion.[423] This may be a limitation, in that only one genetic end point is monitored, although little empirical evidence supports this criticism. A prokaryotic or eukaryotic cell apparently uses a number of pathways at the same time to cope with adducts that are covalently bound to DNA. Therefore, the genetic lesions caused by a mutagen can be detected in assays for many genetic end points, including base-pair substitution and frameshift mutation, deletion, mitotic recombination or gene conversion, unscheduled DNA synthesis, sister chromatid exchange, and chromosomal aberration.[170]

The agar-incorporation method is the standard procedure for the Salmonella/microsome assay, as well as many other microbial tests.[14] The test substance and microbial cells (with or without an exogenous metabolic activation system) are mixed in soft agar and overlaid onto a selective medium in a petri dish. Dimethylnitrosamine and a few other substances are not detected normally as mutagens in the standard agar-incorporation assay, but are detected as mutagens if the microbial cells, test substance, and metabolic activation system are incubated together before the addition of soft agar.[511] This procedure is commonly called a preincubation test. Mutant (revertant) colonies are counted after 2-3 d of incubation. Another bacterial test is the spot test,[14] in which bacteria are spread or overlaid in agar on a selective medium, and the test chemical is applied as a solid or liquid. If the chemical is at least somewhat diffusible in the aqueous media, mutation is detected as a ring of revertants around the test material. Measurement of effect and exogenous activation is very limited in this procedure.

Tests also may be performed in liquid suspension. In the liquid incubation assays, the test substance and microbial cells are incubated in liquid suspension (buffer or minimal growth medium) with or without exogenous metabolic activation. Time and concentration of exposure can be varied, and the number of revertants per survivor can be calculated. However, artifactually positive responses

frequently are reported by investigators who (in the
Salmonella/microsome assay) fail to control the carryover
of histidine onto the selective plates or who incorporate
histidine into the selective medium.

Another test in suspension is the fluctuation test,[144][145]
a variation of the procedure developed by Luria and Delbrück.[260]
The test agent is added to a suspension of auxotrophic
cells in minimal medium supplemented with glucose. The
suspension is diluted out into test tubes or microtiter
wells. Mutagenic agents are recognized by their ability
to increase the number (above the number of untreated
control) of test tubes or wells that contain growing, and
therefore mutant, cells after 72-96 h. In host-mediated
assays,[129][242] test substances are subjected to in vivo
intraperitoneal, intratesticular, and intrasanguineous
host metabolism by injection of the microorganisms. After
an appropriate incubation time, the indicator organisms
are removed from the host animal and assayed for mutagenicity. The test therefore measures effects of the
parent compound and its mammalian metabolites. Another
way to detect effects of some mammalian metabolites of
test chemicals is to use bacterial tests to detect the
presence of mutagens in urine. These assays have detected
a few mutagens that are not detected in the standard
incorporation assay. However, host-mediated assays are
not particularly sensitive, and known mutagens often yield
negative responses.[420] Some conditions require rather
novel approaches. For example, gases (e.g., vinyl chloride)
and some liquids (e.g., methylene chloride) are not detected
as mutagens in the standard agar-incorporation assay,
because they are volatile or hydrophobic. Exposure of the
microorganisms to the test substance in a sealed container
is required to maximize the potential for mutagenic response.[23][360]

FORWARD-MUTATION ASSAYS

Although one of the first assays for mutagenicity was a
forward mutation to streptomycin resistance in E. coli,
forward-mutation assays in bacteria have not been used as
extensively as reverse-mutation assays. A forward-mutation
assay should detect a wider range of mutagens than the
presumably more restrictive reverse-mutation assays, but,
in practice, there is little evidence to support this
expectation.

E. coli Kl2 343/113 has been used for detection of
forward mutation to resistance to 6-methyl tryptophan and
loss of ability to ferment galactose.[289] Forward mutation
to sporulation mutants in Bacillus subtilis and to 8-

azaguanine resistance in <u>Salmonella</u> <u>typhimurium</u> strain
TM677 also has been tested.[265] [423] Liquid incubation is
the most commonly used method.

DNA-DAMAGE ASSAYS

When DNA damage occurs, a number of repair systems can
increase the cell's probability of survival. Several
assays for genotoxicity rely on indirect measurement of
the effects of these repair systems. Two assays (the <u>B</u>.
<u>subtilis</u> <u>rec</u> assay and the <u>E</u>. <u>coli</u> DNA polymerase assay)
measure reduction in the survival of chemically treated
cells that lack at least one DNA-repair enzyme, compared
with cells that have an intact repair system.[198] [373]
The phage-induction assays detect DNA damage that
induces the <u>recA</u> protein, which inactivates phage repressor.
In the absence of repressor, the phage multiply and produce
plaques on Petri plates of bacteria. Genes coding for
particular enzymes may be inserted into the phage chromosome and be expressed. The measurement of plaques[290] or
enzymatic activity[112] is used to indicate the genotoxic
effect of the chemical. The <u>rec</u>, phage-induction, and
polymerase assays are conducted with either spot-test or
liquid-suspension techniques. Exogenous metabolic activation
is functional only in the latter.

FUNGAL GENOTOXICITY ASSAYS

The main reason for using fungi for screening potential
mutagens is that some mutagens that cannot be detected
with bacterial systems might be revealed with fungal
systems. Being eukaryotes, fungi possess many genetic
properties that do not have counterparts in bacteria. In
addition, unrelated microorganisms apparently differ in
susceptibility to the induction of mutation by various
agents. Fungi have their own metabolic activation and
detoxification systems. The yeasts <u>Saccharomyces</u> <u>cerevisiae</u>
and <u>Schizosaccharomyces</u> <u>pombe</u> and the molds <u>Neurospora</u>
<u>crassa</u> and <u>Aspergillus</u> <u>nidulans</u> have been used most
extensively to screen chemical and physical agents for
mutagenicity. Special strains have been constructed to
test large numbers of compounds in screening programs with
standard protocols. Fungi have been used in simple qualitative tests on plates, in quantitative tests with liquid
suspension to determine dose-response relationships, and
in fluctuation tests that require many manipulations.

Some strains have been used in host-mediated assays and in the examination of mutagenic metabolites from tissues. Most strains reveal the types of mutational events that were induced by the mutagen. In addition to endogenous activation, compounds have been tested after chemical activation and activation by liver homogenates.

Over 700 chemical and physical agents have been tested with strains of S. cerevisiae, S. pombe, N. crassa, or A. nidulans. The results are being tabulated and related to chemical structure, physical state, carcinogenicity, and procarcinogenicity by the GENE-TOX Program.[42 199 258 398 520]

SACCHAROMYCES CEREVISIAE

Yeast has numerous advantages as a test organism and is the most suitable eukaryotic microorganism for carrying out genetic manipulations and assays. Among the advantages of the yeast S. cerevisiae are its ability to exist in either a stable haploid phase or a stable diploid phase, its rapid growth, and the ease with which single-cell suspensions can be prepared. Unlike many other microorganisms, some strains of S. cerevisiae are viable with many mutant genetic markers; this makes it possible to construct complex tester strains. Recent advances in recombinant-DNA technology have made it possible to manipulate the genetic material of S. cerevisiae with great sophistication.

Numerous diploid and haploid strains of S. cerevisiae have been chosen for mutation assay systems, but no strain or small group of strains has been accepted universally. Some of the strains previously used in extensive testing programs and some being seriously considered are listed in Table 5-3.

Haploid tester strains contain multiple markers that respond differently to mutagens. Strain XV185-14C contains the markers ade2-1, arg4-17, lys1-1 and trp5-48, which revert intragenically or by formation of UAA suppressors at a number of loci and the marker his1-7, which reverts by mutation at the original site and sites in the gene; the hom3-10 allele was chosen to reveal frameshift mutation, although the nature of the lesion has not been demonstrated directly. Strain XV185-14C has been used in suspension with and without metabolic activation to test the mutagenicity of many chemicals. Larimer et al.[228] have used a related strain, XA4-8C, that lacks marker arg4-17 to measure forward mutation by resistance to canavanine; the strain also contains marker rad2, to maintain sensitivity to at least some mutagens. The strain XL7-10B also has been

TABLE 5-3 Strains of the Yeast S. cerevisiae Used in Short-Term Tests of Mutagenicity

Strains	Genotype	Detected Genetic End Points	References
Haploid:			
XV185-14C	MATα ade2-1 arg4-17 lys1-1 trp5-48 his1-7 hom3-10	Reverse mutations	280, 520
6126/16c	MATα ade1-10 arg4-27 aro7-1 his4-1 trp1-1	Reverse mutations	427
XI7-10B	MATα CAN1⁺ his1-7 lys1-1 ura1	Forward and reverse mutations	227
Diploid:			
D3	$\frac{MATa\ CYH4\ ade2\ his8}{MAT\alpha\ +\ +\ +}$	Mitotic crossing-over	519
D4	$\frac{MATa\ gal2\ ade2-2\ trp5-12\ leu1}{MAT\alpha\ +\ ade2-1\ trp5-27\ +}$	Mitotic intragenic recombination	518
D5	$\frac{MATa\ trp1\ ade2-40\ MAL1\ +}{MAT\alpha\ +\ ade2-119\ +\ MAL4}$	Mitotic crossing-over, intragenic recombination, and reverse mutation	515
D6	$\frac{MATa\ his4\ ade2-40\ ade3\ leu1\ trp5\ cyh2\ met13}{MAT\alpha\ +\ ade2-40\ +\ +\ +\ +\ +}$	Mitotic nondisjunction	345
D7	$\frac{MATa\ ade2-40\ trp5-12\ ilv1-92}{MAT\alpha\ ade2-119\ trp5-27\ ilv1-92}$	Mitotic crossing-over, intragenic recombination, and reverse mutation	516
6117	$\frac{MATa\ +\ +\ cyh2\ met13\ aro3\ lys5\ ade5\ ade2-1\ ura4\ can1}{MAT\alpha\ leu1\ trp5\ +\ +\ +\ +\ +\ ade2-1\ +\ +}$	Mitotic intragenic recombination	427
JD1	$\frac{MATa\ ade2-1\ ser1\ his8\ his4C\ trp5-U9}{MAT\alpha\ +\ +\ +\ his4A\ trp5-U6}$	Mitotic intragenic recombination	85, 416
D₆J₂	$\frac{MATa\ ade5\ +\ aro2\ +\ cyh2\ +\ leu1\ +\ ade3}{MAT\alpha\ +\ lys5\ +\ met13\ +\ trp5\ +\ ade6\ +}$ etc.	Meiotic nondisjunction	344

used to measure canavanine forward mutations and his1-7 reverse mutations.[227]

Forward mutation can be detected when normal haploid strains are exposed to a mutagen and the cells are plated on a medium with a reduced adenine supplement; mutation in any of the ade1 and ade2 loci results in the accumulation of a red pigment and in the formation of easily detected red colonies. By using red ade1 and ade2 strains, one can detect additional mutations in at least five genes as white colonies; these genes control steps in purine biosynthesis that precede the steps controlled by the ade1 and ade2 genes. Adenine mutants with distinct colony colors have been used in mutagenicity testing systems with S. cerevisiae[271] and with other species, including S. pombe (ade6 and ade7 mutants) and N. crassa (ad-3 mutants), as described below.

Although the colored-adenine system does not require selective measures and poses no problems with mutation expression, routine testing of forward mutation with this systems is tedious and requires many plates to detect weak mutagens.

In addition to screening for mutation, some of the diploid strains have been used for detecting mitotic crossing-over, mitotic intragenic recombination, and mitotic nondisjunction (Table 5-3). Strain D3 is hetero-zygous for markers ade2 and his8, which are situated on the right arm of chromosome XV; mitotic crossing-over between ade2 and the centromere produces red colonies auxotrophic for histidine. Strain D4 contains two heteroallelic pairs, ade2-1/ade2-2 and trp5-5/trp5-27; the frequencies of induction of mitotic intragenic recombination are determined by plating the treated cells on media lacking either adenine or tryptophan. Strains D5 and D7 contain the complementary heteroallelic pair ade2-40/-ade2-219, which is useful for deducing the genotype of the resulting recombinational events; the parental ade2-40/ade2-219 strains are white, the ade2-40/ade2-40 sectors are red, and the ade2-119/ade2-119 sectors are pink. Strain D7 also contains the trp5-12/trp5-27 heteroalleles for detecting intragenic recombination and the ilv1-92/ilv1-92 homoalleles for detecting reversion. Strain D6 and strain 6117 detect mitotic nondisjunction; the loss of chromosome VII produces white colonies resistant to cycloheximide. Tests of the other recessive markers reveal whether the white resistant colonies arose by nondisjunction or by double mitotic crossing-over. Other diploid strains used in testing and detecting mitotic intragenic recombination are JD1[85] and BZ34.[297] A strain

D$_9$J$_9$ especially designed to measure meiotic nondisjunction has been tested with a variety of chemical agents.[344]

SCHIZOSACCHAROMYCES POMBE

Strain Pl of the yeast S. pombe has been used extensively to detect forward mutation; it requires adenine for growth and has the genotype h⁻ade6-60 rad10-198. The strain produces red colonies, because mutation of the ade6 (or ade7) locus causes the accumulation of a red pigment, a polymer derived from a precursor in the biosynthesis of adenine. The forward-mutation system of strain Pl is based on mutation of any five genes (adel, ade3, ade4, ade5, and ade9) that control early reactions leading to the formation of the pigment precursor. Thus, mutants are unable to synthesize the red pigment and are scored as white colonies derived from the predominantly red colonies; any mutation that inactivates the adel, ade3, ade4, ade5, or ade9 locus would be revealed. Such mutation includes simple base-pair substitution, addition, and deletion, as well as gross aberration that allows cell survival. Strain Pl also contains the rad10-198 mutation, which causes increased sensitivity to chemical agents and to ultraviolet and x radiation and which generally increases the frequency of induced mutation.[257] [258]

A second forward-mutation system consists of mutating normal strains and detecting mutants that form a red pigment owing to defects in the ade6 or ade7 locus. Like strain Pl described above, the rad10-198 marker can be incorporated in the strain.[258]

Several strains of S. pombe have been used in other test systems that depend on reverse mutation. The auxo- trophic markers in these strains included his52, his7, met4, ade6, and ade7. Most of the revertants arise by mutation at several different suppressor loci, and minor proportions arise by intragenic events at the original locus. Although large numbers of compounds have been tested with these strains, standardized protocols were not used.[258]

NEUROSPORA CRASSA

A report being prepared by Brockman et al.[42] will describe and evaluate the N. crassa test systems that detect gene and genomic mutations. The most extensively used N. crassa test system is the forward-mutation system developed by de Serres and co-workers.[93] In this system,

mutation in either of the two domains of the ad-3 locus
(ad-3A and ad-3B) results in a requirement for adenine and
in the accumulation of a purple pigment, similar to the
pigment seen in some adenine-requiring mutants of other
fungi. Tests are carried out on conidia with a two-
component heterokaryon; one component contains ad-3A and
ad-3B mutations, whereas the other contains the wild-type
AD-3 genes. The recessive ad-3A and ad-3B mutations
produce purple colonies when the wild-type gene mutates.
This test system reveals point mutations and chromosomal
deletions that encompass at least a portion of the AD-3
locus. One advantage of the system is that the recessive
lethal damage is recovered and its frequency can be estimated
from the proportion of heterokaryotic colonies with recessive
lethal aberrations in one of the two components. This
system has been used to test the mutagenic activity of an
extensive number of agents, including those requiring
activation. The procedures for carrying out the tests are
complex and require much technical skill.

A more convenient test system, developed by Ong,[332]
uses strains N23 and N24 for detecting ad-3 reverse
mutations that include base-pair substitutions and presumably
frameshift mutations.

A specially constructed cross (I-41-5 x I-34-8) of N.
crassa has been used to determine the ability of agents to
produce meiotic nondisjunction.[147] The parental strains
were heterozygous for four auxotrophic markers on chromosome 1; prototrophic disomics can be selected by plating
ascospores on minimal medium.

ASPERGILLUS NIDULANS

A large number of strains of A. nidulans have been used
to test for gene mutation, chromosomal mutation, genomic
mutation, and mitotic crossing-over. The majority of
investigations of chemically induced gene mutation in
haploid strains of A. nidulans used one of the following
three systems, which are critically discussed by Scott et
al.:[398] the methionine system, the 2-thioxanthine system,
and the arginine system. The methionine and 2-thioxanthine
systems are forward-mutation systems that detect base-pair
changes and small deletions, whereas the arginine system
appears to be a reversion system; the nature of the
alterations detected in the arginine system is unknown.

In the methionine system, suppressor mutations are
selected on methionine-less medium with strains of A.
nidulans requiring methionine because of blocks in any of
eight genes, usually methGl. No true reversions are

generally observed, and the reversions occur by mutations at five or more distinct suppressor loci. These suppressors are believed to act by the formation of alternative pathways that bypass the original lesions.

The 2-thioxanthine system relies on the observation that normal strains of A. nidulans produce yellow conidia, instead of green conidia, when grown on media containing the purine analogue 2-thioxanthine. Mutants that produce green conidia on 2-thioxanthine-containing medium have deficiencies either of the uptake system or of xanthine dehydrogenase. These deficiencies in the uptake system and xanthine dehydrogenase are due to mutations in eight and seven loci, respectively.

In most investigations with the methionine and 2-thio-xanthine systems, the haploid strain Glasgow biA1;methG1 was used. In addition to being compatible with both systems, this strain carries the biA1 mutation, which increases permeability to external substances.

In the arginine system, revertants of the arginine-requiring strain BIN-252 are simply selected on arginine-less medium. Although the nature of the original mutation and that of the reverse mutation have not been reported, this arginine system has been extensively used by Kovalenko and co-workers in Russia (see Scott et al.[398]).

Käfer et al.[199] have discussed in detail the use of heterozygous diploid strains of A. nidulans for investigating the effects of chemicals on genomic mutation, chromosomal mutation, and mitotic crossing-over. Twenty different diploid-strain heterozygous signal markers have been used by various investigators. Usually, homozygosity or hemizygosity of recessive markers is used to reveal and distinguish mitotic crossing-over and nondisjunction, as in diploid strain P1, which contains the heterozygous signal markers fpaA1 and yA2 on chromosome 1. Strain P1 is green when grown prototrophically and is sensitive to p-FPA, because the markers are heterozygous and recessive. Homozygosity or hemizygosity of the recessive marker fpaA1 or yA2 leads to p-FPA resistance or yellow colonies, respectively. Mitotic crossing-over and nondisjunction can be distinguished by examining other markers that were originally heterozygous on both arms of chromosome 1. Segregants of this strain, which are aneuploid for chromosome 1, can be yellow or green, depending on which of the two chromosomes is involved. Nondisjunctional yellow sectors also should require p-aminobenzoic acid and aneurine and should be resistant to p-FPA. Because the first event in nondisjunction is the production of unbalanced aneuploid sectors, either stable haploid or stable diploid yellow sectors will appear from a poorly growing colony.

Testing can be carried out qualitatively with a plate test
or quantitatively with liquid suspensions.

In addition, less extensively used diploid test systems
include one type that reveals recessive lethals and balanced
translocations and another type that measures the increased
elimination of duplicated segments from duplicated strains.

EVALUATION OF FUNGAL SYSTEMS

Systems using the yeasts S. cerevisiae[520] and S.
pombe[258] and the molds N. crassa[42] and A. nidulans[199 398]
have been evaluated for short-term testing of carcinogens.
de Serres and Hoffmann[91] have evaluated the results of
eight yeast assay tests conducted for the International
Program for the Evaluation of Short-Term Tests.[190 203 257
280 343 417 517]

Comparison of the various fungal systems indicates that
mutagenicity tests that use molds, such as N. crassa and
A. nidulans, require a higher degree of technical skill
than tests that use yeasts, such as S. cerevisiae and S.
pombe, especially for quantitative tests. Forward-mutation
tests that are based on the change in frequencies of
colored colonies due to adenine mutation require the
scoring of more colonies than tests based on selection;
the time and cost of these forward-mutation tests limit
their usefulness in rapid screening. An examination of
the mutagenicity of 40 chemicals revealed considerable
differences in sensitivity, specificity, and accuracy of
eight yeast test systems.[91]

It is generally, but not universally, agreed that
fungal test systems are less sensitive than bacterial test
systems; in almost all cases, a higher dose of the agent
being tested is required to elicit a response in the
fungal systems. Yeast tests are the fastest and least
expensive eukaryotic assays.

No tester strain or small group of strains can be
recommended for routine screening programs. Ideal strains
would be able to detect genetic end points by selection
and respond to agents that damage not only DNA, but also
cell components that control chromosomal disjunction. It
may be possible to use strains with high concentrations of
activating enzymes, thus obviating exogenous activation.
Although many agents may induce mutation in all prokaryotes
and eukaryotes, it is not known whether the pattern of
endogenous activation and the induction of nondisjunction
are similar enough in fungi and mammals for fungal systems
to be reliable in human detection programs. Recent advances
in recombinant-DNA technology may permit the construction

of yeast strains that have mammalian components and mutagenic responses equivalent to those of mammalian cells.

MUTAGENESIS ASSAYS IN CULTURED MAMMALIAN CELLS

Mammalian cell mutagenesis is useful to detect and identify potential chemical carcinogens. Some 200-300 chemicals have been tested in a number of mammalian cell mutagenesis assay systems. Several carcinogens--such as natulan and p,p'-DDE--that are negative or difficult to detect in the Salmonella/microsome assay are mutagenic in mammalian cell assays. Aflatoxin G_2 and chrysene, which are not considered carcinogenic, also are not mutagenic in mammalian cell systems, but are mutagenic in the Salmonella/-microsome assay.[37] In some classes of chemicals, the degree of carcinogenicity and mutagenicity can be correlated--e.g., polycyclic hydrocarbons and nitrosamines in cell-mediated assays.

It is important to emphasize that often doses that induce mutation in mammalian cells are significantly lower than those used in bacterial systems, e.g., a difference of more than several orders of magnitude in the case of nitrosamine and some polycyclic aromatic hydrocarbons.

Since the original publications from the laboratories of Puck and Chu,[62,201] a series of specific-locus mutation assays using cultured mammalian cells have been developed and used to detect environmental mutagens.[148,419] The most commonly used target cells in these assays are from clones of the Chinese hamster V79[62,175] and Chinese hamster ovary (CHO)[201,331] cell lines and mouse lymphoma L5178 cells.[67] These cells are suitable for mutagenesis studies, because they have a high plating efficiency (more than 50%), short generation times (16 ± 4 h), and, in the case of the Chinese hamster cells, a nearly diploid karyotype.[175,201] Cultured human and rodent normal fibroblasts, which have a stable diploid karyotype and can be easily obtained, are of limited use because of their low plating efficiency and limited life span.[25,185]

Mutants in cultured mammalian cells are usually characterized by at least two of the following criteria:[54,60,419]

• The altered cellular phenotype is stable and is transmitted to daughter cells.
• The number of cells with the altered phenotype can be increased by treatment with a mutagen.
• Altered gene products can be associated with the altered cell phenotype.

• The frequency of cells with a recessive phenotype is associated with chromosomal euploidy.

Drug resistance is the best genetic marker because of the ease in selecting mutants with a single-step procedure. The most common are 8-azaguanine and 6-thioguanine resistance, associated with loss of or alteration in hypoxanthine-guanine phosphoribosyl transferase (HGPRT) activity;[54] 5-bromo-2-deoxyuridine (BrdUrd) or trifluorothymidine (TFT) resistance,[67] which results from loss of or alteration in thymidine kinase (TK) activity; and ouabain resistance, associated with an alteration in the binding site of the plasma-membrane sodium-potassium-activated ATPase.[24] Chinese hamster cells are used mainly to depict mutations at the HGPRT and Na-K ATPase loci, whereas mouse lymphoma cells are usually used to assay TK mutations. The gene for HGPRT in humans, mice, and Chinese hamsters is on the X chromosome; thus, cells are monogenic, owing to the presence of a single X chromosome in a male cell and the inactivation of one of the pair of X chromosomes in a female cell.[54 60 419] HGPRT catalyzes the conversion of hypoxanthine and guanine to their corresponding nucleoside-5'-monophosphates. It also catalyzes the conversion of the purine analogues 8-azaguanine and 6-thioguanine to the lethal nucleoside-5-monophosphate.[451] For these reasons, cells with mutations that inactivate the HGPRT gene product grow in medium containing the purine analogues that kill HGPRT$^+$ cells. This is also the principle behind the TK conversion of BrdUrd or TFT to cytotoxic products.[67] Resistance to these analogues is obtained by mutation of cells heterozygous at the TK locus (TK$^{+/-}$) to cells recessive for this gene (TK$^{-/-}$). Both HGPRT$^-$ and TK$^{-/-}$ cells revert to HGPRT$^+$ and TK$^{+/-}$ cells when they undergo mutation and can divide in the presence of thymidine, hypoxanthine, aminopterin, and glycine (THAG). Aminopterin inhibits folic acid-requiring metabolism, making the cells dependent on exogenous hypoxanthine, thymidine, and glycine. Inactive HGPRT and TK cells cannot use exogenous hypoxanthine or thymidine, respectively, and die unless they regain the enzyme activity by spontaneous or induced mutation.

The Na-K ATPase, in the plasma membrane of mammalian cells, is inhibited when ouabain binds to the α subunit that is phosphorylated during catalysis.[24 372] Unlike HGPRT$^-$ and TK$^{-/-}$, the ouabain-resistant phenotype (assigned to chromosome 3 in the mouse)[218] is dominant, stable, and characterized by a reduced uptake of ^{86}Rb and ^{42}K in the presence of ouabain and by reduced binding of ouabain to the plasma membrane.[24] Ouabain resistance can be induced by a variety of mutagenic agents, but not by ionizing radiation and the frameshift mutagen ICR191,[17] whereas the HGPRT and TK loci are responsive to many classes of mutagens, including ionizing radiation and ICR191. HGPRT and TK activities probably can be totally deleted without affecting growth of the cultured cells in nonselective medium, whereas Na-K ATPase activity is vital. Thus, ouabain resistance is a special mutation that probably reflects base substitutions in discrete sections of the Na-K ATPase locus, which affect the binding of ouabain, but do not destroy enzyme activity.[17] That is presumably why the frequency of ouabain-resistant mutants is lower than that of HGPRT⁻ and TK⁻/⁻.[148] [177] The specificity of ouabain resistance may be useful to identify the type of mutation that can be induced by a specific mutagen, but limits its usefulness for the general screening of mutagens that induce mainly frameshift mutation.

Selection of mutants in mammalian cells in culture involves several technical variables, including isolation protocol, phenotypic expression, time before selection, cell density that permits maximal mutant recovery, drug concentration, and culture media.

Expression periods, which presumably include the time required to fix the mutation at the DNA level and the dilution of the wild-type gene product, vary with the cell type and genetic markers.[62] [67] [148] [331] [419] For example, the expression times for HGPRT⁻ and TK⁻/⁻ mutations can vary in different cell types from 5 to 10 d, whereas that of ouabain resistance is 1 to 2 d. Cell density at the time of selection is important in the isolation of HGPRT-defective cells; reduced mutation frequencies occur at high cell densities.[62] [67] [331] This presumably is due to metabolic cooperation mediated by cell contacts that allow the toxic nucleotides to pass from the wild-type cells into the mutated ones.[480] Thus, establishing the critical cell densities is important to obtain accurate optimal mutation frequencies. Optimal doses of selective agents are of extreme importance if outgrowth of wild-type cells is to be prevented.

The adverse effect of many chemicals depends on their conversion to reactive electrophilic intermediates by mono-oxygenases.[157] [283] Most cell lines currently used for mutagenesis studies are not capable of these chemical conversions. Therefore, inclusion of a metabolic activation system in a test system is essential. In mutagenesis assays with mammalian cells, three metabolic activation systems have been used:

- <u>Microsome-mediated assay</u>. Activation of chemicals

in the presence of a subcellular fraction from rodent
liver, supplemented with the necessary cofactors, including
an NADPH or an NADPH-generating system, has been used
extensively in mammalian cells. Many factors affect
activation of chemicals in microsome-mediated assays:
species, sex, organs from which tissue homogenates are
prepared, type of enzyme-inducer used in pretreating
animals, amount of tissue homogenate in the reaction
mixture, time of incubation, and the requirement of
contact or proximity between target cells and metabolic
activation systems.[67 174] A wide variety of chemicals are
mutagenic in a microsome-mediated assay, including polycyclic
aromatic hydrocarbons, nitrosamines, aflatoxins, and vinyl
chloride.[27 67 172 219 222 223]

• Cell-mediated assay. Cell-mediated mutagenesis[176]
uses intact cells for metabolic activation, rather than
disrupted tissue homogenates. Target cells are cocultivated
with metabolically competent nondividing cells (activating
layer), which activate chemicals. This system established
a relationship between the degree of carcinogenicity and
mutagenicity of polycyclic aromatic hydrocarbons, with
lethally irradiated rodent fibroblasts as an activating
layer;[174 176 318] isolated hepatocytes also have been used
with nitrosamines and aflatoxins.[27 197 225] In some
studies, polycyclic hydrocarbons were mutagenic after
their activation in a cell-mediated assay by intact human
cells.[173] A series of studies have indicated that the DNA
adducts and metabolic pathways of benzo[a]pyrene and 7,12-
dimethylbenz[a]anthracene in intact cells are different
from those produced after metabolism by subcellular
fractions.[32 318 412 413] Thus, these studies and those on
the mutagenicity of polycyclic aromatic hydrocarbons and
nitrosamines suggest that the cell-mediated assay reflects
more accurately the metabolic pathway occurring in vivo.

• Host-mediated assay. In the host-mediated assay,
target cells are inoculated into an animal that receives
the chemical treatment. The assay can be performed only
with cell lines that do not kill and are not killed by the
host. Several chemicals--including AF-2, EMS, DMN, DEN,
and MNNG--have been tested in this assay system. These
chemicals induce mutations in the direct test or in cell-
or microsome-mediated assays. Such studies may be useful
in understanding responses--including tissue distribution,
activation, detoxification, and elimination of chemicals--
in whole animals.

Several mammalian mutagenesis systems are used widely
to detect environmental mutagens. For isolation of
mutants, choice of cell lines and genetic markers is of

considerable importance. Chinese hamster cells and L5178Y
mouse lymphoma cells seem most suitable, because mutants
are isolated easily. Forward mutation to obtain resistance
to purine analogues, pyrimidine analogues, and ouabain has
been characterized.

Metabolic activation systems--such as microsome-,
cell-, and host-mediated assays--have been included in
mammalian cell mutagenesis systems. Microsome-mediated
assays have been used to detect many chemicals, including
nitrosamines, polycyclic hydrocarbons, aflatoxins, and
vinyl chloride. Cell-mediated assays seem to be a better
indicator of in vivo metabolic pathways. Microsome-
mediated assays seem suitable for general screening of
chemicals, and cell-mediated assays are more valuable in
the assessment of data.

Mammalian cells in culture permit several end points to
be measured simultaneously in the same cell system. These
include malignant transformations, chromosomal changes,
and DNA damage and repair, as well as specific-locus
mutation.[26]

DNA REPAIR AS A PREDICTIVE INDICATOR OF CHEMICAL MUTAGENICITY AND CARCINOGENICITY

DNA damage has been defined recently by Hanawalt and
his colleagues[152] as any modification of DNA that alters
its coding properties or its normal function in replication
or transcription. Damage can be repaired if it is recognized
by a component of the repair enzyme system that acts to
remove the damage and to restore the original structure of
the DNA.

There are three main types of DNA damage that can be
repaired by cellular processes: missing, incorrect, or
altered bases; interstrand cross-links; and strand breaks.
These types of DNA damage can be induced by some chemicals,
and there is increasing evidence that these chemicals are
carcinogenic. Therefore, procedures that can detect
damage to DNA or its consequences are potentially valuable
to predict carcinogenic activity.[41]

DNA repair can be classified according to three mechanisms
(see Stich et al.[440]):

• Photoreactivation and dealkylation by enzymes that
directly reverse the altered DNA structure to its original
state. This form of repair has been associated mainly
with microorganisms and is thought to occur in mammalian
cells.[443] [444] It is not involved currently in predictive
tests for carcinogenicity or mutagenicity.

• Excision repair involving removal of nucleotides in the neighborhood of DNA damage followed by resynthesis and rejoining of the DNA. Evidence of this form of repair is used in some screening tests.

• Replication and postreplication (recombination) repair believed to occur during semiconservative DNA replication. They are of considerable basic interest[339] and are also used to some extent in screening tests.[198]

Exposure of cells to carcinogens may result in the formation of DNA adducts varying in size from methyl groups to bulky structures, such as metabolites of polycyclic aromatic hydrocarbons and aromatic amines. In vivo, these adducts usually are removed enzymatically and at different rates from the DNA. Because the liver is the main site of activation of chemical carcinogens, the DNA of this organ usually forms more adducts. Direct detection and measurement of DNA damage are thus possible, in principle, by detection and measurement of the bound adduct. Because the number of adducts is usually extremely small, very sensitive methods are required for their measurement.

DNA cross-links may result from linkage of the two strands by bifunctional adducts, in which case the linkage would be detected by any procedure sensitive enough to detect the adduct. Cross-links also inhibit strand separation and may be so detected.

DNA strand breaks may occur through interaction with the activated form of a carcinogen, such as a free radical, or after the action of endonucleases at the site of damage by the carcinogen. Single strand breaks are measured by alkaline sucrose-gradient centrifugation, and double strand breaks by sedimentation in neutral sucrose gradients. More recently, the procedure of alkaline elution from membrane filters has been introduced.

Nucleotide excision and base removal followed by the action of apurinic-apyrimidine endonucleases (AP endonucleases) are the two types of excision repair that currently are thought to occur. A number of nucleotides are excised from the damaged DNA strand. After excision, the correct complementary bases are replaced by polymerase action, with the intact strand as template. Finally, the new strand is attached covalently to the adjacent undamaged old strand by the enzyme DNA ligase.

The repair process can be measured by several techniques of varied complexity. These include measurement of adduct formation and the rate of its disappearance, the detection of enzyme-sensitive sites, and the measurement of strand breaks. Replacement of the damaged region, which is the actual process of DNA repair, has been investigated by other procedures, including the measurement of unscheduled DNA synthesis and the incorporation of BrdUrd by isopycnic centrifugation, the use of bromouracil photolyses, and the use of benzoylated, naphthoylated DEAE cellulose chromatography. Rejoining of the DNA strand has been demonstrated by alkaline sucrose-gradient centrifugation and alkaline elution applied at increasing intervals after exposure to the carcinogen. The return of the damaged DNA to normal size indicates strand rejoining.

DNA DAMAGE

DNA Adduct Formation

The formation of adducts of activated carcinogens (ultimate carcinogens) with DNA has been studied extensively in vivo with the intact animal and in vitro with various cellular and subcellular systems (reviewed by Sarma et al.[387]). The hypothesis that cancer may result from a carcinogen-induced change in DNA has been discussed by Lawley.[232] This process might have a mutational mechanism or could occur by some nonmutational mechanism mediated by interaction with DNA. It is, of course, well known that carcinogens react with a variety of other cellular constituents, including RNA and protein.[282][283] However, the in vivo covalent binding of organic chemicals to DNA recently has been proposed as a quantitative indicator of chemical carcinogens by Lutz.[261] An important disadvantage of this procedure is the requirement for radioactively labeled compounds. However, Lutz pointed out that many newly synthesized chemicals for large-scale use are prepared with an appropriate label, because this usually is required for pharmacokinetic and metabolic studies required in standard toxicity testing. Taking data from the literature, Lutz found an impressive correlation between carcinogenic potency and binding of the compound to DNA of rat liver. The development of the radioimmunoassay of DNA-carcinogen adducts for alkylating carcinogens,[296] aromatic amines,[356] and polycyclic hydrocarbons[356] indicates possible ways in which the DNA binding assay may evolve without the necessity for radiolabeling. The recent work of Harris and co-workers[153] on an ultrasensitive enzymatic radioimmunoassay may have great value in the development of this field.

Damaged Sites on DNA Sensitive to Enzymes

Paterson developed this approach and has reviewed it comprehensively.[347] The rationale of the procedure is to use excision-repair endonucleases that convert defective sites in DNA into single strand breaks that can be measured by alkaline sucrose-gradient centrifugation or alkaline elution. The procedure can be performed in vitro or in vivo. In the in vitro method, the DNA of cells is labeled with [^{3}H]thymidine, extracted, incubated with or without the endonuclease, and denatured in alkali for analysis of single strand breaks. To serve as an internal control, untreated DNA labeled with [^{14}C]thymidine is coextracted with the treated DNA labeled with tritium. The assay also can be performed in vivo by partial cell-wall disruption of the cultured cells immediately after exposure to the carcinogen. This permits intracellular entry of enzymes that recognize lesions in DNA. After endonuclease incubation, the cells are lysed directly on alkaline sucrose gradients, and the operation is carried out as for the in vitro method. In principle, this procedure for the detection of DNA damage can selectively monitor one or more specific types of lesions, depending on the substrate specificity of the endonuclease preparations. Furthermore, the enzymatic assays do not require the cells to be exposed to toxic compounds, such as hydroxyurea and BrdUrd. The procedure has detected DNA damage induced by several types of carcinogens, as demonstrated by Duker and Teebor,[102] but it is limited by the requirement for the pure nuclease and by the lack of knowledge of the susceptibility of different types of DNA damage to the enzymes. It is possible, however, that this method will become more valuable as more becomes known about its properties.

Strand Breaks

As already indicated, strand breaks can be detected and measured by alkaline sucrose-gradient centrifugation and by alkaline elution. Both procedures have been applied to cells from intact animals, as well as to in vitro systems.

Alkaline sucrose centrifugation was introduced by McGrath and Williams,[278] who showed that DNA from irradiated Escherichia coli sedimented more slowly than control DNA after lysis in alkali and that the sedimentation pattern approached that of the untreated DNA at increasing intervals after radiation treatment. Applying the procedure to mammalian cells, Lett and colleagues[246] demonstrated rejoining of x-ray-induced strand breaks in the DNA of leukemic cells. In both cases, the cells were labeled with [³H]thymidine, enabling the presence and amount of the DNA in the sucrose gradients to be monitored. The details of the method have been reviewed by Cleaver.[65] The method was applied to whole animals in vivo by Cox et al.,[74] who labeled the liver DNA with [³H]thymidine by treatment of partially hepatectomized rats during the phase of greatly increased hepatic DNA synthesis. Although this maneuver detected and measured DNA strand breaks in vivo, it is limited to hepatic cells. Zubroff and Sarma[521] greatly improved the method by developing fluorimetric methods for measurement of DNA from fractions from the gradient and permitting study of effects on organs other than the liver. Later, detailed study of the conformation of DNA released from rat liver nuclei by alkaline lysis under the conditions of the in vivo experiments validated the procedure as an index of DNA damage and repair.[341]

Alkaline sucrose-gradient analysis has been used extensively to study DNA damage by a variety of carcinogens in vivo and in vitro. Effects of carcinogenic alkylating agents, including nitroso compounds, on rat liver in vivo have been reported by Farber and colleagues[84 438] and by others.[89 397] Koropatnick and Stich[217] developed an interesting use of the method in reporting the induction of DNA fragmentation in mouse gastric epithelial cells, as shown by shifts in the sedimentation profiles after centrifugation through alkaline and neutral sucrose gradients. The cells were labeled by injecting [³H]thymidine into young mice; the carcinogens were administered by stomach tube. The latter compounds included 4-nitroquinoline 1-oxide, N-acetoxy-2-acetylaminofluorene, and the product of coadministration of methylguanidine and nitrite, which presumably led to formation of the nitrosylated derivative in the stomach. In contrast, the precarcinogens 2-acetylaminofluorene and dimethylnitrosamine had no demonstrable effect on the stomach DNA, but the latter compound did induce strand breaks in the liver. The authors claimed that their procedure had the advantages of in vitro short-term bioassays for carcinogens plus the thoroughness of using whole animals. DNA repair synthesis was shown by unscheduled incorporation of [³H]thymidine. The direct-acting mutagen and pancreatic carcinogen azaserine (O-diazoacetile-L-serine) also was shown to induce DNA damage and repair in pancreas, liver, and kidney cells by Lilja and colleagues.[249]

Alkaline elution of large DNA fragments from cells lysed on filters was devised by Kohn and colleagues[215 216] and has been applied to the study of damaging effects on DNA of carcinogens given to animals in vivo. As with the sucrose-gradient procedures, the DNA measurements have been carried out either by labeling with [^{3}H]thymidine or by fluorometry. The alkaline-elution technique cannot detect, for example, the dealkylation of O^6-methylguanine, but only the seemingly innocuous products that result in depuration. The ratio of O^6-alkylguanine to these other products depends on the chemical used. Parodi and colleagues[342] have developed a procedure for prescreening chemical carcinogens with microfluorimetric measurement of DNA and have tested a small number of N-nitroso compounds and related alkylating carcinogens. They argued that their procedure was superior to alkaline sucrose sedimentation, emphasizing the laborious requirements in the latter procedure for removal of the sucrose, which interferes with measurement. Petzold and Swenberg[351] have reported similar findings with rats neonatally labeled with [^{3}H]thymidine and have extended the carcinogens tested to include 4-nitroquinoline 1-oxide, aflatoxin B_1, benzidine, 2-acetylaminofluorene, and 7,12-dimethylbenz[a]anthracene. They concluded that the alkaline-elution assay is a rapid and reliable assay for assessment of the capacity of a compound to induce DNA damage. Again, there is insufficient evidence to recommend alkaline elution as a general screening procedure, but further work may validate it.

DNA REPAIR

Unscheduled DNA synthesis is observed by the incorporation of precursors into DNA in the absence of semiconservative replication. It was first demonstrated by Rasmussen and Painter[363] in studies on repair of damage induced in cultured mammalian cells by ultraviolet radiation and was later shown to occur as a result of exposure of cells to the chemical carcinogen 4-nitroquinoline 1-oxide.[439] The phenomenon can be demonstrated radiochemically by exposing the damaged cells to a labeled precursor and measuring incorporation into DNA. The precursor usually is [^{3}H]-thymidine, because it is specific for DNA and the nucleic acid does not have to be extracted and purified before the assay. Because incorporation is much greater in semi-conservative replication than in repair synthesis, steps must be taken to eliminate the former process. This often is done by treating the cells with hydroxyurea or using cells, such as lymphocytes and hepatocytes, that may have extremely low semiconservative synthesis. A widely used alternative is the detection and measurement of incorporation of the labeled precursor by autoradiography. The heavier labeling of semiconservative replication usually can be distinguished from the lighter incorporation of repair synthesis. Also, different cell populations can be distinguished by their morphology, whereas radiochemical methods can measure only the bulk DNA from the whole tissue or organ, unless preliminary cell-fractionation procedures have been carried out. However, a simple assay for radioactivity is easier and takes less time.

Attempts have been made in several laboratories to develop relatively simple methods for using unscheduled DNA synthesis as an index of DNA damage and hence as a screening test for carcinogenicity. As with all other tests for chemical carcinogens, cells that can metabolically convert precarcinogens to their active forms must be used,[284] and an enzyme system must be included to carry out this process, as is done in the Salmonella/microsome test.

Stich and co-workers[439] were among the first to show the induction of unscheduled DNA synthesis by chemical carcinogens. In their experiments, nearly nondividing cells were exposed to the test compounds at various concentrations, the highest being half that previously determined to be toxic. Of the 64 compounds tested, 29 were proximate or ultimate carcinogens, 15 were precarcinogens that required toxification, 16 were nononcogenic compounds, and 4 were of unknown carcinogenic potential. All the directly acting carcinogens induced unscheduled DNA synthesis, whereas the nononcogenic agents did not. In general, the precarcinogens were not active, except occasionally after longer exposures and at higher concentrations. In a later publication,[440] the authors found unscheduled incorporation of [^{3}H]thymidine into the DNA of human cells exposed to the precarcinogen dimethylnitrosamine in the presence of a rodent liver S-9 activation system, but, as before, dimethylnitrosamine without the S-9 system was inactive.

Because the liver is the main organ for metabolism of foreign compounds, including carcinogens,[266 490 505] the largest amount of the activated or ultimate forms of the carcinogens should be generated in the hepatocyte. Of course, there are deactivating pathways for proximate and ultimate carcinogens that may deflect the activated products from the cellular DNA; nevertheless, the hepatocyte can be assumed in most cases to be the most effective cell for activation of carcinogens and mutagens. With some exceptions, procarcinogens are activated by microsomal mono-oxygenases that depend on cytochrome P-450. This cytochrome also is present in greater amounts in the liver than in other organs. For this reason, the hepatocyte has been used extensively for carcinogen screening tests based on unscheduled DNA synthesis. Since the successful culturing of rodent hepatocytes in vitro, these cells have been extensively used; more recently, suspensions of isolated hepatocytes have been introduced.

Another system dealing with unscheduled DNA synthesis in hepatocytes is that developed by Gary Williams and colleagues.[491-494 496] This test uses primary rat liver cell cultures and measures unscheduled DNA synthesis by autoradiography. Replicative DNA synthesis is virtually absent, and addition of hydroxyurea to the medium has no detectable effect.[492] In a modified form of the test,[493] fresh liver cells are used, and a longer exposure to the chemical is introduced to permit greater DNA modification and repair, more convenient scheduling of the processing, and simplification of the grain counting by use of an automatic counter. In contrast with the other procedures for measuring unscheduled DNA synthesis, the Williams test has been used with a relatively large number of classes of chemical carcinogens and has proved to be reliable (see Williams et al.[495]).

A test that depends on unscheduled DNA synthesis with HeLa cells has been proposed by Garner and colleagues.[272 495]

Progress has also been made in studying unscheduled DNA synthesis directly in germ cells. Studies on such cells are, of course, much more relevant to genetic risk. The induction of unscheduled DNA synthesis in mammalian germ cells in vivo after treatment with a chemical mutagen was first shown by Sega.[401] Several other reports on unscheduled DNA synthesis in mammalian germ cells have come out of Sega's laboratory since then.[50 400 402-405 428]

With male mice, it is possible to study the occurrence of unscheduled DNA synthesis, taken to be DNA repair, in meiotic and postmeiotic germ cell stages after treatment with mutagenic agents. This is done by making use of the well-studied sequence of events that occur during spermato-genesis and spermiogenesis in the mouse. The last scheduled DNA synthesis occurs in primary spermatocytes, which then mature through a series of germ cell stages, taking between 33 and 36 d to develop into mature spermatozoa in the vasa deferentia.

If the mice are treated in vivo with a suspected mutagen and are also given testicular injections of [^{3}H]thymidine ([^{3}H]dT), then any unscheduled incorporation of [^{3}H]dT into the DNA of meiotic and postmeiotic germ cell stages is an indication that the suspected mutagen was able to reach the germ cells and produce some sort of "repairable" lesions in the DNA. The germ cell stages in which unscheduled DNA synthesis has been found to occur after treatment of males with several different mutagenic agents span from leptotene to midspermatid. Apparently, once protamine has replaced the usual chromosomal histones in the developing spermatid, no further DNA repair is possible (at least until after fertilization).

An advantage of this sort of test is that it is much easier and more rapid than dominant-lethal tests, chromosomal-aberration studies, and specific-locus mutation experiments. Because the test is done in vivo, activation of the test chemical is possible in the germ cells themselves or in other organs that might then release the active compound to the circulatory system and thereby cause an interaction with the germ cells. For most of the chemicals looked at, the measurement of DNA repair in mouse germ cells appears to be a considerably more sensitive biologic end point than measurement of dominant lethals or translocations.

CYTOGENETIC TESTS

When cells are exposed to mutagens, the resulting mutations can be classified as gene mutations or gross chromosomal aberrations. Chromosomal aberrations may occur anywhere in the genome. Because of the difference in size between a gene and the genome, gross chromosomal aberrations occur at a vastly greater frequency than mutations at a single locus. This makes it possible to determine effects of mutagens by observing aberrations in relatively small numbers of cells, and cytogenetic tests have provided a very sensitive method for determining whether an agent can interact with the genetic material.

CHROMOSOMAL-ABERRATION TESTS

Aberrations differ according to the stage in the cell cycle when they are produced. Some mutagenic agents--such as ionizing radiation, 8-ethoxycaffeine, streptonigrin, and bleomycin--can induce aberrations in cells in all stages of the cell cycle. These agents can induce double strand breaks in DNA. If the aberrations are induced in the G_1 phase, before the chromosomes are replicated, full chromosomal aberrations are produced, whereas, if the cells are exposed in the S or G_2 phase, when the chromosomes contain two chromatids, chromatid aberrations are formed. With ultraviolet radiation and most chemicals that do not induce strand breaks, the situation is somewhat different. Although lesions can be induced in the DNA at any time of the cell cycle, aberrations are not formed until lesion-bearing chromosomes enter the S phase. Consequently, these agents are called S-dependent and produce only chromatid aberrations. The results of different types of aberrations vary. For example, a chromosome deletion usually will be lethal to both daughter cells, because parts of both chromatids are deleted, and the acentric fragment will be lost at division. With a chromatid deletion, only one of two daughter cells will contain the deleted chromatid and will be killed; the other cell will contain a normal chromosome. Similar differences in the number of affected daughter cells also occur for viable aberrations, such as symmetric exchanges (translocations), which are important for quantitative assessment of genetic hazards.[115 500]

There are also differences in cellular sensitivity in the different stages of the cycle. In cytogenetic tests, cells in different stages of the cycle must be treated and analyzed. If the study is to be carried out in vivo on cycling cells or in vitro on asynchronous cells, a single treatment will expose cells in all stages of the cycle. An analysis of different stages can be made by fixing cells at different times after treatment, when the cells appear at metaphase, where the chromosomes can be analyzed. With synchronous cells, treatment at different times after initiation of synchronization permits cells in different stages of the cycle to be treated.

Many of the compounds that induce mutations are pro-mutagens that require metabolic activation to be converted to the proximate or ultimate mutagenic form. In in vitro assays, this activation usually is achieved by treating the compound with a liver microsomal system, the S-9 mix (see Chapter 4 for discussion). In vivo mammalian systems, however, require no special provisions for activation. Cytogenetic tests with mammals therefore consist of treating cells in culture with a compound or exposing an animal to it. Because different agents produce effects at different stages of the cell cycle and cause different amounts of mitotic delay that could affect the appearance of the cells at metaphase, multiple posttreatment sampling times are necessary to allow cells exposed in all stages of the cycle to be analyzed. For the best measurement, results should be expressed as the frequency of aberrations per cell, and not as percentage of aberrant cells, which is merely an all-or-none observation. Because different aberrations have different genetic consequences and dose relations, aberrations should be classified as chromosomal or chromatid aberrations. Within each of these classes, the aberrations should be subdivided further as deletions or exchanges. Another class of cytogenetic effect, chromatid gaps, should be presented separately, because the distinction between a chromatid deletion and a gap (achromatic lesion) is arbitrary.

Various types of cells can be scored for chromosomal aberrations. Spermatogonial cells, spermatocytes, oocytes, early embryos, bone marrow cells, and lymphocytes have been used successfully after in vivo treatments of an animal. For short-term cytogenetic analysis, however, an in vitro cell-culture assay is often chosen. Such in vitro assays usually use a peripheral lymphocyte system or a monolayer cell-culture system.

Each cytogenetic test system has advantages and disadvantages. For instance, if a very simple determination of a compound's ability to produce chromosomal aberrations in vivo is desired, a bone marrow assay is probably simplest and least expensive. If, however, genetic hazards to future generations are of primary concern, assays of germ cells would be more appropriate. In in vitro assays of peripheral lymphocytes or cell lines, the cells can be made synchronous or fairly synchronous. Also, the results in vitro (in the case of lymphocytes) can be compared with those with the same cell type in vivo.

The disadvantages of cytogenetic assays are that they are time-consuming and that negative results indicate only that further studies must be conducted with S-9 activation and with multiple fixations to account for possible different sensitivities of stages of the cell cycle. Furthermore, the scoring of 300 cells per point for chromosomal and chromatid aberrations is very difficult, requires much expertise, and is necessary to establish an accurate result.

SISTER-CHROMATID-EXCHANGE TEST

A simpler, quicker, and less expensive cytogenetic test uses sister chromatid exchange (SCE). SCEs are detected in chromosomes that have been treated in such a way that the two sister chromatids of a chromosome differ chemically and thus stain differently. Most chemical mutagens induce SCEs at concentrations lower by a factor of about 100 than those needed to produce significant yields of ordinary chromosomal aberrations. The major exception to this is the small group of chemicals that, like x rays, produce double strand breaks in DNA and induce aberrations at all stages of the cell cycle.

The usual technique by which sister chromatids are made to stain differently from one another is to grow cells for two rounds of DNA replication in the presence of a thymidine analogue, such as BrdUrd. Because of the semiconservative replication of DNA, after two rounds of replication a chromosome will have one chromatid in which the DNA has only one polynucleotide strand substituted with BrdUrd and another in which both polynucleotide strands are so substituted. If such cells are treated with agents that lead to long-lived lesions that will be present during chromosomal replication when the cell is in the S phase, exchanges will occur between the two daughter chromatids. These will be viewed in the chromosomes as switches in the intensity of stain between one chromatid and its sister chromatid.[230][501]

Like other cytogenetic tests, SCE tests can be performed on cells treated in culture or in vivo. For the in vivo method, cells from treated animals can be excised and cultured in vitro in the presence of BrdUrd or the animal itself can be given an injection or infusion of BrdUrd so that SCE can be observed in bone marrow or spermatogonial cells directly. The latter method is one of the simplest and least expensive ways to observe the effects of chemicals in gonads. The test is not limited to mammalian cells, but has been successfully carried out in plants, insects, and fish.

The SCE test requires a metabolic activation system in vitro. In addition, chemicals administered in the G_1 phase that lead to negative results must be retested during the S phase, to ensure that the negative response was not merely an indication that repair had removed lesions before the cells entered the S phase. However, with most chemical agents this is not a problem, because the lesions leading to SCEs are often long-lived. Another disadvantage is that the precise correlation between the amount of SCE and mutational damage that is heritable is not known.

Although the basic mechanism of SCE formation is obscure, the SCE test shows that a chemical attacks chromosomes, affects their replication, or both. Most chemicals that induce SCEs produce a spectrum of lesions in DNA itself. Some of these lesions lead to SCE, and some lead to mutation. The proportions of the different types of lesion and the relative numbers of SCEs and mutations may differ for each chemical.

The SCE test is easy to perform, easy to score, and very sensitive. It has shown that SCEs are induced by the classes of compounds that induce mutations in the Salmonella/-microsome test[276] and by compounds, such as saccharin[503] and diethylstilbestrol,[160][374] that do not.

PLANT SYSTEMS IN GENETIC TOXICOLOGY

There is extensive information on the effects of chemicals on the genetic systems of vascular plants. Genetic studies cover both cytogenetic effects and gene mutations, include data on more than 100 plant species, and span the history of chemical mutagenesis. In fact, one of the earliest reports of mutagenic effects of chemicals was on the induction of chromosomal aberrations in plants.[328] Since then, several hundred chemical and physical mutagens have been studied in plants.

Plant systems do not occupy a prominent position in genetic toxicology. However, they continue to be used in basic mutation research; a wide array of induced genetic end points--including gene mutations,[353] chromosomal aberrations,[143] aneuploidy and polyploidy,[143] mitotic recombination,[16] and paramutation[22]--can be studied in plants.[109 143 323] Moreover, a few systems offer particular advantages for application in genetic toxicology. Specifically, some plant systems appear to be very sensitive to airborne and gaseous mutagens, to be suitable for use as in situ monitors for mutagens in the environment, and to permit studies of the role of plant metabolism in the conversion of promutagens to mutagens.

Five plant systems or types of study have been selected for coverage in this report: plant cytogenetic analysis, chlorophyll mutations, the Tradescantia stamen hair test, the maize waxy locus system, and plant metabolic activation systems. Descriptions of other plant systems may be found in the proceedings of workshops on the use of higher plants as monitors for environmental mutagens[94] and on the use of pollen systems to detect biologic activity of environmental pollutants.[71]

Cytogenetic methods with plant root tips[206]--especially those of Vicia, Allium, and Hordeum--were widely used in the 1950s and 1960s to study the effects of chemicals on chromosomal structure and have played an important part in the development of cytogenetic tests in genetic toxicology. Many chromosomal alterations can be detected in plants,[143] and, in addition to studies of mitotic cells, methods using microsporocytes (i.e., pollen mother cells) have permitted the study of meiotic cells.[263] Although basic research in plant cytogenetics continues, cytogenetic tests in plants have been replaced to some extent in genetic toxicology by mammalian cell-culture tests and tests in whole mammals.

The decrease in the use of plant cytogenetic tests does not mean that there are no instances where plant cyto-

genetics can make contributions in genetic toxicology. It
is reasonable to suggest that there is value in monitoring
for chromosomal aberrations[143][264] or micronuclei,[263][264]
as well as for gene mutations, in plants grown in particular
environments.

Although most in situ monitoring with plants occurs in
controlled environments, it has also been proposed that
measurements of frequencies of chromosomal aberrations in
wild populations can be useful in mutational monitoring.[209-212][461] For example, populations of Osmunda regalis
(royal fern) near a river polluted with industrial wastes
have higher frequencies of chromosomal aberrations than
populations in a less polluted site.[210] However, more
developmental work is required before the monitoring of
natural plant populations can be assessed adequately,
particularly because appropriate control populations are
difficult to identify and more general cytogenetic information
is needed on natural populations.

The detection of mutants that have deficiencies in
chlorophyll synthesis is a method that has been used for
many years in plant-mutation research. The method involves
many genetic loci, because chlorophyll-deficient mutants
can arise by mutation in structural genes that correspond
to several steps in chlorophyll synthesis, as well as in
regulatory genes.[484] Chlorophyll mutations have been
studied in many plants, of which barley[109][287] and
Arabidopsis[109][364] have been used most extensively. Work
with chlorophyll mutations has made many contributions to
mutation research in the elucidation of the mode of action
of alkylating agents,[109] of interactions among mutagens,[286]
and of mutagen specificity.[31][512] The detection of chlorophyll
mutations, however, is used less commonly for mutagen
testing today than might have been anticipated a few years
ago.

A test involving chlorophyll mutations that is currently
finding some use is based on the yellow green-2 ($yg_2$2)
locus in maize.[69][70] Plants that are heterozygous for yg_2
have green leaves. Although only ionizing radiation and
about six chemicals have been studied in the yg_2 system,[355]
the method warrants further study. Also suggested for the
application of chlorophyll mutations in genetic toxicology
is the detection of yellow and dark-green twin spots in a
yellow-green strain of the soybean, Glycine max. The twin
spots, which are inducible by mutagens, are interpreted as
an indication of mitotic recombination.[16][481]

In addition to chlorophyll mutations, other morphologic
and physiologic characteristics have been used in mutational
studies in plants.[70][109] Two characteristics that have

been investigated extensively are stamen-hair color in Tradescantia[466] and the nature of the starch in pollen grains in maize.[109 353]

The stamen-hair test in Tradescantia[113 466] is a specific-locus test in which mutations are detected by changes in the color of cells in the stamen hairs of plants of clone 02 and 4430, which are heterozygous for flower color. The inflorescence, which contains the plant's reproductive organs, is determinate and composed of 18-20 flower buds in various stages of development. In each bud there are six stamens, each of which contains about 50 hairs when mature. The color of the stamen hairs corresponds to flower color, with blue being dominant and pink recessive. In the Tradescantia test, many cuttings with inflorescences are exposed to aqueous or gaseous mutagens. A treatment sample of 300 cuttings will yield enough data to resolve as little as a 10% increase in mutations to pink over the background frequency. The mutation rate is calculated as the number of mutants per stamen hair and can be converted to the number of mutations per meristematic cell.[466] Advantages of the Tradescantia stamen-hair system are that the scoring of mutants is straightforward, that it is sensitive to low doses of radiation and gaseous chemical mutagens,[179 390] and that it is relatively inexpensive, with results available in less than 2 wk. It is suitable for detecting mutagens in the ambient atmosphere,[179 390] and a mobile laboratory has been designed for atmospheric monitoring with Tradescantia in sites throughout the United States.[390] Disadvantages of the stamen-hair system are that mutation scoring must be carried out sequentially over several days immediately after treatment, that large numbers of stamen hairs must be collected and scored each day when the method is used to test for mutagens at low concentrations, and that the system does not distinguish between gene mutations and chromosomal mutations.

Another test that shows promise for in situ use is that based on the maize waxy locus,[109 252 353 355] which determines the presence or absence of amylose in pollen grains. Pollen grains that contain the dominant allele Wx are referred to as "starchy"; they contain starch composed of amylopectin and amylose and stain black with iodine. Pollen grains that contain the recessive allele wx are referred to as "waxy" and do not stain black with iodine, because their starch contains only amylopectin.[355] Forward mutations at the waxy locus can be detected by screening for reddish waxy pollen grains among the black starchy pollen grains stained with iodine. Fortunately, nonviable pollen grains are not confused with mutants, because aborted pollen grains have a distinctive collapsed appearance (Plewa and Wagner[355] and Plewa, personal communication, 1981). Nevertheless, that some reddish pollen grains are not actual <u>wx</u> mutants cannot be disregarded and constitutes one of the limitations of the assay.[127] Besides detecting reddish forward mutants, one may also screen for black starchy revertants among the pollen grains produced by strains of maize that are homoallelic waxy mutants. As in the forward-mutation test, the possibility of phenocopies (nonhereditary changes caused by environmental factors that mimic genetic changes) must also be considered when interpreting results in tests for reversion.[127] Whether the pollen grain has the starchy or waxy phenotype is determined by the genotype of the haploid pollen grain, not by that of the diploid parent plant. Thus, each pollen grain scored in the waxy locus test is a separate individual, and the method permits the straightforward screening of a large population.[353] Obviously, in conducting this test, care must be taken to avoid contaminant pollen from other plants that could be erroneously scored as mutants. Although the waxy test has been used most extensively in corn, waxy mutants can also be studied in other cereals.[9 127 162 322] The waxy locus test in corn typically takes about 6 mo to conduct and analyze under field conditions. However, efforts are being made to refine the test so that it can be conducted under greenhouse or laboratory conditions in less than 10 wk;[355] reducing the time required to perform the waxy locus test involves the use of inbred Early-Early synthetic strains of corn that reach anthesis about 4 wk after planting.[355]

Besides serving as in situ monitoring systems, plants are potentially valuable in environmental mutagenesis, because they can metabolically activate some compounds. In addition to plant activation of promutagens, such as dimethylnitrosamine,[16] that are also activated in mammalian metabolism, the possibility of unique abilities of plants to activate some substances warrants attention. For example, interest in metabolism of promutagens by plants was stimulated by the evidence[140 354] that maize can activate the nonmutagenic herbicide atrazine and some related compounds to substances that are detectable as mutagens in microbial tests. Atrazine was also mutagenic in the waxy locus test in the maize plants themselves.[354]

The environmental implication of the results with atrazine is that application of herbicides, which are widely used in corn agriculture, can lead to mutagenic plant metabolites in crops. More generally, this result suggested that, like mammalian metabolism of promutagens, plant metabolism can be important for human health and that protection of the public from exposure to genotoxic substances requires consideration of possible mutagens that are not produced in mammalian metabolism, but that can be metabolically produced in crop plants. Two approaches for dealing with this problem are the use of genetic toxicology assays in plants and the incorporation of plant metabolic activation into assays with bacteria or other organisms.[140][353][354] In the latter case, plant metabolic activation can be provided by treating the indicator organism with a tissue homogenate from plants that were exposed to the suspected mutagen[140][353] or treating the indicator organisms with a homogenate from unexposed plants with the test chemical and cofactors,[353] in the same manner as with a mammalian liver S-9 metabolic activation system.

MUTAGENICITY TESTING IN DROSOPHILA

Drosophila breeding techniques for detecting physical and chemical mutagens have been used for over 50 yr. H. J. Muller initiated both the mutagenesis work and the development of genetic strains for the rapid and easy detection of mutations, chromosomal rearrangements, and aneuploidy. The reader is referred to several detailed reviews of the many testing procedures available.[5][295][508]

The major advantages in using Drosophila as a test system for environmental mutagens are that it is a sexually reproducing eukaryotic organism with male and female germ cell stages equivalent to those found in mammals, with a generation time of about 12 d and production of hundreds of offspring by a single pair of parents, and that more is known about the genetics of Drosophila than of any other higher eukaryote. Drosophila geneticists have constructed a wide array of tester stocks that detect all classes of gene and chromosomal mutations that are also likely to occur in man. Drosophila has a very active mixed-function oxidase system that is comparable with that of the rat.

THE SEX-LINKED RECESSIVE-LETHAL TEST

The sex-linked recessive-lethal test is the most widely applied test for mutation in Drosophila. It has proved to be sufficiently sensitive to mutagenic activity of chemicals, many of which exert only weak activity at the concentrations used. The test can routinely demonstrate a doubling of the spontaneous-mutation rate. The X-linked recessive-lethal test includes a variety of genetic end points: intragenic changes, small deletions, and chromosomal aberrations that are lethal. It is estimated that any of about 800 genes (of the 1,000) on the X chromosome are subject to lethal mutation.[6] Both direct-acting mutagens and those requiring metabolic activation (promutagens) are detected by this genetic test.[482] Promutagens, however, are most effectively detected in early spermatids, rather than in mature sperm. The breeding procedures of exposed parents are sufficient to ensure the sampling of any desired germ cell stage.

The test (Figure 5-1) is usually performed by treating wild-type males of a standard laboratory stock. When females are the treated parents, particular care must be taken to avoid the accumulation of preexisting lethals. The treatment may be applied to embryos, larvae, or adults by feeding, injection, or inhalation. The males are mated to a tester strain of females. The tester line carries a series of dominant and recessive X-linked genetic markers

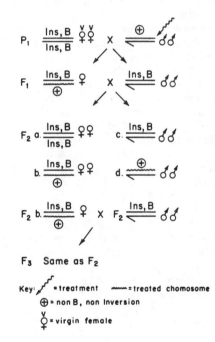

FIGURE 5-1 Diagram of the sex-linked recessive lethal test when the parental male is treated. F_1 cultures that fail to produce male progeny of class (d) are scored as lethal-bearing cultures. Reprinted with permission from Abrahamson and Lewis.[5]

and a complex set of X-chromosome inversions that prevent crossing-over with the treated homologue. The matings are preferably performed as a single pair in order to record induced and spontaneous clusters of identical mutations, but mass matings of 20-30 parents per culture are also used.

The F_1 females from this mating are individually mated with several sibling males (or males of equivalent genotype). Because the F_1 females carry both a treated X chromosome and the tester X chromosome with recognizable genetic markers, two distinct classes of F_2 males are normally expected--wild-type and mutant tester males.

The sex-linked recessive-lethal test is a highly objective scoring procedure with minimal observer bias. Scoring of a few thousand F_2 cultures per day by an adequately trained technician is routine.

A control experiment with untreated males is performed simultaneously. For specific stocks, well-established spontaneous-lethal frequencies exist; thus, on the basis of historical control values (usually 0.1-0.2% lethals) and a small-scale simultaneous control, it should be possible to decide whether the exposure was mutagenic. About 7,000 F_2 cultures are required to determine whether the spontaneous rate was at least doubled by the treatment. Obviously, fewer tests are needed for mutagens that induce very large mutation rates. If a significant increase in recessive-lethal frequency has not been observed in 7,000 tests of the treated group, the treatment is considered to be negative. Finally, it should be stressed that, with 800 different test genes distributed over the X chromosome, unique DNA-mutagen specificities should be detectable.

Several academic laboratories now routinely screen 20-30 unknown compounds per year. The cost of such a nonprofit testing service is about $7,000-8,000 per compound for testing postmeiotic male germ cells at one exposure with the degree of sensitivity described above.

It may be possible to increase the sensitivity of testing considerably and thereby decrease the number of tests and the corresponding cost by using repair-deficient mutant strains. Several laboratories are engaged in validating these systems for the sex-linked recessive-lethal test.

CHROMOSOMAL-ABERRATION GENOMIC-MUTATION TESTS

Valencia et al.[477] analyzed published reports of mutagens that induced reciprocal translocations, partial chromosomal loss as a result of very large deletions, and complete chromosomal loss or gain that resulted in recognized aneuploidy.

Sixty compounds were tested for their ability to induce reciprocal translocations in male germ cells: 26 were classified as positive, 8 as negative, and 26 as inconclusively tested. There were 76 compounds reported in tests for chromosomal breakage involving partial chromosome loss: 27 were classified as positive, 13 as negative, and 36 as inconclusive. Many of these studies involved less sensitive test systems than are now available and were done at a time when screening was not the objective of the experiment.

Nondisjunction studies, designated as involving the production of additional chromosomes (disomic gametes), involved classifying 44 compounds: 15 as positive, 15 as negative, and 14 as inconclusive. Again, screening was not the objective of the work in many cases, and the criterion was more stringent than that used previously.

Cytologic procedures are usually used to detect this array of chromosomal and genomic mutation. Although this is possible in Drosophila, the detection techniques are generally genetic. By the use of appropriate genetic markers in the tester strain, each of the above kinds of change becomes phenotypically recognizable either among the classes of exceptional progeny or as a result of abnormal segregation ratios. Cytologic analysis of these phenotypic exceptions has confirmed the genetically determined abnormality. Thus, these detection systems permit the rapid screening of tens of thousands of progeny or thousands of culture vials (as in the sex-linked recessive-lethal test) for specific abnormalities.

Until recently, the sensitivity of chromosomal-aberration tests for detecting mutagens was considerably lower than that of the recessive-lethal system. Thus, many mutagens that substantially increased lethal frequency were often denoted as poor clastogens (chromosome-breaking agents), whereas the reverse was not the case.

Reciprocal-Translocation Tests

Reciprocal translocation results from the interchange of nonhomologous chromosomal segments, which leads to a disruption of the random assortment of nonhomologues in meiosis. A translocation requires two generations of matings to detect. In practice, exchanges between the two large autosomes (chromosomes II and III) are detected most commonly, whereas those involving the Y chromosome and either or both of the major autosomes are somewhat less common.

After exposure, wild-type males are mated to a tester strain of females whose X chromosomes and autosomes contain appropriate genetic markers in homozygous condition. The F_1 male progeny are singly mated with several females genetically identical with their mothers. The resulting back-cross progeny are examined for the presence of specific phenotypic classes. In the absence of an induced translocation, there are eight classes of progeny present (sex is included as a phenotype). If a translocation was induced, only four or fewer classes of back-cross progeny are usually observed. The specific phenotypes of the surviving progeny denote which type of translocation was present. Confirmatory matings can be carried out, because wild-type male progeny continue to carry the identical translocation transmitted by their F_1 male parent. Only a small number of control matings are necessary, if any, because the spontaneous frequency of reciprocal translocation is very low (0.0001 or less in standard wild-type laboratory stocks). Thus, the finding of four or five independent translocation cultures in samples of several thousand cultures or fewer is adequate evidence of mutagenicity. The mutagenic potential of many mutagens that induce translocations in mature sperm is increased if the treated sperm are stored in the female 10 d or more before fertilization. The translocation frequency of stored sperm is often 10 or more times greater than that of unstored sperm. The spontaneous frequency of reciprocal translocations may also be increased by storage.

F_1 Tests

Most workers prefer to use simpler, less laborious tests to detect induced chromosomal aberrations. Descriptions of three simple single-generation tests follow.

Sex-Chromosome Loss. The most common test can be incorporated into the sex-linked recessive-lethal test or run independently. Breakage of the X or Y chromosome in sperm can lead to complete loss of either of these chromosomes in the fertilized egg or to deletions of major parts of these chromosomes (Figure 5-2). Male X chromosomes carry the recessive body-color gene, yellow ($\underline{y}$), and are usually ring-shaped, rather than rod-shaped. The Y chromosome contains, in addition, the translocated tip of the X with the wild-type, grey allele of yellow ($\underline{y}^+$) on one arm; the other arm of the Y is marked with the dominant eye-shape

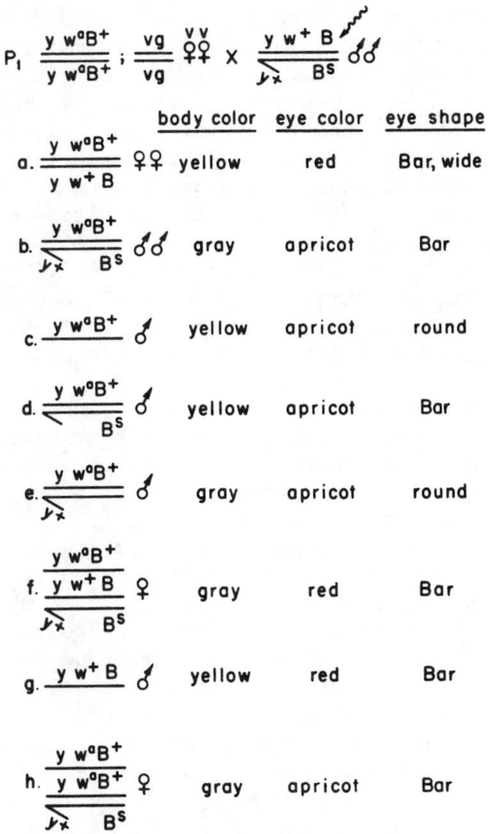

$$P_1 \quad \frac{y\ w^a B^+}{y\ w^a B^+} \ ; \ \frac{vg}{vg} \ \substack{v\ v \\ \text{♀♀}} \quad \times \quad \frac{y\ w^+\ B}{y_x} \ \frac{}{B^s} \ \text{♂♂}$$

	body color	eye color	eye shape
a. $\dfrac{y\ w^a B^+}{y\ w^+\ B}$ ♀♀	yellow	red	Bar, wide
b. $\dfrac{y\ w^a B^+}{y_x \quad B^s}$ ♂♂	gray	apricot	Bar
c. $\dfrac{y\ w^a B^+}{\quad}$ ♂	yellow	apricot	round
d. $\dfrac{y\ w^a B^+}{\quad B^s}$ ♂	yellow	apricot	Bar
e. $\dfrac{y\ w^a B^+}{y_x}$ ♂	gray	apricot	round
f. $\dfrac{\dfrac{y\ w^a B^+}{y\ w^+\ B}}{y_x \quad B^s}$ ♀	gray	red	Bar
g. $\dfrac{y\ w^+\ B}{\quad}$ ♂	yellow	red	Bar
h. $\dfrac{\dfrac{y\ w^a B^+}{y\ w^a B^+}}{y_x \quad B^s}$ ♀	gray	apricot	Bar

FIGURE 5-2 Diagram of a chromosome-loss test for the sex chromosomes when the male is the treated parent. The regular progeny are shown as classes (a) and (b). Class (c) is a presumptive loss of either the X or Y chromosome, but a portion of such a sex chromosome lacking marker mutants may still remain. Classes (d) and (e) represent loss of the y^+ and B^s marked regions, respectively, of the Y chromosome. Class (f) is a rare class and arises from nondisjunction of the X and Y chromosome in the parental male. Classes (g) and (h) are rare classes that arise from primary nondisjunction of the X chromosomes in the parental female. Reprinted with permission from Abrahamson and Lewis.[5]

mutant Bar-Stone (B^S), which also is derived from an X-chromosome rearrangement. Such males are mated to females that are homozygous yellow. The expected F_1 progeny are yellow females and grey, Bar-eyed males. If the X or Y chromosome is lost in the fertilized egg, yellow-bodied non-Bar-eyed sons are recovered. If a deletion occurs that includes either the $\underline{y}^+$ gene on the one arm of the Y or the $\underline{B}^S$ gene on the other arm, the resulting exceptional yellow Bar or grey non-Bar male progeny are recovered. These exceptional types are readily detected. Because each fly in this experiment is a test of the mutational event, very large numbers of flies can be counted in a short time to determine the potential mutagenicity of a compound.

Zimmering and Kammermeyer[514] markedly increased the sensitivity of this test, so chemicals that heretofore were deemed to be incapable of breaking chromosomes now appear to be very active. Zimmering has incorporated the X-linked recessive mutant meiotic[9a] (mei[9a]) into the female tester line. This mutant is defective in excision repair; thus, damaged chromosomes introduced by sperm into mei[9a] eggs are repaired less efficiently than when introduced into eggs of normal females. In addition to increased frequencies of aberrant offspring, Zimmering has shown that marked changes occur in the sex ratio of the progeny of these matings. Sex ratio is only trivially altered when repair-competent females are mated to exposed males. The ratio of F_1 females to males is very nearly 1 when repair-competent females are used. In the repair-defective environment, chromosomal damage induced by weak mutagens or by low concentrations of strong mutagens results in sex-ratio shifts from 1.0 to 0.7-0.5. These sex-ratio shifts are produced by the death of eggs fertilized by sperm that have a damaged ring-X chromosome. Two suspected mechanisms may cause this death. The first is that the broken ring X produces dicentric chromosomes that disrupt mitotic divisions if repair does occur. The second suggests that SCEs are produced in the mei[9] cytoplasm; that leads to the formation of giant dicentric rings, with similar consequences. If the latter mechanism can be demonstrated, it will provide evidence that SCEs can have serious genetic consequences under appropriate conditions.

Because the use of repair-defective mutants in mutation screening experiments is relatively recent, their deployment to other test systems in Drosophila may profoundly influence the sensitivity and costs of such systems.[507]

The Bithorax Test. The bithorax test[248] detects chromosomal rearrangements that involve about 10% of the genome. One break must be within a specific salivary-band region of chromosome III, whereas a second break may be in any part of the remaining genome. When associated with the appropriate genetic breeding scheme, such rearrangements are identified by a wide band of abnormal tissue between the fly's thorax and abdomen. Again, each F_1 fly is a test. Although not all reciprocal translocations are detected, the sensitivity is very great, because many flies can be readily examined (electronic counting devices may reduce the work effort considerably). In addition, cytologic analyses of the abnormal F_1 lines detected both reciprocal translocation and inversions. Treatment may be performed on either sex. DeJongh[87] observed that induced translocations were recovered more frequently than inversions from postmeiotic germ cells, whereas the reverse occurred in premeiotic germ cells. The observation indicates that meiosis leads to selection against translocations while not affecting the segregation of inversion chromosomes.

Half-translocations. Muller and Herskowitz[294] and Parker[340] independently have used attached-X female stocks that detect detachments of the attached-X chromosome. The majority of these detachments were due to translocations between the X chromosome and chromosome 4 when no Y was present in the female. Only half the reciprocal translocation was recovered in a viable fly. Gross deletion of one of the attached-X chromosomes accounts for the remaining exceptional types. The experiment is useful in detecting breakage in oocytes and oogonial germ cells. The most mature oocytes are generally the most sensitive indicators of chromosomal breakage in the female. It should be noted that reciprocal translocations are not readily detectable in oocytes, because meiosis (which is completed after fertilization) usually results in loss of the reciprocal products and death of the zygote--a problem that is not encountered when postmeiotic germ cell stages of the male are treated.

NONDISJUNCTION TESTS

The nondisjunction test developed by Craymer[75] involves an X:Y translocation stock that is mated to a standard female line with appropriate genetic markers.

After normal chromosomal disjunction in the parental stocks, all zygotes receive aneuploid sex chromosomes and a normal euploid maternal complement; as a result of this genetic imbalance, they die before eclosion. Different phenotypic classes of exceptional progeny routinely are recovered from nondisjunction in the female, gross deletion of the paternal X:Y chromosome, complete loss of the XY chromosome, and primary nondisjunction in the paternal male. Thus, only exceptional progeny develop. The total number of zygotes produced can be estimated. Hundreds of thousands of gametes are under test, but only a minority (the exceptional types) are viable. The system has been used by Foureman[125] to study radiation and ethyl methanesulfonate-induced damage in males and is being used as a screen for other potential nondisjunction-inducing chemicals.

Traut[463] has developed a test that permits the recovery of aneuploids induced in females. Like that of Craymer, this test is extraordinarily sensitive, because only the abnormal progeny, the aneuploids, survive; the normal progeny do not. In addition to detecting sex-chromosome nondisjunction, Traut's scheme also detects chromosome II aneuploids. The untreated male strain with its marked X and Y chromosomes contains (in place of a normal chromosome II) the isochromosomes 2L and 2R. Segregation products of these chromosomes will lead to nonviable zygotes when normal female oocytes have been fertilized; however, if nondisjunction (or an isochromosomal rearrangement) occurs in the oocyte, two complementary unbalanced gametes can produce a chromosomally balanced zygote—two biologic wrongs correct each other. Traut calculated that the spontaneous frequency of aneuploidy is 2×10^{-4}, on the basis of 3.2×10^6 individuals theoretically produced but not counted.

MAMMALIAN TESTS

As is apparent from the earlier part of this chapter, there is no shortage of tests to determine whether a given chemical can induce mutation. Yet, even if a chemical is found to be mutagenic in some tests, the ability to predict human mutation and possible genetic damage remains undeveloped. Data collected on humans by population monitoring perhaps could identify a potent mutagen, if the complexities of poorly controlled exposure and many possible confounding variables could be overcome; however, chemicals discovered to be harmful directly in humans would probably have inflicted great damage on many persons before their danger was discovered. Mammalian tests for mutagenicity provide a way of doing controlled in vivo experimentation in the same phylogenetic infraclass (Eutheria) as humans and thereby greatly reduce the amount of interspecies extrapolation necessary in making predictions about human genetic risk from a chemical.

An understanding of gametogenesis in the mouse is of great importance in interpreting the results of mutation experiments. Some germ cell stages are more sensitive to genetic damage than others, and the relative sensitivity varies markedly with the mutagen. Stages of long duration are more relevant to genetic-risk estimation than more transient stages, unless the latter are extremely susceptible.

The stem cells in male mice first appear 3 d after birth. Testes of adult mice contain germ cells in many different stages of development, ranging from stem-cell spermatogonia to mature spermatozoa. It has long been known that, if male mice receive a high exposure to many chemicals or radiation, they often become sterile after a few weeks, but then regain fertility. The length of the sterile period depends on the chemical and the extent of exposure to it. The reason for this delayed transitory sterility is that some types of differentiating germ cells are easily killed by the chemical (or radiation). In the case of radiation, the most resistant cells are spermatozoa, spermatids, and secondary spermatocytes,[327] which are at the end of the sequence of differentiation, and stem cells, which are at the beginning.[326] Usually, when a sterile period occurs, mice are fertile until the maturing germ cells have survived treatment, and sterility persists until the stem cells are replenished and more spermatozoa develop.

The duration of various stages of spermatogenesis in the mouse has been of great value in interpreting mutation experiments. Offspring sired more than 7 wk after exposure[377] and for the entire remaining reproductive life span of the male are derived from treated spermatogonial stem cells. For estimates of genetic risk in the male, stem-cell spermatogonia are very important. Other germ cell stages of adult male mice persist for only a few weeks. By persisting so much longer, stem-cell spermatogonia can accumulate a much larger dose when the dose rate is low. Male gametogenesis in rodents is believed to be roughly equivalent to that in man, although, of course, the time scale is much longer in man.

There are no reproductive stem cells in female mice. All primary oocytes are already present about a week before birth. Many of these remain in an arrested diplotene stage of meiosis for many months before ovulation or loss by atresia. Stages of primary oocyte development are defined by the cytologic appearance of the oocyte and its follicle.

Because the germ cell stage of longest duration in the female mouse and human is the arrested diplotene oocyte, this might appear to be the stage of maximal hazard in risk estimation. However, of the few chemicals (all of which are mutagenic in screening tests) that have been tested for mutagenic effect at this stage, none has yielded a significant increase over the spontaneous-mutation rate. This stage has also shown no mutagenic effect of radiation. So it remains possible that other germ cell stages in the female, despite relatively short duration, might nevertheless produce more mutations; and these stages have not yet been adequately tested.

Tests for mutagenicity are often divided into those for gene mutation and those for gross chromosomal aberration (that is, structural changes in the chromosomes that can be seen with a microscope). Likewise, mammalian tests can be divided into those which measure the frequency of mutations in only a small part of the genome (for example, at a few genetic loci) and those which measure the frequency in the whole genome. Some tests focus on mutations merely as events to be counted in making quantitative comparisons; others focus on the total damage caused by mutations in some part of the body, with the result that mutation frequencies are expressed per genome. All tests measure forward mutations, and, unless otherwise noted, all use the laboratory mouse, which is genetically the best understood experimental mammal.

SPECIFIC-LOCUS TEST

This method is the most extensively used for detecting the induction of gene mutations and multilocus deficiencies at specific genetic sites. Although several mammalian tests could be described as specific-locus tests, the designation is used here to refer specifically to the seven-locus form of the test developed by Russell.[382] In this test, each mouse that is exposed to the test agent has the normal allele for both genes at each of seven specific loci scattered throughout the genome. The exposed animals are mated to test-stock mice that are homozygous for a recessive mutation at each of the seven loci. When a mutation occurs at one of these loci in the treated germ cells, the resulting offspring manifest an easily recognized mutant phenotype. Such a presumed mutant is bred. Mutant stocks are usually set up for later analysis. Six of the mutations are detected by specific changes in coat color, the other by an extreme reduction in size of external ear. Mutations at some of the loci often have associated dominant effects, such as a marked reduction in body size.

Because mutations can be noticed so easily with this technique, the large samples of offspring that are often required to draw conclusions can be examined quickly. An additional advantage is that two of the genetic loci are tightly linked, with a recombination frequency of only 0.16%.[375] This provides a way of determining which treatments induce large multilocus deficiencies. Important merits of the specific-locus method include the ease of examining individual offspring, the existence of extensive experimental data for comparison, and the existence of massive historical control (801,406 offspring tested in the male and 204,639 offspring tested in the female). The historical control in the male is based on data collected in three laboratories.[377] Because the phenotypes are apparent, these mutations can readily be used in complementation studies (for example, L. B. Russell[375]) to learn more about the nature of the mutations and the genetic regions in which they occur.

The specific-locus method is particularly useful in making comparisons of the effects of dose, dose fractionation, sex, cell stage, and other factors on the mutational response in mammalian germ cells, as well as comparisons of the relative responses to different chemicals. Most of what is known about the induction of gene mutations and small deficiencies in germ cells of mammals by radiation and chemicals has been learned in such comparative studies.

Almost 30 chemicals have been studied with this test, and most of these were previously known to be mutagens (often potent) in at least some short-term tests. The samples tested are often large enough to exclude a high mutation frequency in spermatogonial stem cells; for nine chemicals, the induced-mutation frequency in these cells has been shown to be less than 4 times the historical control mutation frequency (at the 5% significance level). Therefore, these nine chemicals were considered negative in spermatogonial stem cells in this test by GENE-TOX criteria[377] (see also Table 6-2). It is, of course, possible that each of the nine chemicals induces mutations at an undetectably low frequency. Nonetheless, one possible interpretation of these data is that stem-cell spermatogonia are much more resistant to mutation induction than one might expect from results of short-term tests. Resistance could depend on the efficiency of detoxification and repair systems. Other interpretations of negative results are equally likely for some of the chemicals, and some of these are discussed in the GENE-TOX report on this test,[377] in Chapter 6, or in both.

A few chemicals have been found to induce specific-locus mutations in spermatogonial stem cells, and ethyl nitrosourea (ENU) is extremely effective. At the highest dose studied, an average of 1 of 141 offspring has a mutation at one of these loci[380]--this is 134 times the spontaneous-mutation frequency.

Although it is possible that chronic exposure reduces the mutation frequency, the low mutation frequencies found for chemicals other than ENU have made it difficult to test this question. One notable exception is procarbazine, with which the first demonstration was made of a fractionation effect in mice.[106] A pronounced fractionation effect has recently been demonstrated for ENU.[380][383] Ten fractions of 10 mg/kg administered at weekly intervals yielded only 13% as many mutations as a single injection of 100 mg/kg. The dose-response curve also suggests an accelerating curve (positive second derivative) at low doses. Furthermore, unscheduled-DNA-synthesis studies and ENU-binding studies show that the amount of ENU interacting with DNA in the testes is linearly related to acute dose over the range of 10-100 mg/kg. Regardless of the cause, a nonlinear dose response and a fractionation effect mean that one cannot extrapolate linearly from large, unfractionated doses. Rat data show that fractionated doses produce a phenomenon similar to that which occurs in E. coli, in which O^6-alkylguanine is rapidly removed, owing to the increase in an acceptor protein.[485]

ELECTROPHORETIC MUTATION TEST

A recently developed version of the specific-locus test detects electrophoretic protein variants at at least 21 loci.[194-196] It is based on early test-system development by Malling and Valcovic[270] and Soares.[424] A significant increase in the mutation frequency for ENU has been demonstrated with this test.[195] Two inbred strains of mice are used that differ at 10 loci whose protein products are electrophoretically demonstrable. In addition, mutations resulting in the loss of any of 11 other proteins common to the two strains can be detected. Males of either strain are exposed to the test substance, and, at the desired time after exposure, they are mated with females of the other strain. Later, all parental and F_1 animals are examined for the biochemical characters of interest. Gene products in red-cell lysates and kidney homogenates are analyzed with gel electrophoresis. Almost all F_1s survive the surgical procedures used to get samples and are thus available for further breeding analysis. Untreated control groups are examined in the same way.

The strain of origin can be identified for mutations involving the 10 demonstrable protein differences between the strains. It is not known how many genes are responsible

for the other group of 11 gene products, but it is thought
that the number is probably not much larger than 11.
Variants are tested for heritability; in most cases, this
is in effect a test of allelism, too.

Important merits of the electrophoretic mutation test
include the likelihood of eventually being able to determine
the molecular basis of many of the mutations. Moreover,
some of the same genes are being studied in human populations.[315] Three times as many loci are being screened as
in the specific-locus test, and this number will probably
increase. This larger number of loci compensates somewhat
for the much longer time required to observe each F_1
animal. Other methods of studying mutagenesis with
biochemical techniques have been applied to a limited
extent or are being developed. Technologic advances may
make such approaches more efficient.

DOMINANT-SKELETAL-MUTATION TEST

Because both the specific-locus test and the electrophoretic
mutation test deal with mutation in only a tiny portion of
the genome and their effects are difficult to relate to
first-generation genetic damage in humans, neither method
is useful in estimating absolute genetic risk (as opposed
to estimating relative risk with the doubling-dose approach).
Ehling[105] developed the dominant-skeletal-mutation test
and the dominant-cataract-mutation test,[221] which permit
risk estimates for first-generation genetic damage. Selby
and Selby[408 409] extended the skeletal-mutation work by
showing that the observed mutations are transmitted to the
next generation. Mice of one inbred strain are exposed to
a test substance and then mated to mice of another inbred
strain at the desired time after treatment. After F_1
offspring have produced their own offspring, the skeletons
of the F_1 offspring themselves are prepared for examination
by clearing and alizarin staining. If the skeleton of an
F_1 has abnormalities that are thought likely to result
from a dominant mutation, the skeletons of its offspring
are examined to see whether the effects have been transmitted.
Statistical comparisons can permit confirmation that a
mutation causes particular effects. The damage caused by
individual dominant skeletal mutations can be evaluated
with regard to whether similar damage in humans would
result in a serious handicap. To extrapolate from induced
dominant damage in one body system (the skeleton) to total
dominant damage, UNSCEAR[473] multiplied by 10 and the BEIR
III Committee[303] multiplied by 5-15 when they used such
data in estimating the genetic hazard to humans from

radiation. Other relevant information, such as the shape
of the dose-response curve, can be used to extrapolate
downward from the experimental dosage to human exposures.
When this was done for radiation, correction factors from
specific-locus experiments had to be used,[303] [473] because
they were not yet available for dominant skeletal mutations
themselves.

The general approach of studying dominant-skeletal-
mutation frequencies is of two forms, the one just described
being the breeding-test method. Although slow and tedious,
the breeding-test method yields an estimate of first-
generation genetic damage based on proven mutations and
produces a collection of mutants, some of which are useful
models of genetic disorders in humans. It seems likely
that the breeding-test method would be used only if a more
solid estimate of genetic risk were essential for a particular
test substance. A much quicker application of the dominant-
skeletal approach[407] forgoes the breeding test and concentrates
on detecting skeletal malformations, which on the basis of
earlier work[409-411] have a high probability of being
caused by dominant mutations. Conclusions are based on
presumed mutations, whose induced frequency is found by
subtracting the control frequency from the experimental
frequency.

Although the dominant-mutation frequency per locus is
probably extremely low,[399] the proportion of F_1 offspring
with a dominant skeletal mutation is much higher than the
proportion with a specific-locus mutation, because of the
presumably large number of genes at which mutations can
be detected. In comparison with the specific-locus test,
the much greater time required to observe each F_1 is to
some extent made up for by this higher frequency. Additional
merits of the sensitive-indicator approach are that it
deals with dominant mutations and that the damage seen can
be related quite easily to human disorders. Dominant
skeletal mutations represent a spectrum of events: gene
mutations, small deficiencies, and heritable translocations (at least 3 of 37 mutations).[408] (Skeletal
abnormalities are also frequently seen in human chromosomal
syndromes.)

CATARACT-MUTATION TEST

The rationale for studying the induction of dominant
cataract mutations in mice is the same as that for dominant
skeletal mutations. The test[108] [221] uses a breeding-test
method. Cataracts are observed in dilated eyes with a
slit lamp. The observation time for each mouse is much

less than that required for skeletal analysis. However, as would be expected if the phenotype is representative of a much smaller proportion of the genome, the frequency of induction is much lower; in fact, it is even lower than that of specific-locus mutations. Important merits of the cataract-mutation test are that it measures first-generation genetic damage and that it incorporates a breeding test, thereby eliminating nonmutant variants from consideration.

SPOT TEST

In comparison with the preceding mammalian tests, the mouse spot test[378] is rapid. It involves exposing embryos that are heterozygous for a number of coat-color markers to the chemical of interest and looking for spots of color in their otherwise black fur 3 wk later. (Embryos are exposed in pregnant animals.) With the exception of a few types of spots that are excluded because they may result from abnormal differentiation or cytotoxic effects, spots are thought to result from a broad spectrum of somatic mutations. These changes would have occurred at a time in each mouse when about 200 precursor pigment cells could have undergone mutation to result in a visible spot at the time of scoring. Because mutations at four loci (in the version of the test used most) can be detected in each cell, each mouse examined for spots represents about 800 loci tested.

Because the test is performed in vivo, metabolic conditions should parallel the human condition more closely than they would in either in vitro mammalian tests or nonmammalian tests. The spot test can detect intragenic mutations, small or large deficiencies, deletions of entire chromosomes (either from breakage or from nondisjunction), and somatic crossing-over.[378] Because germ cells are not tested and because some of the induced mutations detected in somatic cells would not be compatible with survival of offspring, had they occurred in germ cells, it is difficult to make quantitative risk estimates for genetic effects. The major role of this test is to screen substances to determine which ones may be potent mutagens in mammals. Potent chemicals in this test would then have high priority for being studied in germ-line mutagenesis tests. Comparison of the GENE-TOX reports for this test[378] and the specific-locus test[377] shows good agreement. Almost all chemicals positive in the spot test are positive either in stem-cell spermatogonia or in post-stem-cell stages or both. So far, no chemical has been negative in the spot test and positive in the specific-locus test. Because these tests monitor many of the same loci, quantitative comparisons of results are also possible. For almost all chemicals that are positive in both tests, the ratio of spot-test to specific-locus-test "unit" mutation rate (per locus per mole) is between 1 and 10.

GRANULOMA-POUCH ASSAY

Another relatively rapid in vivo test for somatic mutation is the granuloma-pouch assay.[268] Granulation tissue growth is initiated in rats on the inside of a subcutaneous air pouch by injecting croton oil. The rats are then exposed to the test substance. Two days after treatment, the animals are killed and the granulation tissue is dissociated enzymatically. Mutation frequencies are expressed as the frequencies of cells resistant to 6-thioguanine or ouabain. A comparison of the mutational responses after systemic and local administration of the test substance yields important knowledge about the formation and distribution of the proximate mutagen. As with the mouse spot test, the mutations are not germinal mutations. Few chemicals have been tested with this assay; three chemicals (benzo[a]pyrene, N-methyl-N'-nitro-N-nitrosoguanidine, and procarbazine) had positive results.[267,268]

DOMINANT-LETHAL TEST

This test[146] deals primarily with gross chromosomal damage. The dominant-lethal test is widely used and is usually performed on exposed males. Nongenetic maternal effects make it much more difficult to study induction of dominant lethality in females. Exposed male rats or mice are mated at weekly (or shorter) intervals to cover the span of spermatogenesis of interest. Females usually are killed for uterine examination around day 14, and the numbers of total implantations and fetal or embryonic deaths are recorded. The corpora lutea are also counted sometimes. The proportions can be analyzed statistically to see whether dominant lethality has been induced, and appropriate formulas are used in calculating the percentage of dominant lethality.[107,146]

Most dominant lethals probably result from multiple chromosomal breaks in the germ cells. Frequencies are typically much higher in postspermatogonial stages,[104] and often there are characteristic patterns of dominant lethality with regard to different stages of sperm development.[104] The results can be very useful in determining

whether mutagens reach the testes, because postspermatogonial stages are inside the blood-testis barrier. If
they respond to the mutagen, the stem-cell spermatogonia,
which are almost certainly outside the barrier,[415] surely
were exposed to the test substance. Dominant-lethal test
results can thus be helpful in interpreting negative
results in a specific-locus test. Dominant-lethal test
results are also important in deciding the degree of
chromosomal damage in some germ cell stages. Because
dominant lethal mutations cannot result in living offspring,
dominant lethals have a rather indirect bearing on estimates
of human genetic risk. Furthermore, the test suffers in
sensitivity, because of the normally high frequency of
spontaneous embryonic death. Thus, whereas a positive
result may be very significant, a negative one should not
be taken as very useful. Nonetheless, the ease of carrying
out the test leads to its frequent use.

If the dose-response curve and pharmacokinetics for a
given chemical were understood, dominant-lethal data might
prove useful in setting an upper limit on risk from gross
chromosomal effects, as has already been done for radiation.[303]
A recent major finding regarding the dominant-lethal test
is that the strain of the female to which the exposed male
is mated can markedly affect the results obtained with
some chemicals.[138] Use of some particular strains may
thus make the test more sensitive for identifying induced
chromosomal damage in postmeiotic male germ cells.

HERITABLE-TRANSLOCATION TEST

This test is usually much more sensitive, but considerably
more expensive and slower, than the dominant-lethal test,[134]
and it deals with a clearly defined type of mutation that
is transmitted to and scored in viable offspring. Males
are exposed to the test substance and mated to untreated
females. Male progeny (usually derived only from postspermatogonial treatments) are tested for translocations
by the fertility test or the cytogenetic test. In the
fertility test, males are tested, usually with a sequential
procedure, to determine fertility rates.[137] Animals
suspected of having a translocation (because of decreased
fertility) are then subjected to cytologic examination.
All F_1 males are examined in the cytogenetic translocation
test.[7] Most translocation carriers have characteristic
multivalent associations in diakinesis-metaphase I spermatocytes, which produce many unbalanced gametes because of
blockage in spermatogenesis.

Because the heritable-translocation test measures

transmissible mutations in postmeiotic cells, it may prove
useful in risk assessment for gross chromosomal aberrations.
Heritable translocations can cause morphologic damage in
carriers themselves,[20][187][408] and not just in offspring
of some of them, as had earlier been thought.[367] In view
of this, much more must be learned about the fraction of
heritable translocations that are also dominant mutations
causing morphologic damage. It should be noted that some
chemicals induce a high frequency of dominant lethals, but
only a very low frequency of heritable translocations.[139]

ANEUPLOIDY TESTS

Convenient methods[376] exist in the mouse for detecting
whole-chromosome aneuploidy, as determined by sex-chromosome
loss and nondisjunction. These methods are possible
because XO female mice and XXY male mice are viable.
Genetic markers are used that make it apparent from the
phenotype of offspring whether they are aneuploids.
Experiments can easily be designed to measure induction of
sex-chromosome loss or nondisjunction in either sex.

Some or all events leading to sex-chromosome loss or
nondisjunction are either not inducible in or not recoverable
from some of the germ cell stage.[376] However, very few
chemicals have been tested, and none in all germ cell
stages. Sex-chromosome loss has been shown to be induced
by triethylenemelamine in spermatids and spermatozoa,[55] by
isopropyl methanesulfonate in primary oocytes within 6 wk
of being ovulated,[136] and by hycanthone methanesulfonate
in primary oocytes within 1 wk of being ovulated.[384]

MICRONUCLEUS TEST

Several assays in mammals permit a determination of the
incidence of micronuclei;[393] of these, the only one
sufficiently developed to be a standard assay is the in
vivo mammalian bone marrow polychromatic-erythrocyte
assay.[155] Micronuclei are formed from chromosomes or
chromosomal fragments that are not incorporated into
daughter nuclei at the time of cell division. Thus, this
very rapid test serves as an in vivo somatic cell screening
test for finding genotoxic chemicals that might break
chromosomes or cause nondisjunction in germ cells. It has
been applied to more than 150 chemicals.[156]

SPERM-MORPHOLOGY TEST IN MICE

In the most common use of this test,[510] epididymal sperm of exposed mice are examined to determine the proportion of sperm with abnormally shaped heads. Scoring is rapid. As with some of the other tests described, however, the relationship of this end point to heritable mutation is unclear. It is even uncertain what relationship it has to somatic mutation. What is clear is that genotoxic agents are spermatotoxins. Positive correlations[510] between results of this test and results of some of the tests for heritable mutations suggest that many test substances found to be positive in the sperm-morphology test induce chromosomal aberrations, gene mutations, or both. The sperm-morphology test has also been adapted to several other mammals, including humans.

The role of this test is as a screening procedure that must be supported by some other tests when results are positive. Its biggest limitation is the uncertainty of whether the variants in sperm result from mutation. A few mutations have been induced that produce a high proportion of sperm abnormalities in F_1 sons. It is unlikely that fertilization with a malformed sperm constitutes an increased genetic hazard to the fertilized egg.[509]

GENOMIC MUTATIONS IN THE VOLE

The field vole, Microtus oeconomus, has X and Y chromosomes with unique patterns of heterochromatin, which means that they can easily be identified in spermatids. Thus, by simple microscopic examination of testes, spermatids with XX, XY, YY, or no sex chromosome can be identified (the latter with less certainty because a poorly stained cell can mimic one without sex chromosomes). Diploid spermatids can be identified not only on the basis of their two sex chromosomes, but also because they are large cells.

Tates[453] has reported that nondisjunction and diploid spermatids have been produced by MMS, p-fluorophenylalanine, vincristine, procarbazine, carbendazim, and bleomycin (in addition to radiation), but curiously not by colcimid, a well-known polyploidizing agent. If this system can be validated, its simplicity and low cost could make it a candidate for use in routine testing for genomic mutations.

OTHER TESTS

Two other tests that are being developed deserve brief mention, because of their potential for determining whether a test substance can induce gene mutations in mammalian germ cells. One is an immunologic technique for identifying biochemical mutations in sperm;[269] the other, it is hoped, will detect induced mutations at many loci that cause subtle changes in the dimensions of bones.[121] The first of these still requires proof that the presumed mutations occur in viable sperm. The second could be exceedingly useful, if it yields a much higher mutation frequency than can be obtained with other tests; but it is not known whether individual mutant mice can be identified reliably.

COMBINATIONS OF TESTS

There are many possible ways in which mammalian tests can be combined to yield more information per mouse. For example, if one is willing to decrease the rate at which offspring are evaluated in specific-locus tests, the same offspring can be observed for cataracts or other effects. The dominant-cataract-mutation test, in its present form, is done in this way.[221] Also, male parents used for dominant-lethal tests on postspermatogonial stages can be used for other tests on spermatogonia.

THE DATA BASE IN MUTAGENICITY TESTING

By any standards, the task of adequately testing all chemicals to which there may be substantial human exposure is formidable. Millions of chemical substances are known.[122] The U. N. Environment Program[467] has estimated that approximately 500,000 of these are in use, with about 10,000 produced in quantities of 500-1,000,000 kg per year. The number of chemicals in commercial use in the United States has been estimated at 70,000.[170] [273] According to Fishbein,[122] more than 25,000 of these are produced in large quantities, and 700-3,000 new chemicals are introduced each year. Despite considerable variation in the estimates of numbers of chemicals, it seems reasonable to assume that the U.S. population may be exposed to at least 50,000 chemicals.

Great variation exists both in production of chemicals of commerce and in their potential for important human exposure. Although one could suggest with some justification that chemicals produced in the largest quantities require the most thorough toxicity testing, considerable health effects can be associated with chemicals produced in small quantities (e.g., some drugs and food additives) and chemicals that occur primarily as natural substances (e.g., mycotoxins). Production volume is therefore only one factor that determines human exposure and possible toxic risk.

Just as there are difficulties in estimating numbers of chemicals to which people may be exposed, estimating numbers of chemicals that have been assayed for mutagenicity is not totally straightforward. One approach may be to compile a list of chemicals from the total literature that is cited in relevant computerized bibliographic information-retrieval systems. For example, the number of chemicals represented in all the literature holdings of the Environmental Mutagen Information Center (EMIC) can provide some indication of the extensiveness of the data base in mutagenicity testing. However, the value obtained in this way is subject to interpretation. Some tests may be unpublished or reported in literature that is not represented in the EMIC data base, which is incomplete for years before 1969; such tests would cause an underestimation of numbers of chemicals tested. Other factors suggest that a number based on the EMIC holdings actually may be an overestimate; for example, some of the chemicals represented in the EMIC files undoubtedly have been tested inadequately, and inclusion in the EMIC data base indicates only that a particular literature citation exists and that the chemical has been tested. On some of the chemicals, there may be no available data, as in the case of chemicals mentioned only in abstracts. Despite these limitations, the numbers of chemicals cited in the EMIC files provide an approximation of the genetic-toxicology data base.

There are 11,167 chemicals with Chemical Abstracts Service (CAS) registry numbers represented in the 35,000 citations that EMIC has cataloged since 1968 (EMIC, personal communication, 1981). This number is based on the literature for all genetic-toxicology tests, including tests for DNA damage, mutation, chromosomal aberration, and a variety of other effects on mitotic or meiotic mechanisms. Roughly 50-75 new CAS numbers are added to the EMIC file each month. In addition to the 11,167 chemical substances, the EMIC data base contains 2,500 chemical names that lack CAS registry numbers; some of these may be duplicates of the recognized chemicals. Overall, it seems fair to say that there is a genetic-toxicology literature for 11,500-14,000 chemicals.

A major effort to evaluate genetic-toxicology test systems and the associated data base has been undertaken by the U.S. Environmental Protection Agency through its GENE-TOX Program. In this Program, scientists experienced in the use of most of the major mutagenicity tests are evaluating the published literature on mutagenicity testing.

Through this evaluation, guidelines are being proposed to establish criteria for an adequate test in each of the major assays.

The number of chemicals that have been tested adequately by current standards is much smaller than the total number for which there is a genetic-toxicology literature. Although the work of the GENE-TOX panels is not complete, it seems likely that there are 2,500-3,000 unique chemicals that have been tested adequately in at least one assay according to GENE-TOX criteria (EMIC, personal communication, 1980). Most of the GENE-TOX assay-system work groups have already finished their literature evaluations. As of November 1980, 2,487 chemicals were listed as adequately tested. One assay system for which the evaluation of papers was still incomplete, however, was the Salmonella/-microsome test. It is anticipated that this assay will contribute 300-400 chemicals that have not been adequately tested in other assays. These data, heterogeneous and incomplete though they are, are useful in several ways. They provide information that is part of a regular test program, such as we suggest in Chapter 9. They can provide ancillary information useful for interpretation of doubtful or ambiguous results from regular test programs, and they may provide information that will enable the development of better test programs.

The distribution of the genetic-toxicology data base among assay systems is indicated in Table 5-4, which presents numbers of chemicals that have been tested in each assay and numbers of literature citations based on the literature holdings of EMIC and the classification of chemicals with respect to adequacy of tests by GENE-TOX criteria (EMIC, personal communication, 1980). It should perhaps be pointed out that the sum of the numbers presented in the table is not a useful indicator of the extent of testing. Some of the descriptors used for assays are not mutually exclusive, and the same test may be entered more than once. In addition, many chemicals have been tested in several different assays. Although they should not be summed, the individual numbers presented in Table 5-4 can be used to indicate the extent of the data base for a variety of important assay systems. Some spaces in the table are blank, because schemes used for classifying assays are not always parallel, and some of the numbers therefore are not readily retrievable from the computerized files. Obviously, information like that presented in Table 5-4 continually changes; the table is current as of the end of January 1981.

TABLE 5-4 Distribution of the Genetic-Toxicology Data Base among Assay Systems[a]

Organism/Assay	Chemicals Represented in EMIC Literature Holdings	Chemicals Adequately Tested by GENE-TOX Criteria	Literature Citations in EMIC Data Base (All Publications)	Literature Citations in EMIC Data Base (Publications with Original Data Only)
I. All genetic-toxicology tests	>11,200	>2,670	34,030	22,218
II. Classification by organism				
A. Bacteria	--	--	5,102	3,595
1. Bacillus subtilis:	822	--	384	274
Gene mutations	--	--	103	59
Repair--rec assay	--	--	73	30
2. E. coli	2,607	--	2,058	1,559
Gene mutations	--	~150	507	--
WP2/WP2uvrA	1,958	~120/150[b]	150/105	84/60
Repair:				
polA test	--	--	52	35
recA test	--	--	78	42
3. Salmonella typhimurium	3,280		2,117	1,195
Gene mutations				
Salmonella/microsome test (5 standard strains)	2,533	>724	1,430	884
Other (forward-mutation assays)	--	--	20	--
B. Fungi	--	--	2,104	1,407
1. Aspergillus	275	124[c]	161	111

TABLE 5-4 continued

Organism/Assay	Chemicals Represented in EMIC Literature Holdings	Chemicals Adequately Tested by GENE-TOX Criteria	Literature Citations in EMIC Data Base (All Publications)	Literature Citations in EMIC Data Base (Publications with Original Data Only)
2. Neurospora	195	166[c]	289	161
Gene mutations	--	102[c]	75	23
Forward mutation	--	--	--	--
Reversion	--	--	--	--
Nondisjunction	--	70[c]	13	7
3. Saccharomyces cerevisiae	908	443	958	611
Gene mutations	--	--	308	107
Mitotic crossing-over	--	--	112	29
Mitotic gene conversion	--	--	59	23
4. Schizosaccharomyces pombe	83	~58	144	84
C. Mammalian cell cultures	200—300	136	5,419	3,904
1. Chinese hamster cells	781	--	1,255	816
V-79 cells:	345	--	442	282
Gene mutations	191	184	259	168
Cytogenetic effects	--	--	85	56
CHO cells:	272	--	409	--
Gene mutations	49	18[c]	164	100
Cytogenetic effects	--	--	144	97
2. Human cells	1,562	51?	2,805	1,990
Lymphocytes/leukocytes	--	51?	1,151	892
3. Mouse cells	962	--	1,311	988
L5178Y lymphoma cells	231	48[c]	180	105
Other	--	--	1,131	883
4. Rat cells	503	--	425	335
5. Syrian golden hamster cells	314	--	252	194

D. Drosophila melanogaster	922	--	1,451	867
1. Sex-linked recessive lethals	646	388	708	444
2. Heritable translocations	32[d]	17[d];56[c]	125	81
3. Nondisjunction/sex-chromosome loss	--	66[c]	109/128	69/79
E. Vascular plants	--	354[c]	4,136	3,160
1. Allium--cytogenetic effects	--	--	483	427
Allium cepa only	--	144	326	286
2. Arabidopsis--gene mutation	--	78	169	82
3. Glycine	--	35	57	43
Gene mutations	--	--	45	--
Mitotic recombination	--	--	5	4
4. Hordeum	--	--	531	411
Gene mutations	15	20	--	--
Cytogenetic effects	61	61	--	--
5. Pisum	--	--	203	161
Pisum sativum only	254	--	143	115
6. Tradescantia	100	--	93	46
Gene mutations--stamen hair system	--	33	22	--
Cytogenetic effects	--	12	--	--
7. Vicia	--	--	493	483
Cytogenetic effects	--	83	--	--
8. Zea	156	22	187	129
Gene mutations	--	--	--	--
F. Mammals				
1. Chinese hamster	--	--	171	91

TABLE 5-4 continued

Organism/Assay	Chemicals Represented in EMIC Literature Holdings	Chemicals Adequately Tested by GENE-TOX Criteria	Literature Citations in EMIC Data Base (All Publications)	Literature Citations in EMIC Data Base (Publications with Original Data Only)
2. Mouse	2,036	--	2,480	1,646
a. Gene mutations--germ cells (specific-locus test)	--	25[c]	48	--
b. Gene mutations--somatic cells (spot test)	--	27	24	6
c. Cytogenetic effects--somatic cells	--	--	--	--
d. Cytogenetic effects--germ cells (excl. heritable translocations)	--	--	>91	>48
e. Cytogenetic effects--heritable-translocation test	32[c]	17[c]	89	72
f. Dominant lethals	--	--	502	245
g. Sperm abnormalities	--	152[c]	39	19
3. Rat	1,641	--	2,136	1,586
a. Dominant lethals	--	--	193	180
b. Sperm abnormalities	--	--	15	12
4. Syrian golden hamster	343	--	92	73
III. Classification by genetic end point				
A. DNA repair	--	--	861	503
1. Differential-killing assays--bacteria	--	611[c]	241	157
2. Unscheduled DNA synthesis	--	<244	309	169
3. Other	--	50	--	--

B. Gene mutations

1. Microbial tests	--	--	>1,839	>1,085
2. Mammalian cell cultures	--	--	>764	>408
3. Drosophila melanogaster	--	388	>1,006	>626
4. Plants	--	349	>127	--
5. Mammals	--	--	>969	>481
C. Mitotic recombination--all species	--	--	--	62
D. Cytogenetic effects				
1. Plants	--	--	>271	>215
2. Drosophila	--	--	554	333
3. Mammalian cell cultures	--	66[c]	856	--
4. Mammals				
a. Bone marrow	--	29[c]	>438	>253
b. Spermatogonia and spermatocytes	--	28	--	--
c. Lymphocytes/leukocytes	--	53[c]	--	--
d. Oocytes	--	19[c]	--	--
5. Micronucleus tests	220	--	>191	127
a. Plants	--	--	>32	--
b. Mammals	>150[c]	~160	>159	100
6. SCEs	--	163[c]	>544	>320
7. Dominant lethals	--	143[c]	739	>379

a. Source of information is Mrs. E. S. von Halle of EMIC, unless noted otherwise.

b. Brusick et al.[45]

c. GENE-TOX abstracts from meeting of December 3-5, 1980.

d. Generoso et al.[134]

6

STRATEGIES FOR RISK ASSESSMENT: THE CHOICE AND USE
OF TEST SYSTEMS TO ESTIMATE HUMAN GERMINAL MUTATION

There are two major, separable problems in assessing
human genetic risks. The first is the extrapolation of
results of mutagenicity tests to estimates of human
germinal genetic damage. The second is the estimation of
the impact of known genetic damage on future generations.
The first topic is the subject of this chapter. The
second is addressed in Chapter 7.

The characteristics of many mutagenicity tests are
outlined in Chapter 5. Although the choice of tests and
test data for human extrapolation is principally a scientific judgment, practical considerations also influence
this choice. Some short-term tests are inexpensive, as
well as able to identify weak mutagens. In contrast,
germinal tests on mice are too expensive and time-consuming
to be applied in the mutagenicity testing of most chemicals,
even though results with mice are presumed to be more
relevant to man. The contrast between the sensitivity and
practicality of short-term mutagenicity tests and the
biologic relevance to man of germinal mouse tests constitutes a serious dilemma in choosing tests whose results
are to be extrapolated to humans. Thus, before extrapolation
of test data to human effects can be undertaken, the most
appropriate test systems must be carefully evaluated. The
organization of this chapter reflects this approach.

Large-scale mutagenicity testing is already under way.
More than 12,000 chemicals had been tested by early 1981,
mostly in Salmonella or mammalian cell-culture systems.[11]
Data are accumulating rapidly, and regulatory agencies
must decide what test data are most appropriate for
predicting risks to human health.

The rapid development of test systems resulted from the
great increase in fundamental knowledge of genetics and
mutation. The information gained from fine-structure and

molecular analyses in microorganisms is being extended and applied to higher eukaryotic cell systems and to whole animals. Continued improvements in our understanding of mutagenesis and in test systems are to be expected. It is therefore important that recommendations as to which test systems to use be flexible enough to accommodate new knowledge. Unlike knowledge of experimental mutagenesis, knowledge of induced human germinal mutation has increased only minimally. With the exception of one cytologic study of irradiated testes,[39] there has been no direct demonstration of induced germinal mutations in man. Therefore, without a biologically common end point, as in human-animal comparisons in carcinogenicity testing, it is necessary to extrapolate from mutagenicity test results to identify potential human genetic damage.

Extrapolation from experimental organisms to man has considerable justification as a qualitative measure, but quantitative extrapolation is uncertain. There is neither sufficient uniformity among systems nor sufficient basic knowledge for confident quantitative extrapolation to human mutation. Even closely related species differ substantially in metabolism of mutagens and promutagens and in repair capacity. Extensive information on these metabolic and biochemical characteristics is available on only a few mammals, and only a few strains have been studied; their similarity to man is presumed, but largely unknown. The correspondence between human and mouse germ cell stages and mutational responses is not well understood. Dominant-lethal tests in mice have shown large differences that are specific to particular strains and chemical mutagens.[137] Skeletal and cataract mutations in the mouse have been used to estimate radiation effects in man;[221 303] but radiation exposure of the gonad is directly and easily measured, and that is not true of most chemicals. Molecular dosimetry of chemicals, although of great promise, is not yet sufficiently developed for wide use. The ability to produce monoclonal antibodies has improved to the point where it is feasible to consider antibodies against specific DNA adducts. Such a technique, once perfected, could provide a precise measure of human dose to correlate with data from experimental animals.

As discussed in Chapter 7, there is no feasible way to extrapolate from results of mouse tests to an estimate of the total impact of a mutation-rate increase in the human population, nor to make more than a crude and uncertain estimate of the increase in serious genetic defects in the first few generations. Yet this inability does not mean that all mutagens should be treated equally. Short-term tests can identify substances that are potential mammalian mutagens, and mutagens differ greatly in potency in such systems. Compromise approaches between a purely qualitative description and a rigorous quantitative assessment of genetic damage are needed. Among such approaches, rank orders and ratio statements about mutagens seem promising for reaching manufacturing and regulatory decisions.

EVALUATION OF RISKS AND HAZARDS

One possible way to identify hazards and risks is to consider the problem as a sequence of steps. Testing and evaluating potentially mutagenic chemicals could proceed through the following steps:

1. Hazard Identification. The first step is to determine whether a substance is mutagenic. For this purpose, inexpensive and sensitive short-term tests have been developed and are extensively used. This report discusses the general features of these tests and proposes a specific mutagenicity screening program to detect potential mammalian mutagens.

2. Hazard Characterization. Once chemicals have been identified as mutagens, they can be classified according to their relative potency and spectrum of effects. The activity of mutagenic chemicals varies markedly, as does the nature of the damage they cause.

3. Risk Estimation. In this step, the effect per unit of exposure is estimated. For genetic effects, there are two components: estimation of damage to germ cells, and estimation of impact on future generations. To estimate genetic risk, results from germinal tests in the mouse can be used to extrapolate to possible human effects.

4. Risk Assessment. This is a calculation of a potential effect based on the potency of the mutagen and taking into account the known or expected human exposure.

5. Risk-Benefit Analysis. Mutagenic risks are weighed against other risks and against actual or anticipated benefits of a chemical.

The first three items are the subject of this report; risk-benefit analysis and risk assessment are beyond the scope of the Committee.

As one proceeds through this sequence, the information becomes less precise. Hazard identification of mutagens has become very successful in the last decade, because of the development of excellent short-term tests. When extensive data are available, hazard evaluation is possible. If sufficient mammalian data have been collected, crude risk estimates can be made.

Whether and how a mutagenic chemical can be used depend on a number of considerations, some tangible, some not. One factor is the amount of the chemical that would be used; chemicals intended for wide use with considerable human exposure demand greater attention. The age of a person at the time of exposure also matters: the older the person, the less the potential genetic harm. The concentration of the chemical that is likely to get into the body is important, as is its route of entry (e.g., by ingestion or breathing). The mutagenic strength of a substance may permit a choice between two mutagens of equal benefit. In a risk-benefit analysis, such factors as the following can be considered: How important is the substance? How large is the segment of the population that would be expected to benefit? Is it possible that the benefits outweigh the risks, as in the case of a mutagen used to treat a serious disease? Can the mutagen be replaced by a nonmutagen or a weaker mutagen?

Risk estimation remains in a primitive state. Without direct human information, extrapolation from test organisms is necessary. The test organism of choice for risk estimates is the mouse, but extrapolation from mouse to man cannot be made with confidence and precision. Even more difficult is the translation of genetic damage occurring in germ cells to the effects on the welfare of future generations. As the number of generations since exposure increases, our ability to predict genetic damage diminishes. Nevertheless, in the belief that a rough estimate of uncertain validity is better than none, we suggest procedures for estimating human heritable effects.

SCREENING

Screening is the principal method of hazard identification for a mutagen assessment program. As described in Chapter 5, microbial and cell-culture systems not only are sensitive to weak mutagens, but can detect a variety of genetic end points--base-pair substitution, frameshift mutation, deletion, and chromosomal rearrangement. There is no way of knowing what fraction of all potential human mutagens would remain undetected in a combination of such tests, but there is reason to believe that the fraction is likely to be small.[11 170 288] For example, almost all chemicals that induce mutations in Drosophila and the mouse have been found to be mutagenic in short-term tests (see Table 9-4, Chapter 9). We conclude that a battery of short-term tests can be used with confidence to identify potential mammalian mutagens and that more expensive tests on whole animals are neither necessary nor desirable for initial screening.

A screening program is presented in Chapter 9. If a chemical is mutagenic in several tests in a screening battery, the presumption that it is mutagenic in man is strong, despite the absence of mammalian data. However, if a chemical is nonmutagenic in several sensitive test systems, it can be presumed to be nonmutagenic in man. Intermediate results--weak mutagenic activity or inconsistent results--require more careful, extensive testing, whose justification would depend in part on the projected benefits of the substance in question.

CRITERIA FOR SELECTION OF TEST SYSTEMS

The choice of a test system depends on whether it measures the same end points that are of concern to man. This usually means that the system should detect three major classes of mutation--genic, chromosomal, and genomic. Only with additional justification would other end points, such as chemical damage to DNA and mammalian cell transformation (neoplastic transformation), be recommended as part of a mutagenicity test battery. Such systems can be validated by demonstrating that they predict mutation.

A test system should be as relevant as possible, while meeting the requirements associated with practical application on a large scale. Relevance is based on similarity to man in the following five categories:

• The metabolic processing of the agent. The mechanisms of activation and detoxification should be as similar as possible to those in man. A minimal battery of tests should include the opportunity for appropriate metabolic activation on the basis of accumulated testing experience. A postmitochondrial supernatant from rat liver is most commonly used today.[181] Because in principle it would mimic the human situation, human material would be preferred, but it is not practical, both because of the difficulty in obtaining material and because humans cannot be given the chemicals used for metabolic induction in the rat.

• The structure and chemical nature of the chromosomal target. Eukaryotes are preferable to prokaryotes, especially for assessing chromosomal breaks and aneuploidy. Preference is based on the assumption that eukaryotic tests give more biologically pertinent results when mammalian damage is the ultimate level of concern. The principal reason for this is similar chromosomal structure among the eukaryotes.

• The processing of DNA damage. The processes of repair and other modes of mutation avoidance should resemble those of man.

• The transmission of the mutation. Tests on germinal tissue are preferable to those on somatic cells.

• Correspondence of germ cell stages. Some germ cell stages are more sensitive to mutagenesis than others. In humans and other mammals, stem-cell spermatogonia persist from within a few days of birth throughout the reproductive lifetime, and the postspermatogonial germ cells persist for a much shorter time. In female mammals, the stage of by far the longest duration is the arrested primary oocyte. The short-lived germ cells have much less time to accumulate a dose; accordingly, they would require markedly higher mutational responses to acquire equal importance in hazard evaluation or risk estimation. For these reasons, stem-cell spermatogonia and arrested primary oocytes in experimental organisms are regarded as the most relevant for human risk assessment.

The tests chosen necessarily represent a compromise: relevance, sensitivity, cost, and other considerations must be balanced against each other. There are reliable and practical tests for genic and chromosomal mutations, and a testing program must include assays for both kinds of damage. However, there are as yet no validated short-term tests for genomic mutations, although several are being developed; as one becomes practical and is validated, it should become part of a mutagenicity screening program.

In the choice of tests to be incorporated into a screening system, the following criteria are of importance:

• The number of chemicals that have been tried in a given test.
• The classes of chemicals tested.
• Concordance of results with chemicals previously subjected to other tests.
• The genetic end points assayed by the test.
• The expense of the test and the speed with which it can be performed.
• The number of laboratories that have performed the test and the reproducibility of results among laboratories.
• The diversity of phylogenetic groups represented collectively in the test systems.

• The sensitivity and specificity of the test.

According to the mutagenicity assessment program outlined in Chapter 9, classification of a chemical as a presumed mammalian mutagen permits an acceptable degree of confidence that it would cause some genetic damage in man. This presumption could be rebutted by definitive toxicokinetic evidence that the substance does not reach the germ cells or for other reasons is not effective. If a chemical is not mutagenic in the screening system, it is presumed not to be a mutagen. Genomic mutagens, which cannot yet be effectively identified in short-term tests, remain outside this presumption. The sensitivity and wide range of end points of a well-selected screening scheme make it unlikely that any substance not found to be mutagenic in the scheme would be found to be mutagenic in a mammal. However, if a mammalian germ-cell test is positive, this is sufficient to classify a chemical as a mammalian mutagen.

For many substances, mutagen assessment will not have to proceed beyond screening. But if a chemical is both mutagenic and of great societal benefit, further testing is warranted to refine estimates of genotoxic activity. The screening program outlined in Chapter 9 does not distinguish between weak and strong mutagens, but this distinction is important. Mutagenic potency may well determine whether a manufacturing or regulatory decision can be reached at this stage. It is desirable to denote the strength of the mutagenic response in individual test systems. Because the screening program is not designed to address the question of potency, we have devised a rough logarithmic scale for ranking chemicals by their strength of muta-genicity in a test system. As there are differences in carcinogenic potency between saccharin and aflatoxin, so there are differences in mutagenic activity between weak and strong mutagens. Such distinctions may be important in making societal decisions.

BEYOND SCREENING: TESTING WITH THE MOUSE

Chemicals that are weakly or inconsistently mutagenic (the two properties tend to go together), but of specific benefit, may be tested further in mice. The mouse has been the experimental organism of choice in mammalian genetics, and mutagenicity tests with mice have been developed most extensively. A positive result in a mouse mutagenicity test is of great importance, because it is direct evidence of a germinal mutagenic effect in a mammal. But the difficulty is that mutagens that show small effects in short-term tests are likely to yield negative or inconclusive results in mouse tests. Then, as discussed elsewhere, the decision as to the likely effect in the human is difficult.

In the past, the specific-locus test in the mouse has often been used in connection with radiation and chemical mutagens. This system detects recessive gene mutations and small deletions at particular marked chromosomal sites. Much of the information about mammalian radiation mutagenesis has come from this test. In fact, the specific-locus test was a major source of data for estimates of radiation risk by BEIR III[303] and UNSCEAR.[473] It has also been useful for determining whether heritable gene mutations are induced in mammalian germ cells by specific chemicals. When positive effects have been found, it has been useful for evaluating the effects of such variables as exposure concentration, sex, and cell stage on the frequency of mutation induction.

The specific-locus test is not intended for human risk estimation. The seven loci sampled may not be representative of the whole genome. To continue the example of the appendix to this chapter, a mutation rate of 0.000003 per seven loci corresponds to 0.009 for 20,000 loci, if this is taken as the haploid gene number. This is nearly 1% per zygote, not a negligible number. It would be desirable to have methods to measure mutations in the entire genome, or in an entire chromosome, such as are used in Drosophila. Such methods are being developed in mice, but are not yet suitable for routine use.

For risk estimation, it is desirable to choose phenotypes that mimic human genetic diseases. Dominant phenotypes are most important, because these constitute the bulk of the human effects in the first 5-10 generations. Skeletal mutations (and more recently cataracts) have been used as the basis of radiation-risk assessment[303] and permit the measurement of dominant effects and sampling of a larger fraction of the genome. Testing a class of mutants that produce particular phenotypes, such as skeletal anomalies, is independent of the uncertainty of how large a fraction of the genome is being tested, but replaces one uncertainty with another. The question then becomes: "What fraction of genetic damage is expressed in the form of skeletal defects?" Both skeletal and cataract mutation systems need extensive use to correlate results with those of other test systems. The induction of similar phenotypes in other small mammals would also be valuable for comparative purposes. It is important that mouse strains other than the few currently in use and more known chemical mutagens be studied in these assays.

Detailed comparisons of induced skeletal and eye anomalies in the mouse with human skeletal and eye defects are desirable. Systems for measuring heritable translocations in postspermatogonial cells in the mouse have been developed and can be extended to estimate the risk to corresponding human stages.[134]

Ideally, if mouse experiments are to be used to estimate the rate of induction of gene or chromosomal mutations, chemicals should be tested at enough doses to establish a dose-response curve. However, if the purpose is simply to confirm that a chemical is mutagenic in a mammal, then a single positive result at a single dose is sufficient. A large dose (close to the maximum that is tolerated by the animal) can be given, and the concentration-time relations can be adjusted so that other toxicity does not unduly influence the mutant yield.

The main difficulty in interpretations based on one data point is the implicit assumption of linearity between the high-dose exposure of mice and the anticipated low-dose exposure of humans. Figure 6-1 illustrates the difficulty. If the single dose is at D_1, the low-dose extrapolation gives a reasonably correct value. If the curve is accelerating in this region, the true effect may be overestimated. The greater concern, however, is that a high dose, like D_2, will be given. In this case, the

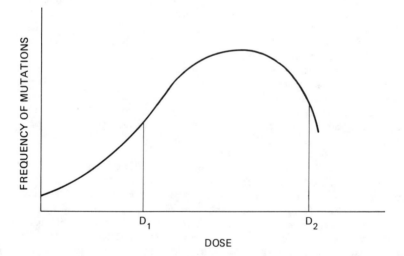

FIGURE 6-1 A possible dose-response curve. A single-dose experiment at dose D_1 would yield approximately the correct prediction of the low-dose effect, whereas an experiment at dose D_2 would lead to an underestimate.

effect may be greatly underestimated, or a compound may be classed as nonmutagenic when it is really mutagenic. This is the basis for the GENE-TOX recommendation[377] that in specific-locus experiments the highest dose used should not cause a sterile period so long that the males are not yet fertile by 81 d after treatment. A sterile period indicates germ-cell killing, and the usual explanation of downward curvature at high doses is that differential cell killing hides the mutation effect. Curves of this shape are often found in mutation tests in several organisms. The phenomenon is well established; it is not well understood. In tests on mice, the only instance of a negative slope at high doses was seen after a very long sterile period.

It has been suggested[379] that the finding of no mutant mice among a specified number of progeny can be used to establish an upper 95% confidence limit of a dose that yields no mutations. The calculations, which are illustrated in the appendix to this chapter, are simple and direct, but must be interpreted with extreme caution if based on data at one dose point.

Such an interpretation could lead to serious errors if the dose-response curve had leveled off or turned downward at a dose lower than that applied (see Figure 6-1). It might not add greatly to the expense to test a lower dose for the possibility of an effect greater than linear interpolation from the original high-dose data would predict. However, full assurance that the slope is positive may require an experiment with many mice and thus vitiate the main object of the single-point, high-dose experiment--to provide a low-cost estimate of the upper limit of the risk. The absence of a sterile period would be reassuring, but there are possible reasons other than cell-killing for a plateau or downward curvature.

Experiments with ethyl nitrosourea at high doses, even though there is a long period of sterility, show that linear extrapolation would actually overestimate the effect at low doses, particularly if the low doses are given at a low rate. This is reassuring. Yet, if a new chemical for which no other mouse information exists is being tested at a high dose to give a large extrapolation factor, there is always the possibility that the curve has a long plateau or downward curvature. There is precedent for such curves from x-ray and neutron studies. Finding no mutants might also have some other explanation, such as failure of the chemical to reach the germ cells of the mouse. The test may not include the sex and cell stages that are most sensitive and relevant. The purpose, of course, is to predict possible human effects, and one

cannot be certain how similar mouse and man are. For
these various reasons, the Committee is reluctant to
accept negative mouse results from such an experiment in
the face of positive results from other tests.

SOME COMPARISON OF MOUSE AND DROSOPHILA RESULTS

There is a large body of data on chemical induction of
mutations in Drosophila for comparison with mouse data.
It would be valuable for making estimates of human germinal
risk to know the strength of a correlation between Drosophila
data and those on the mouse. It is instructive to compare
the results of tests of the same chemical in the two
organisms. For the present discussion, we use qualitative
comparisons only: a chemical either produced or did not
produce a significant increase in the mutation rate.
Table 6-1 presents a comparison of results with 17

TABLE 6-1 Results of Tests for Heritable Translocations in the
Mouse of 17 Compounds That Produced Translocations or X-linked
Lethals in Drosophila[a]

Compound	Mouse	Drosophila
Cyclophosphamide	+	+
Ethylene oxide	+	+
Ethyl methanesulfonate (EMS)	+	+
Isopropyl methenesulfonate	+	+
Methyl methanesulfonate (MMS)	+	+
Mitomycin C	+	+
Nitrogen mustard	+	+
Procarbazine	+	+
TEM	+	+
Tris(1-aziridinyl phosphine oxide) (TEPA)	+	+
Tris(1-aziridinyl phosphine sulfide) (thio-TEPA)	+	+
2,3,5-Tris(1-aziridinyl)-$\underline{p}$-benzoquinone (Trenimon)	+	+
Aflatoxin B_1	–	+
Cadmium chloride	–	+
Caffeine	–	+
Captan	–	+
$\underline{N}$-Methyl-$\underline{N}$'-nitro-$\underline{N}$-nitrosoguanidine (MNNG)	–	+

a. All treatments were to postspermatogonial stem-cell
stages. + = significant increase over the controls;
- = no significant increase over controls. Data from Bishop and
Kodell[34] and Lee et al.[240]

TABLE 6-2 Comparison of the Results of 17 Compounds Tested in Both the
Mouse Specific-Locus Test and the Drosophila X-linked Lethal Test[a]

| | Male Mouse | | Drosophila | |
Compound	Postmeiotic Cells	Premeiotic Cells	Postmeiotic	Premeiotic
Ethyl nitrosourea (ENU)	+	+	+	+
Mitomycin C	inc	+	+	+
Procarbazine	+	+	+	+
Triethylene melamine (TEM)	+	+	+	+
Propyl methanesulfonate	inc	+	+	n.t.
Butylated hydroxytoluene (BHT)	inc	−	−	−
Cyclophosphamide	+	n.t.	+	−
Ethyl methanesulfonate (EMS)	+	−	+	+[b]
Methyl methanesulfonate (MMS)	+	inc	+	+
Hycanthone methanesulfonate	inc	−	+	−[c]
Myleran busulfan (Myleran)	inc	−	+	−
Benzopyrene	inc	−	+	−
Methyl nitrosourea (MNU)	+	inc	+	+
Diethyl nitrosamine (DEN)	inc	−	+	+
Sodium bisulfite	inc	−	n.t.	n.t.
Irradiated wheat	n.t.	−	n.t.	n.t.
Caffeine	n.t.	−	+	n.t.

a. + = higher than historical control frequency of 43/801,406 at 5% significance
level; inc = inconclusive, which means neither + nor −, and samples evaluated after
high exposure range from 911 to over 20,000 offspring; n.t. = not tested; − = induced
mutation frequency after high exposure is lower than 4 times the historical control
mutation frequency at the 5% significance level. Data from Russell et al.,[377]
Russell,[380] Lee et al.,[240] and P. Selby (personal communication).
b. Statistically significant increase (5% level) over concurrent control, or
significantly greater than 0.5% mutation frequency.
c. Less than a 0.2% induced frequency (equivalent to spontaneous frequency) with
a sample size of 7,000 or more tests at approximately 800 loci per test.

chemicals that produced X-linked lethal mutations in
Drosophila with results of the mouse heritable-translocation
test. Five compounds that were negative by the heritable-
translocation test in the mouse produced lethals in
Drosophila. In all cases, the numbers of mice tested were
not large, and translocations might have been detected in
mice if larger samples had been used.

Table 6-2 shows an additional comparison between treated
male mice and Drosophila for 17 compounds. Of the five
compounds that produced a statistically significant increase
in specific-locus mutations in mouse stem-cell spermatogonia,
four were tested and produced significant effects in
premeiotic cells in Drosophila. All five compounds were
mutagenic in postmeiotic Drosophila cells, as were the
three compounds tested in postmeiotic mouse cells. Of 11
compounds declared negative or inconclusive in premeiotic
mouse cells (stem cells), four were significantly mutagenic
in corresponding gonial stages in Drosophila. Within this

latter group of 11 compounds, eight gave positive results in Drosophila postmeiotic cells and two were untested. Of the seven chemicals in this table that were positive in mouse postspermatogonial stem-cell stages, all were mutagenic in Drosophila postspermatogonial stages.

From these data, it is clear that more chemicals are positive for postmeiotic than for premeiotic stages in both mouse and Drosophila. However, there are irregularities and complications; for example, ENU is more mutagenic in premeiotic than in postmeiotic stages. We must remember that the premeiotic stages correspond to the human stages of much greater duration and are therefore more relevant. Unfortunately, data on females are sparse.

SEMIQUANTITATIVE RISK ESTIMATION

Although long-term health and other social risks associated with a mutagen cannot be assessed quantitatively with confidence, there are intermediate assessments between a fully quantitative estimate (e.g., in terms of number of years of life lost or number of severe genetic impairments in future generations) and the fully qualitative statement that a chemical is or is not a potential mammalian mutagen. Such intermediate assessments are referred to as "semiquantitative." This distinction is analogous to the EPA weight-of-evidence approach,[475] which this Committee regards as reasonable, in view of the tests and data from which the evidence is derived.

Semiquantitative risk assessments may consist of rank-order statements or ratio statements. The more quantitative assessment uses ratios of mutagenicity. It would be useful to know, for example, that chemical A is consistently 10 times as mutagenic as chemical B. Unfortunately, chemical activity among different tests is often inconsistent, and such ratios are likely to vary greatly.

An alternative is simply to rank chemicals in order of their mutagenicity in test systems. There is often a rough consistency in such rankings,[66] and that suggests a similar ranking of mutagenic potential in man. There are exceptions, however, to consistency in rank order between the mouse and other test systems. Such inconsistencies are to be expected since the route of entry and pharmaco-kinetics can have important influences on the detected mutagenic effect. Nevertheless, there are overall consistencies and in Chapter 9 we suggest dividing mutagens into classes corresponding to tenfold increases in potency in each test system.

A number of schemes for combining ranks have been

suggested for genotoxic chemicals. In one system,[430] carcinogens are ranked by several criteria. Scores are assigned for number of species affected, number of histologically different types of neoplasms, spontaneous incidence of neoplasms in appropriate control groups, amount and duration of treatment required for a specified response, malignancy of induced neoplasms, and genotoxicity in a battery of short-term tests. In a similar scheme for mutagenicity tests,[44] the degrees of response in the different test systems are weighted, with systems phylogenetically closer to man given greater weight. In this way, mutagens are given scores. Advantages of such a scheme are that it is easy to apply and that it is consistent if its rules are adhered to. Disadvantages are that the scheme is arbitrary and that there is no expectation that any specific test could be assigned a weight unambiguously.

RISK ESTIMATION PROCEDURES THAT HAVE BEEN SUGGESTED

There are two approaches to assessing genetic risk from test data. One is to attempt to find some pattern of mutagenesis among different organisms that would permit extrapolation to man. The other is to use data from the mouse. We first discuss attempts to arrive at risk estimates by the former approach.

THE ABCW RELATIONSHIP

One approach to extrapolating from submammalian data to potential mammalian damage is based on the claim that the rate of occurrence of radiation-induced mutations per gene is proportional to the amount of DNA in the genome.[4] The rough proportionality extends over organisms differing by a factor of more than 100 in amount of DNA--for example, fungi and mice. That the relationship is not peculiar to radiation effects was demonstrated in studies with ethyl methanesulfonate (EMS) that showed a similar proportionality between mutation rate and genome size.[154] The ABCW relationship came as a surprise, because structural genes were expected to be the same size in all organisms. Although recent evidence of noncoding regions of DNA, of intervening sequences, and of repeated sequences suggests some basis for an increase in target size in higher organisms, the basis of the ABCW relationship remains unclear.

The ABCW relationship is far from exact. There are wide variations in rates of mutation among different loci in the same organism, so the relationship depends somewhat on the loci used. Furthermore, mutation rates differ among tissues and among stages. Despite the uncertainties about the ABCW relationship,[391] the generality of increasing mutation rate with increasing genome size is clear. The uncertainties do not refute the ABCW correlation, but they do undermine the strict proportionality.

RADIATION EQUIVALENTS

An alternative approach to risk estimation is to relate the mutagenicity of a chemical to the amount of radiation that would produce an equal effect. This approach is best exemplified by the concept of a rem-equivalent chemical (REC). A REC is the dose (concentration times time) that produces an amount of genetic damage equal to that produced by 1 rem of chronic radiation.[98] REC was introduced, not as a basis of risk estimation, but as a guide to setting standards.[40][80] There were already accepted radiation standards, and it was thought that chemical risks could be considered by the same standards if the chemical damage could be correlated with that from radiation.

A major criticism of this approach is that chemicals produce a spectrum of lesions different from those produced by radiation. For example, most radiation-induced mutations include a great deal of chromosomal breakage, but some chemicals induce a large proportion of base changes and other point mutations. Moreover, the relative frequencies of different types of damage differ for different chemicals and for different germ-cell stages. In addition, although radiation exposure can be measured directly in all tissues and cells, that is not yet the case with chemicals. For all these reasons, the REC method is not now useful as a risk-estimation procedure.

Various refinements of the REC concept have been suggested, such as the use of rad-equivalents.[111] The chemical dose would be determined from the chemical damage to the DNA or other macromolecules and related to the radiation dose that causes a corresponding degree of biologic damage. However, despite its novelty and theoretical attractiveness, the procedure suffers from most of the difficulties that make the REC concept inapplicable for risk estimation.

MOLECULAR DOSIMETRY

Molecular dosimetry offers a promising approach for more precise and reproducible dose measurement, thereby

making extrapolation a more plausible exercise.[1-3] [237-239]
Molecular dosimetry is based on the idea that extrapolation
should be related to the effect of the chemical mutagen on
DNA, for example by formation of DNA adducts. It is
limited by lack of basic understanding and especially by
technical difficulties in identifying the adducts. It
currently requires that the chemical of interest be
radioactively labeled and form adducts. It at least shows
that the chemical reached the target.

Molecular dosimetry can be used to create a net of
chemical bridges among test mammals and between mammals
and lower eukaryotic systems. This can be illustrated
with a simple example:

	Nonmammalian Organism	Experimental Mammal	Man
Dosimetry	A	B	
Mutation rate	C	D	E

In this example, D is some observed end point in the
mammal--specific-locus mutation rate, skeletal anomalies,
cataracts, or heritable chromosomal damage. The values
for D and E are assumed to be the same, although our
confidence in the extrapolation would be increased if the
observations in D involved several strains of several
mammals. There is some possibility of direct dosimetry in
man. With molecular dosimetry, the DNA damage in A and B
can be measured in the same way. This corrects for
differences in mutagen metabolism and mutation processes
in the two organisms. B is measured directly in the
spermatogonia or oocytes. The mutational end point, C, is
whatever is most appropriate for the particular test
organism.

For a particular chemical or group of related chemicals,
the functional relation

$$D = f(A,B,C) \qquad (1)$$

is sought. D, the mutation rate in experimental mammals,
is expressed as a function of two dosimetric calculations
and an estimation of submammalian mutation rate. Once
dosimetry and mutation rate are correlated, the mammalian
mutation rate can be used to express that in man. In
simple cases, perhaps at low doses, D may be proportional
to BC/A, but this is not to be expected in general.

Until direct human dosimetry and germinal mutation-rate
measurement are possible, we have to develop and study
such testing bridges. It is not expected that a single

test organism will suffice in such a scheme; instead there
will probably be a network of several test systems. Only
by confirming a pattern with diverse organisms can we
become confident of extrapolations. As confidence in the
above equation increases, it might be possible to bypass
the expensive test D and rely on the other three measurements
to estimate human risk. There remain many difficulties.
For example, data on experimental organisms, including the
mouse, show that one cannot assume that the product of
concentration and time is a constant.

With the great diversity of chemicals and the various
modes of action, it is very likely that scaling (extrapolating) equations like Equation 1 will differ for different
chemicals. Thus, decisions on how genetic-risk estimates
are to be extrapolated to man will have to be made in
different ways for different chemicals. This point of
view is reflected, at least implicitly, in the recently
published EPA proposed guidelines for mutagenicity risk
assessments.[475]

HUMAN RISK ESTIMATES FROM MOUSE DATA

Because genetic effects in man cannot be reliably
predicted from submammalian tests, another alternative for
quantitative risk estimation is to rely on data on the
mouse. Despite reservations about the sensitivity of
mouse tests and the statistical power of experiments with
small numbers of animals, an in vivo mammalian system
incorporates the more relevant biologic and metabolic
factors necessary to make quantitative human risk estimates.

As discussed later, the great bulk of phenotypic effects
that would occur in the first half-dozen generations after
the occurrence of mutations are caused by dominant gene
mutations and chromosomal mutations (mostly translocations).
The former are best estimated at present by phenotypic
classes, such as skeletal mutations and cataracts (discussed
in Chapter 5). These dominant so-called gene mutations
really constitute a heterogeneous category. Some success
has been achieved in explaining the molecular basis of
cataract mutation (e.g., Carper et al.[51]). They probably
consist of gene mutations, small chromosomal changes (such
as deletions), and gross chromosomal changes. The proportions of these may be different with different mutagens.

About one-fifth of human dominant diseases listed in
McKusick's compendium[279] have skeletal effects, but the
true proportion of all dominant mutations having skeletal
effects is probably closer to one-tenth.[473] About half
the dominant skeletal mutations in mice have severe

effects,[473] the rest probably being innocuous. So a
direct, although crude, way to estimate the frequency of
human first-generation serious effects is simply to
multiply the mouse skeletal rate by 10 and then to
multiply the product by 0.5. That calculation assumes
that all dominant phenotypes increase in the same proportion
as those affecting the skeleton. Yet the component due to
deletions and other chromosomal changes may be different
for different phenotypes. Nevertheless, with a large
enough number of genes contributing to skeletal defects,
it is reasonable to assume that these defects consist of
many types, as do dominant phenotypes in general. In
using the extrapolation factor of 10, should one take the
frequencies of the different human traits into account?
It is probably better not to, inasmuch as the incidences
are strongly influenced by the fitness of the individual
traits and therefore are not proportional to their mutation
rates. Needless to say, the figure of 10 is only a crude
estimate, and the BEIR Committee accepted a range of 5-15.

There is considerable evidence that the great majority
of induced skeletal changes are heritable. The normal
procedure of subtracting the control rate from the induced
rate corrects for phenocopies. When this procedure is
used for risk estimation, there should be a sufficient
number of doses to establish the shape of the dose-response
relationship, and the germ cell stages most relevant to
man should be exposed--namely, spermatogonia in males and
oocytes in females.

Confidence in the estimates of human dominant disease
and skeletal defects may be increased by obtaining independent
estimates based on essentially the same procedure, but
with cataracts as the dominant phenotype.[108 220] Although
neither skeletal defects nor cataracts are very precisely
measured phenotypes, the risk estimates for radiation
based on them are in reasonable agreement.

Other recent evidence[325] suggests that tumor susceptibility
in mice may be inherited in a dominant, Mendelian fashion,
thus possibly providing another phenotypic effect to
correlate with a corresponding human condition. Urethane
has been shown to produce a large increase in lung tumors
in the progeny of treated mice. The tumor susceptibility
is consistent with dominant inheritance with about 40%
penetrance. The most striking result is the high frequency
with which the tumors are induced. It is possible that
this is a property of a particular mouse strain and is not
generalizable to humans or even to other strains of mice.
But it is important that these experiments be repeated
with other strains and other chemicals.

The conclusion from this discussion is that there is

not yet an acceptable way to assess the damage directly
caused by a chemical in human germ cells. The absence of
human data makes it necessary to use experimental mammals;
the mouse is used now, although it should be possible to
compare skeletal, cataract, and cytogenetic tests on other
small mammals. Confidence in dominant-mutation tests in
rodents will increase as diverse chemicals are tested in
other small mammals and are found to be concordant.

CANCER DATA IN ESTIMATION OF MUTATION RISK

The BEIR Committees[302] [303] emphasized the difficulty of
providing any quantitative assessment of human mutation
risk. The mouse data were regarded as the best available,
but the requisite information that would permit building a
bridge to man was missing. For this reason, the Committees
regarded as their most robust conclusion that radiation
doses could be related to natural background radiation.
Specifically, the 1972 Committee said: "Our first recommendation
is that the natural background radiation be used as a
standard for comparison. If the genetically significant
exposure is kept well below this amount, we are assured
that the additional consequences will neither differ in
kind from those which we have experienced throughout human
history nor exceed them in quantity." This conclusion was
reiterated in BEIR III.[303]

For chemical mutagens, there is no easily measured
background exposure; for some newly manufactured compounds,
the natural background in the past was obviously zero. It
may some day be possible to determine the extent to which
the spontaneous-mutation rate is caused by chemicals in
the body, but it is not likely that there will be any
information nearly as reliable as that on radiation in the
next few years.

One difficulty with genetic-risk estimation is that the
end point is diffuse, both in the diversity of effects and
in their time distribution. Cancer-risk estimation differs
sharply, in that there are distinct end points. The
expectation of survival and death rates associated with
different kinds of cancer are much better known. It is
simpler for an increase in cancer incidence to be expressed
in quantitative units, such as years of life lost, than for
this to be done for genetic disorders, although there have
been recent attempts to do it. Furthermore, there is a
correlation between exposure to a carcinogen and the
development of cancer in humans and experimental animals.
Corresponding information on genetic effects does not

exist. Nevertheless, there are problems with cancer, too; e.g., latent periods and promoters complicate the analysis.

For many chemicals, carcinogenicity tests will be done, regardless of whether the chemicals are tested for mutagenicity in higher organisms. If it is decided in a risk analysis that carcinogenicity is a sufficient reason for deciding the extent of a chemical's use, then more mutagenicity tests are not warranted. However, if the assembled mutagenicity data are not definitive, an additional risk estimate for genetic effects may be needed. This is particularly important for genotoxic chemicals, such as genomic mutagens, that may not be carcinogens. We therefore conclude that, although carcinogenicity tests cannot replace determinations of genetic effects, positive results in cancer tests may at times obviate genotoxic testing. For important chemicals on which no mammalian testing has yet been done, the decision as to whether it is better to do a mutagenicity test or a carcinogenicity test must take into consideration the degree of confidence in quantitative results of the tests. Some chemicals of great importance may require estimates for both end points, as has been the case with radiation.

APPENDIX

Let p be the true proportion of mutants induced by the high-dose treatment. Then the probability, Pr, of observing no mutants among N progeny is $(1 - p)^N$. Equating this to 0.05 (or some other chosen probability value) and solving for p gives the upper limit of the true value of p at this probability. Here are a few numbers for a probability of 0.05:

N	p	Np
100	0.0295	2.95
300	0.00994	2.98
1,000	0.00299	2.99
3,000	0.000998	2.99

The limiting value of Np is 2.9957 (i.e., -ln 0.05), so there is a simple rule of thumb: if no mutants are found, a mutation rate leading to an expectation of three mutants is excluded at the 5% probability level.

For example, suppose that 1,000 mice were observed and

no mutants were found. The upper limit for the number of expected mutants is 3, or a true mutation rate of 0.003. If the extrapolation factor (ratio of the mouse dose to the expected human exposure adjusted for stage sensitivity, dose rate, and other relevant factors) is taken to be 1,000, the 95% upper confidence limit on the mutation rate for the lower human exposure is 0.000003.

7

STRATEGIES FOR RISK ASSESSMENT: RELATION
BETWEEN MUTATION RATE AND HUMAN WELFARE

Chapter 6 considered the estimation of the human germinal mutation rate. Because of the paucity of information from direct human observation, it is necessary to extrapolate from studies of experimental organisms, cell cultures, and the like. The results of extrapolation are uncertain. But estimation of human mutation rates is only half the problem. It is also necessary to assess the impact of mutation on human welfare.[319]

Our knowledge of the quantitative impact of an increased mutation rate is sparse. A typical statement is that of Trimble and Smith,[464] who acknowledged that we do not have a satisfactory answer even to such a simple question as: "Suppose the mutation rate were doubled; would the effect on human health be serious or trivial?" This chapter discusses the reasons for this pessimistic assessment and ways in which the uncertainty might be lessened.

The human risk estimate may be absolute or relative. An absolute estimate might be of the number of persons expected to have genetic diseases in the future, whereas a relative estimate would be of the expected increase, expressed as a fraction of the normal incidence. If we know the normal incidence, we can convert the absolute effect into the relative, and vice versa.

The extent to which genetic disease contributes to human misery has been variously estimated. Often, 10% is given as the fraction of disease that is genetic. Yet it is clear that this figure depends heavily on what we mean by "genetic." If we count only well-understood dominant and recessive traits that adhere strictly to Mendel's rules, the proportion is considerably less than 10%. If we include all disorders that have some genetic component, the proportion is much higher than 10%. We need to divide the data into finer categories. Even if the genetic component of human disease and disability could be measured precisely, that would provide only part of the information needed for mutation-risk assessment. We also need to know how much of the genetic burden is caused by mutation. This requires a different kind of analysis and is the principal subject of this chapter.

Suppose we have estimated (by such methods as were discussed in Chapter 6) that the overall human mutation rate has been increased by a specified percentage. To make a rational assessment of the impact of the increase, we would need to know:

- The naturally occurring incidences of diseases, abnormalities, and other impairments that are, at least in part, genetically caused.
- The extent to which these incidences are determined by recurrent mutation (i.e., mutation occurring repeatedly over time).
- The increases in incidences at various times in the future as a consequence of an increased mutation rate.
- The medical and social impact of these increased incidences.

Chapter 6 described methods for estimating the increase in the rate of dominant mutations from environmental chemicals on the basis of data on skeletal defects and cataracts in the mouse and estimates of the fraction of all severe human diseases that affect the skeleton or cause cataracts. Thus, we are in a position to make a tenuous estimate of the percentage by which the rate of human dominant mutation would be increased by some environmental mutagen. If penetrance is complete, the mutant genes will be expressed in the next and in ensuing generations until (as described in Chapter 3) they are eliminated by a decrease in the survival or fertility of their carriers.

UNSCEAR[473] based its quantitative risk estimates mainly on severe dominant diseases. Recessive and complexly inherited diseases were regarded as too poorly understood and too diluted by time to be considered. The BEIR reports[302][303] included disease of complex inheritance by making arbitrary assumptions about the extent to which the incidence is mutationally caused and about the time distribution. We agree with the policy of placing major emphasis on severe dominant mutations, but will treat the subject in a more systematic way.

It is clear from Chapter 3 that the increase in incidence of recessive diseases after an increase in mutation rate would be spread out over a very long time and that the effect on a single generation would be very small indeed.

The impact of heterozygous effects of a nonspecific sort would probably be larger. Most human disease and abnormality of genetic origin are not monogenic, however, and we must give some consideration to conditions of complex etiology-- such as congenital abnormalities, hypertension, diabetes, cancer, mental disease and mental retardation. There is room for a considerable range of opinion as to the role of genetic factors in their etiology, but it is generally agreed that both genetic and environmental factors are involved. Some single genes cause susceptibility to heart disease, cancer, mental retardation, and depressive disorders, but in no case is a single gene responsible for more than a small fraction of the total incidence. A number of genes, to say nothing of a variety of environ- mental factors, are involved.

However, it does not suffice to determine the extent of genetic causation. Even if a disease is genetically caused, its incidence can be largely unrelated to the mutation rate.[123] The most thoroughly understood examples, involving a trait that is maintained by superior fitness of the heterozygote, are sickle-cell anemia and thalassemia, both of which are hemoglobin diseases.[245][487] In each case, the homozygotes are often severely anemic, whereas the heterozygotes have had an advantage in the past over "normal" homozygotes because of resistance to malaria. If such a system comes to equilibrium in an area where malaria is rampant, the incidence of anemia is determined by the balance between the harmfulness of the gene in the homozygote and its beneficial effect in the heterozygote. The mutation rate is largely irrelevant; it adds only a trivial number of mutants to those maintained by superior fitness (resistance to malaria) of the heterozygote.

The number of human diseases known to be maintained by this mechanism is very small, being limited almost entirely to hemoglobinopathies, although several more diseases are suspected. It is not known whether this mechanism applies to more than a small fraction of genetic diseases. There are other types of interaction involving genes at several loci that could provide a mechanism for maintaining disease incidence. Another reasonable possibility is that many diseases that seem too frequent to be mutationally maintained are the result of balanced selection in the past. For example, with a near-starvation diet, such as our ancestors must have experienced from time to time, a mild form of diabetes might have been advantageous as a carbohydrate-conserving mechanism. Even if largely genetically determined (which is by no means always the case), these traits would not be substantially increased if the mutation rate increased.

What we need to know is the contribution of recurrent mutation to the incidence and burden of genetic disease. The proportion of the incidence that is caused by recurrent mutation, which would be responsive to an increase in the mutation rate, has been designated the "mutation component."[81 302 303]

THE MUTATIONAL COMPONENT

We shall make two simplifying assumptions. The first is that genetic effects and environmental effects are independent. The second is that the genes responsible for an effect are at equilibrium frequencies. The second assumption can be relaxed, but we use it here for initial clarity.

We let I stand for the impact of the trait (impairment, disease, or disability). Because the impact is proportional to the incidence, it is convenient to let I also stand for incidence. Note that the proportionality constant will differ for different traits. As a linear approximation, the impact can be written as

$$I = a + bu, \qquad (1)$$

where u is the mutation rate and a and b are constants. This assumes that the incidence increases linearly with the mutation rate. Then a is the incidence from causes other than mutation and b the increment in incidence per unit increase in mutation rate. The mutation component, M, is

$$M = bu/(a + bu). \qquad (2)$$

This is the fraction of the incidence (or impact) that is proportional to the mutation rate, whereas $a/(a + bu)$ is the fraction that is due to other causes (complex gene interactions or environment). If the mutation rate is increased from u to $u(1 + k)$, the incidence will eventually increase to $a + bu(1 + k)$; the incidence will have increased from I to $I(1 + Mk)$. Thus, this definition of M has the desired property: it measures the proportion of the incidence or impact that is mutational in origin.

If the relationship between the impact and the mutation rate is linear, as assumed, then, if there is an increment, Δu, in the mutation rate, the increase in impact, ΔI, is given by:

$$\frac{\Delta I}{I} = M \frac{\Delta u}{u}, \quad \text{or } M = \frac{u}{I} \frac{\Delta I}{\Delta u}. \tag{3}$$

If the relationship is not linear, an alternative definition, applicable to small changes in the mutation rate, is:

$$M = \frac{u}{I} \frac{dI}{du} = \frac{d \ln I}{d \ln u}. \tag{4}$$

It was shown[81] that for a wide variety of gene interactions the mutation component is 1 for a detrimental trait determined solely by balance between mutation and selection. If the trait has a quantitative basis, the principle still holds true. For example, if the disease is expressed only when a particular threshold of the underlying variable is exceeded, the mutation component is still 1. The dominance of the gene also does not matter; even a rare recessive disease has a mutation component of 1.

If the trait is caused partially by the environment, the mutation component is given by the broad-sense heritability of the trait. For a quantitative trait, the broad-sense heritability is the fraction of the variance of the trait that is genetically determined. For a rare qualitative trait, it is (to a satisfactory approximation) the fraction of the incidence that is genetically caused. Thus, when we do not know the exact genetic basis of a disease, we can estimate its mutation component by heritability measurement--by correlation and concordance between identical twins. For example, if the concordance of identical twins (preferably reared in different homes) is one-half for some rare trait, this is the estimate of the broad-sense heritability. There is always the problem that measures of heritability based on correlations between relatives are inflated by environmental correlations. In this report, however, we are concerned more with the societal consequences of underestimating the mutation component than of overestimating it, so environmental correlations are not as serious as in most genetic analyses.

So far, we have considered selection to be directional: a trait is harmful, whatever its degree of expression, so selection always acts to reduce the incidence of the trait. In many human quantitative traits, an intermediate value is optimal; for example, it is better to be somewhere near (or somewhat below) the population average for blood pressure than to be too low or too high. This means that a mutant gene that produces a small increase in blood pressure is advantageous in a person with very low blood pressure, but disadvantageous in a person with high blood pressure. The effect of mutation for such a trait is more to increase the variability of the population than to shift the mean. But because too much variability is harmful, the effect of mutation is harmful, as it is when the effect of selection is directional. For such traits, it can be shown that the mutation component is about half the heritability.[81] If the optimum is at the mean, the mutation component approaches one-half; but, as the optimum and mean diverge (as with blood pressure), the mutation component moves toward 1. Thus, for traits in which selection is toward an intermediate value, the mutation component is between one-half and 1 times the heritability.

There is a problem with this analysis. As mentioned earlier, it is possible for a trait to be determined completely genetically--and hence to have a broad-sense heritability of 1--and still not depend on the mutation rate. We can get some further insights by using another kind of heritability, narrow-sense heritability. Roughly, this is the proportion of the phenotypic variance that is genetically transmitted from parents to children.

Narrow-sense heritability is also measured from correlations between relatives. Broad-sense heritability includes all the genetic variability and is best measured by the correlation of identical twins, whose differences are entirely environmental. Narrow-sense heritability is measured by correlations between unilineal relatives, i.e., persons related in such a way that they cannot share two alleles. Narrow-sense heritability is 2 times the parent-child correlation (or concordance) or 4 times the correlation of half-siblings. This is because parent and child share half their genes and half-siblings one-fourth. One of the best ways to measure this in the human population is by the correlation between children of identical twins.[298] Although legally these children are cousins, genetically they are half-siblings; because they are reared in different homes, the environmental correlations are reduced. Very few such data exist; they could be obtained, but not easily or inexpensively.

Table 7-1 shows typical relationships between the mutation component and heritability. The traits are all assumed to be rare. It is clear that, by measuring the two kinds of heritability, we can get considerable information about the mutation component. Some examples of simple situations are given for illustration only; if we know the Mendelian basis of a disease, we do not need to

TABLE 7-1   Relationship Between Heritabilities and Mutation Components

Broad-sense Heritability	Narrow-sense Heritability	Mutation Component	Paradigm	Example
High	High	High	Rare dominant	Achondroplasia
High	Low	High	Rare recessive	Phenylketonuria
High	Low	Low	Heterozygote advantage	Sickle-cell anemia
Low	Low	Low	Environmental	Smallpox

measure heritability, so this analysis is for use with traits whose genetics are not understood.

If both heritabilities are high, there is a high mutation component. If both are low, the mutation component is low. If the narrow-sense heritability is low, but the broad-sense heritability is high, the mutation component is indeterminate. Note that the increased impact of a mutation-rate change may be very small (line 3 in Table 7-1) or, if large, would be spread over a very long period (line 2). For example, the narrow-sense heritability of a rare recessive gene is nearly zero; and its expression is diluted over hundreds or thousands of generations.

We can summarize these conclusions as follows: If narrow-sense heritability is high (and broad-sense heritability is high a fortiori), the trait has an equally high mutation component. An increase in mutation rate will eventually lead to a proportional increase in impact. If broad-sense heritability is high, but narrow-sense heritability is low, the mutation component is indeterminate. However, an increase in mutation rate will not have an appreciable effect for a very long time, if ever. If broad-sense heritability is low (and narrow-sense heritability necessarily is low), the trait is at most very slightly responsive to a change in mutation rate. If there is a change in impact, it will be spread over a very long time.

If we are concerned with genetic effects expressed in the next 5-50 generations (the next 150-1,500 yr), the most important data are those on narrow-sense heritability.

EFFECT OF DEPARTURE FROM ASSUMPTIONS

This discussion has proceeded as though the population were at equilibrium, either with mutation balanced by selection against deleterious genes or with some form of balancing selection (in which a particular gene is favorable in some combinations and deleterious in others). But the environment is changing much faster than the gene frequencies approach equilibrium, so one of the key assumptions used in deriving formulas for assessing the mutation component is invalidated, and the consequences must be examined.

The equations relating mutation and selection to incidence are complex and contain many uncertain and changing variables. One factor of ever-increasing importance is the effect of improved standards of living. The environment of modern man is much less hostile than that of his primitive ancestors; indeed, we benefit from our technologic success to a degree unthinkable by our grandparents. The control or eradication of infectious disease is one major success. Less directly, improved standards of living permit people with genetic disease or weakness to survive, thus decreasing selection pressure. Although environmental improvements do not affect all deleterious genes equally, mutant genes are generally less harmful than in the past. This gradual reduction applies to both survival and fertility. As a consequence, the net effect of environmental improvement is that mutant genes are more persistent in the population.

Figure 7-1 is a qualitative illustration of this concept (the upper part is a repeat of Figure 3-6 in Chapter 3). In the early generations after a pulse of new mutation, the impact is large, but very rapidly diminishes as the most harmful mutants are eliminated. Then there is a very long period when mutants with mild effects or recessive inheritance continue to exert their influence after the severe dominant mutants have been eliminated. If the environment improves, the average impact of the mutant genes diminishes. There will be an imperfect but positive correlation between the diminution in social impact of a mutant gene and its effect on fitness. The total hatched area of the lower graph is somewhat less; if the curves were extended indefinitely, the areas would be approximately equal. However, in the future the environment may not continue to improve, but may fluctuate between improvement and decay.

These figures depict the effects of a pulse of mutations, lasting no more than a single generation (about 30 yr). If the mutation rate increases by, say, 50%, it is likely, with the rapid increases in genetic knowledge, that methods to detect this will be developed within 30 yr. If not, these kinds of calculations can easily be extended to a mutation increase of longer duration.

We have suggested earlier that greatest attention be

given to severe, dominant mutations, because their impact occurs in a few generations, whereas the milder and recessive mutants are spread over such a long time that their impact on a single generation would be lost in the noise of fluctuations in other factors that influence the incidence and impact of human disease. A second reason for concentrating on dominant mutation is that, although we can predict short-range environmental changes with

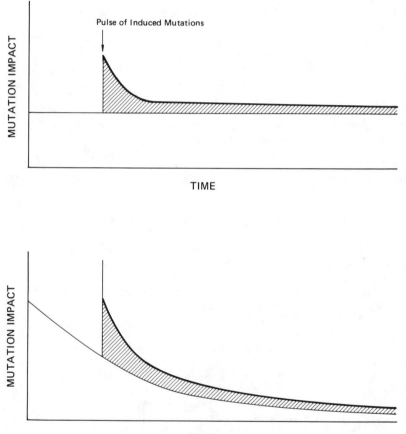

FIGURE 7-1 Top, distribution of impact (hatched area) after a burst of new heterogeneous mutation. The environment is assumed to remain constant. Bottom, distribution of impact with steady improvement in environment, at a rate that is higher than that of approach to mutational equilibrium.

limited confidence, we are utterly incapable of predicting what the world will be like 200 yr or more from now. One prediction can be made, however: changes brought about by all the unpredictable factors will surely dwarf the effects of mutant genes induced in the present generation. Partly for this reason, we have not placed much emphasis on predicting the equilibrium effect of a continuous increase in the mutation rate. It is extremely unlikely that any such equilibrium will ever be attained. In principle, the per-generation effect of a permanent doubling of the mutation rate is the same as the total effect over all time of a single-generation doubling of the mutation rate. But the former depends much more on equilibrium assumptions.

CONGENITAL MALFORMATIONS AND IMPAIRMENTS

Some 2-4% of newborn persons have an abnormality that constitutes a serious burden.[29][184][445] The numbers are uncertain, partly because records are insufficient and partly because classification into severity categories is subjective. Table 7-2 gives some representative risks to relatives of affected persons. The values range from 3% to 5% for children and siblings. The values are higher for deafness, because there is a larger component of simple Mendelian recessive cases than for most congenital impairments. The fact that for most of these traits the rate in siblings is not higher than in parents argues against any important contribution from recessive genes.[63] (A higher sibling correlation for recessive traits is caused by the fact that siblings often resemble each other for rare recessive traits, whereas parent and child rarely do.) Additional evidence of the relative unimportance of recessive genes comes from the absence of an increase in the proportion of consanguineous marriages among the parents of those affected. It should be mentioned, however, that several well-established recessive diseases produce congenital malformations; but these are rare.

Taking the numbers in this table as typical, we can estimate the narrow-sense heritability of these conditions as twice the recurrence rate for children, or between 6% and 14%. The average interval until the first expression of the trait is the reciprocal of this range, or about 7-17 generations. An upper limit on the mutation component is given by the concordance of identical twins. This ranges from 15% to 50% for traits on which data are available. There are many reasons to suspect that these numbers overestimate the mutation component considerably.

TABLE 7-2   Approximate Average Risks to Persons with an Affected
Relative[a]

Condition	Incidence General Population	Relative of Affected Person		
		Parent	Sibling	Monozygotic Twin
Cleft lip or palate	0.001	0.03	0.03	0.25
Clubfoot	0.001	0.03	0.03	--
Hip dysplasia (males only)	0.002	0.05	0.05	--
Pyloric stenosis	0.003	0.04	0.04	--
Anencephaly and spina bifida	0.008	0.04	0.05	--
Heart defects	0.006	0.03	0.03	--
Deafness	--	0.07	0.10	--

a. Data from Bonati-Pellié and Smith,[36] Carter,[53]
and Leck.[233]

One reason is that identical twins have a common prenatal
and postnatal environment. A second is that the incidence
of abnormalities is increased by twinning itself. A third
is that the incidence, to the extent that it is genetic,
may depend on balancing selection, rather than mutation.
    We conclude that the ultimate rise in the incidence of
congenital anomalies after a doubling of the mutation rate
would be considerably less than the 15-50% suggested by
the identical-twin concordances, but there is little
information as to how much less.[53] From the narrow-sense
heritability estimates, the mean period between an increase
in the mutation rate and the first expression in an affected
person would be at least 7 generations. The effect of a
pulse of mutation would be to cause a slight increase in
the incidence of congenital anomalies in the future. The
effects would be spread over many generations, and the
increase in a single generation would be very slight.
    Serious, quantitative discussion of specific conditions
is premature. We are concerned mainly with overall numbers.
But it is instructive to consider one example to show the
complexities that ultimately will have to be taken into
account. Pyloric stenosis is a failure of the pyloric

TABLE 7-3 Risk of Pyloric Stenosis in Persons with
Relatives Who Had Pyloric Stenosis

Sex of	Risk in Relatives of Index Person[a]			
Index Person	Brother	Son	Sister	Daughter
Male	0.07	0.05	0.03	0.02
Female	0.10	0.19	0.04	0.07

a. Data from Carter.[53]

valve (between the stomach and the intestine) of the
newborn to function properly. That failure prevents food
from passing beyond the stomach. Before World War I, the
condition was usually not recognized, and a child who had
it died. Today, it is readily diagnosed and repaired
surgically. The operation became widespread in the 1920s,
so now it is possible to observe children of persons who
have had such an operation. The risk of pyloric stenosis
in these children and in the siblings of affected infants
is given in Table 7-3. One more item of information is
needed to understand these data: males are affected
considerably more often than females. The usual interpretation is that there is an underlying quantitative
distribution of liability to the condition and that those
who exceed a threshold of liability manifest the condition.
The threshold is higher in females than in males; therefore, the incidence is higher in males. Furthermore,
because a higher liability is required for expression of
the trait in females, relatives of affected females are
affected more often than relatives of affected males.[120]
A realistic assessment of mutation components of specific
diseases will have to take such complexities into account.[189]
The conventional method is to measure the heritability of
the liability to the trait, rather than the heritability
of the trait itself.

Included among the various conditions discussed here
are many that have been shown to be inherited as simple
Mendelian dominants and recessives. For these it is not
necessary to resort to empirical data to estimate the
mutation component; it can be determined from simple
Mendelian principles. With increasing knowledge, the
present heterogeneous groups will gradually be broken up
into separate entities with a possibility of a much deeper
genetic, biochemical, or physiologic understanding.

Nevertheless, for the purposes of the present analysis, crude averages of heterogeneous quantities are useful.

CYTOGENETIC EFFECTS

Aside from conditions that are inherited as simple Mendelian dominants, the most completely understood class is that comprising chromosomal and genomic mutations. Blood cells from newborn infants were examined for chromosomal abnormalities in several studies. A recent compilation from the United Nations is summarized in Table 7-4. This list is an underestimate, because detection of abnormalities depends on the sensitivity of the method and the skill of the observer. Abnormalities that are below

TABLE 7-4   Incidence of Chromosomal Anomalies Among the Newborn

Type of Abnormality	Frequency per 100 Live Births
Sex chromosomal anomalies	
XXY `}` Males	0.093
XYY `}` Males	0.093
Other	0.086
XXX `}` Females	0.096
X `}` Females	0.010
Other	0.034
Total sex chromosomal anomalies (among newborns of both sexes)	0.21
Autosomal anomalies	
Aneuploidy	
G trisomy (Down's syndrome)	0.124
Others	0.022
Total	0.15
Balanced rearrangements	0.20
Unbalanced rearrangements	0.06
Total	0.62
Estimated total clinically important	0.3-0.4

the resolution of the system will be missed, and some of these are medically important. Some of the abnormalities are mild or harmless. The XYY genotype, which is sometimes associated with antisocial behavior and an increased risk of being incarcerated, produces no serious consequence in most instances. Likewise, balanced rearrangements are usually without symptoms.[458] Their main consequence is to produce descendants with unbalanced combinations; but these appropriately are counted among the unbalanced types in the generation in which they occur. If such symptomless and mild types are omitted, the total incidence of serious chromosomal abnormalities is reduced to 0.3-0.4 per 100 live births.

The range of phenotypes from these causes is great. Some, like trisomy 13 and 15, produce gross deformities and lead to death in infancy or early childhood. Others, such as trisomy 21, lead to mental retardation and a number of anatomic abnormalities, but are compatible with long life. The social burden of such conditions may be large, not only for the individual, but for the family and for the public if institutional care is required.

Chromosomal abnormalities also are a common cause of abortion. It is estimated that at least 50% of spontaneous abortions are caused by chromosomal aberrations. Nevertheless, less weight is given to these, because their social impact is much less than that of postnatal death or severe disease.

DISEASES AND MALFORMATIONS OF
ADULTHOOD AND OLD AGE

Most of the disabilities of adulthood and the major causes of death have some genetic component--for example, cardiovascular disease, kidney failure, cancer, and mental illness.

The concordance rates for identical twins are often high, but this does not necessarily imply a high degree of genetic determination. The old problem of separating the influences of a common genotype and a common environment still exists. Furthermore, the genetic component may not be mutationally maintained. Some form of balanced selection, perhaps in the distant past, may be responsible for a high incidence. For these reasons, twin concordances must be regarded as upper estimates of the mutation component.

Recurrence rates in children and other first-degree relatives would yield estimates of the more useful narrow-sense heritabilities. Again, common environmental factors are likely to confound the results. For example, Japanese

who live in Hawaii and San Francisco have a much lower
frequency of stroke than those living in the regions of
Japan from which the migrants came[180]--strong evidence
that environmental factors are important in the etiology
of stroke.

High concordances between identical twins and first-
degree relatives are reported for schizophrenia and manic
depressive psychoses. There is evidence of simple dominant
and possibly X-linked inheritance of manic depressive
psychosis in some families, but the extent to which the
total incidence is mutationally maintained is not clear.
The best data for assessing the mutation component of
schizophrenia come from Scandinavian studies[205] in which
the biologic and foster parents of adopted children who
developed schizophrenia were studied. The incidence among
adopting parents was no higher than in the general population,
but in about 10% of the cases one of the biologic parents
developed schizophrenia. These studies come closer than
others to separating genetic from environmental causes,
and the results, taken at face value, suggest a mutation
component of about 10%. More data are needed to establish
the true value.

Diseases of adulthood and old age are different from
diseases of childhood in one highly relevant way. Severe
diseases of childhood can be expected to have a strong
effect on the Darwinian fitness of those afflicted. Such
conditions are kept at a low frequency in the population,
because they reduce survival to adulthood or fertility.
Most diseases of adulthood occur after the usual age range
of reproduction. To the extent that the disease occurs
postreproductively, there is no effect of the condition on
fitness. Natural selection is not influenced by what
happens to people after they have reproduced. The situation
is not always this extreme: most genes have multiple
effects, and some of these may affect people at earlier
ages, so there may be corresponding, but weaker, selection
at earlier ages.

Because of weak selection, adult diseases can have a
high mutation component, and yet a mutation-rate increase
will have very little effect for many generations. For
example, if the selection against a partially dominant
mutant gene is 0.01, the mean persistence of this mutant
in the population before it is eliminated by selection is
100 generations, or 3,000 yr. Consequently, most of the
deleterious genes in the population arose a long time ago;
only 1% are new mutations. The great prevalence of
postreproductive genetic disease is caused mainly by the
inefficiency of natural selection in removing the causative
genes and possibly by the beneficial nature of some of the

genes in earlier ages. We therefore should expect that an increase in mutation rate would have little immediate effect on adult disease. Whatever effect it has would be spread over a very long time; the impact on a single generation would be slight.

Thus, there are two reasons why the impact on the first few generations after a mutation-rate increase can be small. One is the set of factors mentioned earlier: if the trait is recessive, if the penetrance is low, if there is a large environmental component, or if the genes interact in complex ways, the effect in immediate generations is slight, even though the condition is severe and strongly selected against. The other reason is the one cited in the preceding paragraph: the trait is weakly selected against because of late onset or for other reasons, so it takes many generations to reach equilibrium.

The same considerations apply to human quantitative traits with an intermediate optimum. Experiments with Drosophila and other animals have shown that for such traits the contribution of a single generation of mutations to the genetic variance of the trait is very small, perhaps about 0.001.[421] This means that a change in mutation rate would be reflected extremely slowly in an increased variability of the population. Hence, if we can judge from experimental organisms, an increase in human mutation rate would affect such traits only very slowly. The effect of a pulse of mutations on any one generation would be slight indeed.

All these considerations suggest that the policy of concentrating on dominantly inherited diseases, as in the BEIR and UNSCEAR reports, takes into account the major effects of mutation in immediate generations. The harm to one generation from neglecting other factors is very small. We can hope that better understanding of the more subtle effects will occur before any substantial harm has been done by neglecting them.

CANCER

Although all cancers have some features in common, they are a heterogeneous group from the standpoint of etiology. Predisposition to some cancers is inherited in simple Mendelian fashion. Conspicuous among these are "cancer families" with very high incidences of particular malignancies. But these are monogenic cancers, which individually and collectively account for only a small fraction of the total cancer morbidity and mortality--a few percent at most.[214]

The childhood tumors, such as Wilms's tumor and retinoblastoma, are a special group. They occur in infancy or
childhood and apparently have a uniform incidence among
all racial and geographic groups. Some cases are clearly
inherited; others are sporadic. One hypothesis is that
the malignancy results from two mutations. If both
mutations are somatic, that accounts for the sporadic
cases. In retinoblastoma, mutations frequently affect
only one eye. In the hereditary cases, one mutant gene is
inherited from a parent and the second occurs somatically;
usually both eyes are affected. If this simple hypothesis
is correct, the mutation component is the fraction of
hereditary cases, estimated to be about one-third of all
cases.[214]

Some malignancies are strongly associated with particular
types of chromosomal breakage. Others are associated with
deficiencies in immune processes, which may themselves be
caused by mutant genes. Others are caused by diseases,
such as xeroderma pigmentosum and ataxia telangiectasia,
which cause unusual sensitivity to radiation because of
deficiencies in DNA repair.[348] The great bulk of malignancies
have no simple associations or pattern of inheritance.
For example, female first-degree relatives of women who
have had breast cancer have a risk of breast cancer 2-3
times as great as normal, but the data do not fit any
simple hypothesis. For most cancers, heritability is
rather low. Therefore, the mutation component is likely
to be low. There may be a mutation component acting
through both germinal and somatic effects. If the two-
mutation hypothesis for childhood tumors is correct, an
environmental chemical could increase not only the frequency
with which the first mutation would be inherited but also
the frequency with which the second, somatic mutation
would occur. Most calculations concerning retinoblastoma
assume that the second mutation is almost certain to
happen somewhere in the retina, provided that the first,
inherited mutant gene is present.

In one strain of mice, treating the parents with
radiation or urethane produced an increase in cancers,
primarily in the lung, in the progeny. These were inherited
as though they were dominant mutations with about 40%
penetrance*. Whether these results can be generalized to
other species, or even to other strains of mice, will not
be clear until more experiments are done.[325]

Although it appears likely that the mutation component
of cancer is small, this does not imply that the mutation
process is unimportant in carcinogenesis. The full
relationship between somatic mutation and carcinogenesis
is not known, but the presence of many similarities

between the processes argues strongly that they may be fundamentally related. Whatever the case, it is clear that a very high fraction of agents that cause cancer are mutagenic in sensitive test systems.

THE PRESENT INCIDENCE OF GENETIC DISEASE

In one sense, the incidence of genetic impairment is 100%. None of us is without some genetic deficiency and all of us will die, mostly from a cause that includes a genetic component. From this viewpoint, it is meaningless to ask the total incidence or the total cost. Can we be more specific? We are interested here in the contribution of recurrent mutation to genetic impairment. This implies that we should classify genetic diseases by their mode of inheritance.

The first attempt to identify and enumerate all genetic defects in a well-defined population was by Stevenson[437] in northern Ireland. Stevenson's data were used in the periodic UNSCEAR reports.[469 470 473] The only other report of comparable completeness was done by Trimble and Smith[464] in British Columbia. Table 7-5 summarizes the data and presents modifications suggested by UNSCEAR.[473]

Unfortunately, the most important discrepancy between the Irish and Canadian studies is in the dominant category—probably the most important, in view of the prompt expression of dominant mutations. One cause of disagreement is that the earlier Stevenson study classified as

TABLE 7-5 Estimates of the Frequency of Genetic Disorders

| Category of Disorder | Frequency, per 100 Live Births | | |
	Stevenson	Trimble and Smith	UNSCEAR
Dominant	3.32	0.08	} 1.0
X-linked	0.04	0.04	
Recessive	0.21	0.11	0.1
Chromosomal	--	0.20	0.4
Congenital malformations	1.41	4.28	} 9.0
Other multifactorial disorders	1.48	4.73	
Total	6.46	9.44	10.5

dominant a number of conditions that would now be classified as multifactorial. Furthermore, a number of the conditions in Stevenson's list are quite mild and not major health hazards. However, the Trimble and Smith study did not include a number of diseases of later onset that the methods of the study would not disclose. There are two sets of data that purport to answer the same question, but disagree by a factor of about 40 in the most important item. No surveys have been done in the United States or other countries. As discussed in Chapter 10, the study of genetic defects in human populations is encouraged.

UNSCEAR took 1% as a reasonable value of the incidence of dominant impairments (see also Sutton[447]). A proper analysis would include data on the age of onset and degree of severity of the various dominant impairments. For example, five conditions make up a total of nearly 0.5%, or half the dominant group: hypercholesterolemia, Huntington's disease, polyposis of the colon, polycystic disease, and otosclerosis. The major impact of all these is on adults, often past the reproductive age. Therefore, the selection against them is much weaker than might be suspected from considerations of severity alone. Whether they are maintained in the population by balanced selection or by mutation balanced by very weak selection is not known. In either case, the impact of a mutation-rate increase would either be very little or be diluted over a long period.

It has been suggested[81] that it might be possible to assess the proportion of the total incidence of dominant impairments that is due to mutations in the immediate past generation by comparing parent-child and child-parent regressions. If a group of affected parents are selected and their children are examined, new mutations are not included. If affected children are selected and their parents are examined, new mutations are included. A higher concordance in the second case is an indication of the presence of new mutants and may be used to estimate this important part of the mutation component. Whether the procedure will be useful in practice is unknown. Without any solid information, the BEIR Committee[302] guessed that the fraction of the total dominant damage expressed in the first generation is about 0.2. We cannot suggest a more precise estimate.

By far the most accurately determined incidences are those of gross chromosomal abnormalities--both chromosomal mutations (involving changes in chromosome structure) and genomic mutations (changes in chromosome number). A large fraction of the total impact of these is on the first two or three generations. The kinetics of expression of X-linked recessive impairments are much like those of dominant mutants, except that on the average their expression is delayed 3 times as long. This is because in any single generation only one-third of the mutant X chromosomes are in males, where the trait is expressed.

AN EXAMPLE OF RISK CALCULATION

There is insufficient information to calculate accurately the consequences of a change in the mutation rate. To do this, we would need (in addition to information on the rate change itself) the current incidence of the different classes of genetic disorders, the mutation component for each, a measure of the extent to which each disorder is expressed in future generations, and some factor for weighting the classes by severity. However, we are not totally ignorant. A calculation based on reasonable guesses may be useful as a guide for calculations when better data are available and as a rough estimate of the direction of present judgments of risk assessment.

For purposes of illustration, we assume that for one generation there are additional mutations equal to K times the spontaneous rate; that is, the total rate is (1 + K) times the previous rate.

Let us assign symbols as follows:

$I(x)$ = normal incidence of disease category X,
$M(x)$ = mutation component of category X,
$E(x,g)$ = probability of expression of a disorder of category X at g generations after the mutation,
$C(x,g)$ = social cost of a disorder of category X at g generations after the mutation.

The added risk caused by a pulse of mutations equal to K times the spontaneous rate for one generation is expressed:

$$\text{risk} = K \int\!\int I(x)M(x)E(x,g)C(x,g)dg\ dx.$$

It is more convenient to adopt a simpler model and assume that the generations are discrete. The formula then becomes:

$$\text{risk} = K \sum_{xg}\sum I_x M_x E_{xg} C_{xg}.$$

An actual calculation could proceed as follows. We use the incidence data from the UNSCEAR report[473] as given in

Table 7-5. The dominant, X-linked, recessive, and chromo-somal classes are assumed to have a mutation component of 1. (Actually, the value is somewhat less if environmentally caused or multifactorial diseases are mistakenly classified in these categories.) The mutation component for congenital malformation and other multifactorial traits is taken as 0.10. The basis for this was explained earlier by the data in Table 7-2.

To obtain an estimate of E(x,g), we use a simple formula that assumes a uniform probability, $1/p_x$, for elimination of trait x:

$$E_{xg} = (1 - 1/p_x)^{g-1}(1/p_x) = (p_x - 1)^{g-1} p_x^{-g},$$

where p is the persistence of the mutant gene, that is, the average number of persons who carry it before the gene is eliminated from the population. We have taken the values of p to be 4 for dominants and X-linked defects, 100 for recessives, 1.25 for cytogenetic traits, and 10 for the congenital abnormalities and multifactorial traits that are mutationally maintained. These are crude estimates based on the severity and mode of inheritance of the traits.

We have not made any attempt to attach a social cost to these conditions. That would call for expertise, time, and facilities for a detailed medical study, none of which the Committee has. Hence, we ignore the severity and simply count total incidences.

The estimates of genetic disorders in future generations are shown graphically in Figure 7-2. The normal, baseline value is 10.5 per 100 live births. After a mutation doubling, the increased frequency per 100 live births is 0.66 in the first generation, 0.33 in the second, 0.22 in the third--reaching 0.014 in the twentieth and 0.004 in the hundredth. The total, integrated effect for all time (assuming no environmental changes) is 2.4, more easily obtained by simply summing the incidences in Table 7-5 weighted by the mutation component.

Although the numbers in this calculation are uncertain, the graph shows quantitatively some of the points mentioned qualitatively in Chapter 3. The largest impact is in the first few generations. The effect then decreases very rapidly as the dominant and cytogenetic effects are eliminated. About half the total impact occurs in the first half-dozen generations. After that, the effect in any generation is very small, but there is a long tail. If the diseases had been weighted by severity, the piling up in the early generations would be still greater.

The contribution of dominant, X-linked, and cytogenetic

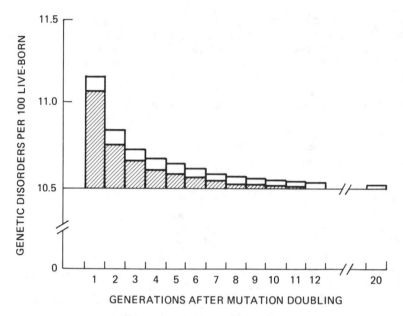

FIGURE 7-2 An example of the increase in genetic disorders after a single generation of a doubled mutation rate (K = 1). The normal incidences are taken to be those of the UNSCEAR column in Table 7-5. The mutation component is taken to be 0.1 for congenital malformations and other multifactorial conditions and 1 for the other categories. The mean persistence times are taken as 4 for dominant and X-linked, 100 for recessives, 1.25 for chromosomal, and 10 for congenital anomalies and multifactorial traits. The normal frequency is 10.5 per 100 live births. The contribution from dominant, X-linked, and cytogenetic disorders is hatched. Because recessive diseases make almost no contribution, the white areas are mainly congenital malformations and other multifactorial conditions.

conditions is hatched in Figure 7-2, to show that the great bulk of the effect in the early generations is from these sources. The white area is from congenital anomalies and multifactorial traits and is the most uncertain. The recessive component is too small to show on the graph. After about 10 generations, the dominant and X-linked components are largely finished, and the main contribution is from congenital anomalies and multifactorial traits. The total contribution (if the environment does not change) of dominant, X-linked, and cytogenetic conditions

is 1.4 of a total (for all effects measured to infinity)
of 2.4, or about three-fifths. About one-fourth of the
total effect is in the first generation and two-thirds in
the first five generations.

CONCLUSION

Although a simplified example, Figure 7-2 conveys the
general understanding of the effects of increased mutation
in human populations. The major early component is from
dominant and X-linked diseases and from cytogenetic
anomalies. Half the total damage from these conditions
occurs in the first three generations after a pulse of
mutations. The other large early component consists of
congenital anomalies and multifactorial diseases. This
category is much less certain, because both the mutation
component and the persistence of these conditions are much
less well understood. The total contribution of recessive
diseases is only 4% of the total effect and is diluted
over hundreds or thousands of generations.

Mutation-risk assessments based on dominant diseases
and cytogenetic anomalies would account for more than 80%
of the first-generation effects and for most of the effects
in the first five generations. On the basis of the
assumptions of this chapter, and subject to revision as
new information appears, the first-generation impact is
about one-fourth the total tangible impact, and about two-
thirds occurs in the first five generations. Because
dominant and cytogenetic effects are the most important in
the early generations after radiation exposure and are the
best understood, we agree with the BEIR and UNSCEAR
committees, which placed major emphasis on these two
categories. Effects of polygenic conditions can be
included in future estimates as their mutation components
become known.

8

TESTING AND MONITORING HUMAN POPULATIONS

There are essentially no positive data on the induction of mutations in human germ cells by external agents. Even the enormous study[396] of children whose parents had been irradiated in the Hiroshima and Nagasaki bombings revealed no statistically demonstrable genetic effects of the irradiation. Nor have children whose parents were irradiated medically or occupationally shown any effects. Therefore, one cannot rely on epidemiologic data to identify chemical agents that pose a genetic risk, particularly because the exposed populations are often small, the doses are variable and hard to measure, the patterns of exposure are complex, and (as emphasized in Chapter 3) there are no unique, easily observed mutant phenotypes--there is usually no way to determine whether a phenotype is caused by mutation or by another mechanism. Even if a mutant phenotype were detected, there would be doubt about when the mutation occurred and whether it was produced by an environmental agent or was spontaneous.

Because data on mutagenesis in humans are meager and it is difficult to measure mutation in humans directly, it would be particularly useful to have measures of mutational effects on man. Many of these points have been discussed in conferences and by individual authors.[78 171 313 314 320 448 483]

Although human populations cannot be deliberately exposed to potential mutagens to measure mutagenicity, there are circumstances in which direct observation is possible--mostly in occupational exposure, ingestion of food additives, and administration of therapeutic drugs. The typical approach is to identify an exposed group and a suitable control group for comparison of some genetic effect. The experimental design is thus similar to that used with other organisms.

The situation is different when a population is to be monitored to detect an increase in mutation over time, with no particular mutagen suspected. The population then serves as its own control, the rate at one time being compared with the rate at another.

It is the general goal of population monitoring and testing to develop efficient systems that require few persons and resources; that goal is far from achievement. In considering tests that might be applicable to humans, as opposed to experimental mammals, some limitations will be obvious. No test is acceptable that requires adminis-tration of hazardous materials, such as radioactive compounds or other known chemical mutagens. Biologic materials are limited to body fluids, such as blood and urine, and cells, such as blood cells, hair follicles, and sperm. These strictures rule out some useful tests that are applied to other organisms and to cell cultures.

Tests used or under development for humans are summarized below and listed in Table 8-1. These have been classified as germinal or somatic. Germinal mutations have been of greater concern, because they are transmitted to future generations and will constitute an unknown but possibly large health burden. Somatic mutations are probably of major importance in carcinogenesis, but otherwise may be of little significance. However, as the table indicates, information on rates of somatic mutation can be obtained from observations on far fewer persons than that on rates of germinal mutation. Also, the period between exposure to a mutagen and a detectable genetic effect is typically much shorter for somatic mutations. It must be emphasized, though, that there is little basis for predicting quan-titative effects in germ cells from observations on somatic cells.

DNA

DNA ALTERATIONS

DNA is available in human sperm and in white blood cells. From these sources, it should be possible to obtain DNA to detect changes resulting from agents, such as alkylating agents, that react chemically to cause mutations. In experimental animals, this can be done easily with radioactive tracers.[238] Very sensitive and precise radioimmunoassays being developed may greatly improve quantitative assessment, so that this technique could be applied to experimental animals and man. No practical chemical assay has been developed that can be

TABLE 8-1 Tests for Mutation in Human Populations

Test System	Somatic/ Germinal	No. Persons Needed to Detect Effect[a]	Period from Exposure to Effect[b]	Duration of Test Effect[c]
DNA:				
Alkylation	S,G	Small	Short	Short
Repair	S	Small	Short	Short
Chromosomes:				
Lymphocyte cultures	S	Small	Short-medium	Long
Micronuclei	S	Small	Short-medium	Long
Sister chromatid exchange	S	Small	Short	Medium
F$_1$ aberrations	G	Medium	Long	Long
Two Y bodies	G	Small	Short	Short
Proteins:				
Amino acid substitutions	[^G_S]	Large Small	Long Medium-long	Long Long
Enzyme activity	S	Small	Short	Long
Alkylation	S	Small	Short	Short
Body fluids:				
Urine, blood	S	Small	Short	Short
Urinary metabolites	S	Small	Short	Short
Cancer in exposed	S	Medium	Long	Long
Reproduction:[d]				
Sperm morphology	G	Small	Short-medium	Medium
Fertility	G	Medium	Medium-long	Medium-long
Phenotypes in F$_1$	G	Large	Long	Long

a. Small, 10 or fewer; medium, fewer than 1,000; large, tens of thousands
b. Short, 1-20 d; medium, up to 9 mo; long, greater than 9 mo.
c. Short, several weeks; medium, several months; long, several years to decades.
d. Effects on reproduction may include nongenetic effects.

applied to human sperm. Such tests are theoretically possible, but would probably be useful only in testing for exposure in specific cases, such as in occupational exposures to particular substances. Because of this limited potential use, the tests would have to be extremely sensitive.

DNA REPAIR

DNA that is damaged by radiation or chemicals can often be repaired by removal of the damaged area and replacement with new nucleotides. If the new nucleotides are radio-active, the extent of repair can be measured.[64][365] Measurement of DNA repair, usually designated "unscheduled DNA synthesis," also has been suggested as an indicator of exposure of chromosomes to mutagenic agents. This system has not been used to detect damage in persons exposed to mutagens. A report that the in vitro induction of un-scheduled DNA synthesis in lymphocytes of normal persons is positively correlated with chromosomal aberrations in circulating lymphocytes suggested that unscheduled DNA synthesis is associated with mutation, although it is difficult to predict the nature of the association.[350] If a useful test could be developed, it should be very efficient in detecting risk, because the unit of observation is the individual.

CHROMOSOMES

CHROMOSOMAL CHANGES IN LYMPHOCYTES

The appearance of structural aberrations in chromosomes of peripheral lymphocytes is a sensitive indicator of exposure to agents that break chromosomes directly.[115][117] This technique has been especially useful in studies of populations exposed to ionizing radiation.[21][38][46][116][254][426] Some chemicals are known to cause similar effects in experimental organisms. Relatively small numbers of persons are required to show a moderate effect, and many of the aberrations are detectable long after the exposure.[21][46][426]

Structural alterations in chromosomes are influenced by variations in laboratory procedure, handling of blood samples, etc. It is imperative that control samples be processed concomitantly with samples from an exposed or other population of interest and that samples be scored blindly. For comparable results among laboratories, procedures must be rigidly followed. With those restrictions, observation of chromosomal aberrations in peripheral lymphocytes constitutes a very sensitive and effective end point for detecting genetic effects in small numbers of persons.

One cannot yet attribute a specific amount of genetic damage to a given amount of chromosomal damage. Indeed, the chromosomal damage itself may be of little health significance, although it is reasonable to assume that whatever agents cause chromosomal rearrangements in these particular cells also cause rearrangements and other genetic effects in germ cells and other tissues. Further research will be required to substantiate the predictive value of chromosomal aberrations.

Most chemicals do not break chromosomes directly; instead, they produce lesions in DNA that lead to the formation of chromatid aberrations when lymphocytes are later stimulated to enter the S phase of the cell cycle. Because DNA lesions can be eliminated in noncycling peripheral lymphocytes before cells are stimulated in culture, the use of chromosomal aberrations in lymphocytes to monitor small exposures to most chemicals is as yet problematic.[499]

MICRONUCLEUS TEST

Acentric fragments often are not incorporated into daughter nuclei at anaphase, but rather appear as micronuclei in the cytoplasm separate from the cell nucleus after cell division. The appearance of such micronuclei is a convenient manifestation of earlier chromosomal breakage, with loss of the distal fragment. Micronuclei can thus be used as an index of chromosomal breakage.[392] Schmid[394] has developed the bone marrow micronucleus test for use in experimental animals.

Adaptation of the original micronucleus test to circulating lymphocytes has made it feasible to consider this test for screening of human populations.[73][155] The test showed a positive dose-response relationship with x rays and mitomycin C, although in the former case the response was small below 100 R. The micronucleus test needs more study before it can be used to monitor populations. It should be useful for small numbers of persons and hence be especially valuable.

SISTER CHROMATID EXCHANGE

One of the most sensitive and easily scored tests of chromosomal response to some chemicals involves sister chromatid exchange (SCE).[52][229][231][501][502] Many mutagens cause an increase in SCE, generally at exposures much lower than required for chromosomal aberrations. An apparent advantage of SCE as a test system is the sensitivity. Using x-ray exposure, Evans and Vijayalaxmi[118] observed 30 SCEs for each chromosomal aberration induced. The mechanism of SCE is not fully understood, but it involves long-term

alteration of DNA. Sufficient substances have been tested
for an increase in SCE to be accepted as evidence of an
increase in risk of mutation.

The use of SCE in cases of in vivo exposure of human
beings has been limited, but is rapidly increasing.[128] [131]
[169] [224] [253] [362] These studies have shown that the chromosomal damage responsible for increased SCE persists for
weeks or months and in one study[128] for years. In the
latter study, increased SCE was found in children of
exposed workers, presumably from in utero exposure or from
later exposure to contaminated clothing, etc. The effect
of increased SCE on health is not understood, but it
appears to be a most important monitor for identification
of persons with probably exposure to some mutagens.

SCE production is probably caused by S-phase-dependent
chemicals. Consequently, DNA repair phenomena that remove
lesions from DNA before lymphocytes are stimulated to
enter the S phase can influence the yield of SCEs just as
they can influence the yield of chromosomal aberrations.
Thus, DNA repair processes and other factors that influence
SCE production still make the mechanistic interpretation
of SCE production complicated when one is monitoring human
populations for small exposure to chemicals.[230]

CHROMOSOMAL CHANGES IN OFFSPRING

Changes in the number or structure of chromosomes
account for nearly half the spontaneous abortions and for
many of the congenital defects in liveborn children. One
in 200 newborn persons has a detectable chromosomal
abnormality.[186] [188] An increase in this incidence could
be detected in a moderate sample if it were carefully
chosen. A drawback is the very long time--40 yr or more--
that could elapse between parental exposure and the birth
of affected offspring.

Aberrations in newborn persons consist of both numerical
changes (due primarily to nondisjunction) and structural
deletions and rearrangements (due to chromosomal breakage).
There has been no unambiguous demonstration in human
beings that mutagens can cause nondisjunction. An
additional problem, insofar as monitoring is concerned, is
that the trisomies and monosomies seen in newborn persons
also cause increased risk of abortion. Therefore, only an
unknown fraction survive to birth.

In spite of these drawbacks, monitoring of chromosomal
abnormalities in the newborn is technically feasible. The
information so obtained would be valuable with respect to
risk if the population base were large--several thousand

persons, with an equal number of controls. The test would thus be insensitive to effects of small exposures in small populations.

It has been argued that monitoring of abortuses would be very effective because of the high rate of chromosomal abnormalities in abortuses.[188] If the problem of uniform ascertainment could be resolved, such monitoring would be very effective for detecting changes in frequency of various types of abnormality.

Y BODIES IN SPERM

A large segment of the long arm of the Y chromosome in man comprises constitutive heterochromatin and is characterized in interphase mitotic cells and in human sperm by the presence of a Y body that is C-band positive and strongly fluorescent with quinacrine mustard stains. The human XYY male has two fluorescent Y bodies (YFF) in somatic cells, but only one Y body (YF) in sperm. This observation is not unexpected, inasmuch as XYY males are usually fertile and produce only XY or XX offspring; that suggests that a mechanism during spermatogenesis prevents the extra Y chromosome from being incorporated into mature sperm.

The YFF human sperm test has been applied to patients who have received x irradiation or chemotherapy for treatment of cancer. Shortly after initiation of therapy, the YFF count is normal (<2%), but it rises substantially over a period of weeks or months and then returns to normal or nearly normal.[202]

In addition to the abovementioned agents, DBCP and formaldehyde have been tested. DBCP is strongly positive, whereas formaldehyde is negative in males with known inhalation exposure to these compounds.

The YFF test reflects nondisjunction of the Y chromosome. It is reasonable to assume that agents that are YFF-positive would also cause nondisjunction of autosomes. The frequency of YY sperm appears to be a very promising means of detecting genomic mutations in man. The Committee suggests that the feasibility of human YFF screening be determined because of the obvious advantage of directly testing chemical exposure that may cause genomic mutation in human sperm. However, even in this case, a YFF test in human sperm should be restricted to screening for occupational exposure to possible genomic mutagens that have been identified in animals.

Unfortunately, the YFF test cannot be used in mice, because their Y chromosome is not heterochromatic. It could be applied experimentally in primates, but, because of the expense of such studies, a concerted effort should be made to find a small mammal with fluorescent Y bodies for routine screening for agents that cause nondisjunction, which is one class of genomic mutation. Refinement of the test--e.g., total DNA measurement per sperm head in YFF sperm--would distinguish between aneuploid-producing and polyploid-producing agents. In the field vole, XX, XY, and YY spermatids are easily detected (see Chapter 5).

PROTEINS

AMINO ACID SUBSTITUTIONS IN PROTEINS

The primary structure of proteins is determined by genes, and changes in protein structure indicate corresponding changes in gene structure. Because of the amount of protein required to detect a structural change, this approach has thus far been useful only in studying germinal mutations, as expressed in the offspring of persons exposed to mutagens. In this approach, a number of proteins are studied in one blood sample.[315] [316] For example, 50 proteins X 10,000 persons X 2 chromosomes per person = 1,000,000 loci tested. Electromorphs are the most common mutation tested. If the rate of mutation to a detectable electromorph is about 10^{-6}, some tens of thousands of persons would be required to detect a doubling of the control mutation rate. Such results are of great interest, but present technology does not favor this approach as a monitoring procedure. The use of high-resolution gel electrophoresis may make the picture more favorable, however. As with all tests of progeny of exposed persons, there is the disadvantage that the mutagen exposure may have occurred years before the birth of the mutant offspring. Several efforts have been made to develop methods sufficiently sensitive to detect mutant proteins in single cells. This would permit the measurement of somatic mutation rates and would therefore be very useful in assessing exposures.[433] [446] Monospecific antibodies against several of the mutant human hemoglobins have been prepared, and rare hemoglobin S- and C-positive cells are found in normal persons.[433] [434] The procedure has not been adapted for routine testing. Such a measure of somatic mutation would be a powerful addition to the techniques for population monitoring.

In a related approach, variants of the enzyme lactate dehydrogenase X (LDH-X), which is found only in sperm, have been detected in mouse sperm with the use of monospecific antibodies to rat LDH-X.[15] The frequency of variants increases on treatment with procarbazine. Presumably, the expressed phenotype reflects the genotype of the gonial cells, rather than of the haploid sperm, but the evidence is direct for an effect in germ cells. Such a system might well be adapted for use in human subjects.

MUTANT ENZYMES

One of the most useful systems in the study of cell biology has been the hypoxanthine phosphoribosyltransferase (HPRT) locus, an X-linked locus in mammals. Mutations to loss of activity of this enzyme cause resistance to the guanine analogues 8-azaguanine and 6-thioguanine. Thus, wild-type HPRT$^+$ cells can be selected against by incorporation of one of these analogues. Conversely, HPRT$^+$ cells can be selected for in the presence of hypoxanthine-aminopterin-thymidine medium. It should be possible to select for HPRT$^-$ cells in normal HPRT$^+$ persons with one of the analogues, and this was one of the first systems used to detect spontaneously occurring mutants in freshly cultured cells from humans.[88][388]
The frequency of 6-thioguanine-resistant cells has been reported to be about 10^{-4} among peripheral blood lymphocytes of normal persons. The frequency is generally higher among cancer patients on therapy with known mutagens. This system therefore offers the possibility of detecting somatic mutations through selection in lymphocyte cultures. However, the extent to which some variations are phenocopies, rather than mutations, remains to be explored. Recent and more refined experiments have given much lower mutation rates, more consistent with other estimates.[442] The variables that influence the results remain to be elucidated, but the possibility of measuring mutation in somatic cells and documenting the nature of the mutant cells makes this a promising system.

ALKYLATION OF PROTEINS

Alkylating agents react with many cell constituents, including DNA (where mutations often result) and proteins. Although the reaction with proteins has no proven genetic or physiologic consequences, it is a measure of exposure and hence of genetic risk. The protein that is most easily isolated is hemoglobin. The alkylation of hemoglobin, which can be measured by sensitive chemical assays, is therefore a useful reflection of recent exposure to alkylating agents. This approach has been used to measure exposure to ethylene, which must first be converted metabolically to ethylene oxide.[111] [335] [406]

Although this system is very agent-specific and requires additional study, it may prove useful where identity of the agent is known, as in occupational exposures.

BODY FLUIDS

MUTAGENICITY ASSAY OF BODY FLUIDS

A presumption of increased mutational risk can be made, if it can be shown that mutagens are circulating in the blood or are present in other body fluids. This is most readily done by testing the mutagenic activity of blood or urine in microbial systems[513] or in vitro cell-culture systems.[56] [243] Such an assay does not require knowledge of the exposure details or of the metabolism of the environmental agents, although thorough study of any agent would include these. Addition of β-glucuronidase to the sample permits identification of some substances that are made nonmutagenic by conjugation as glucuronides.

The efficacy of testing the mutagenicity of urine has been demonstrated on several occasions. Large-scale screening of persons not known to have been exposed to chemical carcinogens has verified that urine samples typically are not mutagenic in the Salmonella/microsome test. Where positive tests have been obtained, the persons have proved to be on medication with agents known to be mutagenic.[285] The test has also been positive for persons accidentally exposed to the known mutagen epichlor-hydrin.[243]

Although it is not possible to equate mutagenicity of body fluids with actual mutation in the host, it is reasonable to assume that such persons are at increased risk of mutation. An increase in mutagenicity can be detected in individuals, making the test especially useful in assessing exposure of small groups. Two drawbacks are the inability to measure cumulative exposure and the inability to translate the results into a quantitative risk, either for individuals or for populations. Neverthe-less, this test shows promise of being important in evaluating human exposure to many mutagens.

EXCRETION OF ALKYLATED METABOLITES

Alkylation of cell constituents leads to unusual components that may not be completely metabolized, but may be excreted. Löfroth et al.[255] noted the excretion of methylated purines after exposure to dimethyl sulfate and proposed that these compounds originated from methylated nucleic acids. Their presence thus indicated an increased risk of mutation.

A monitoring system based on excretion of metabolites is likely to be useful only when the mutagenic agent is known, as in occupational exposures; and the effect will persist only as long as the exposure. Nevertheless, such an approach may have value in special situations. There is no way to translate such observations into a measure of risk.

CANCER AND CANCER EPIDEMIOLOGY

It is widely believed that mutation is an important part of carcinogenesis.[213] At the very least, many mutagens greatly increase the risk of cancer. In addition to the concern about cancer rates themselves, increases in cancer should trigger concern that mutations in general have increased.

Cancer typically has a long latent period, which will complicate the identification of the agent responsible. There also are many problems involved in setting up cancer registries that are representative of a defined population. Nevertheless, careful epidemiologic investigations have identified responsible agents, especially for cancers of unusual types.[281] Monitoring of cancer incidence through registries or other means is worth while, both for direct information on cancer and for possible information on mutational risk.

The monitoring system most relevant to health, and indirectly to mutagenesis, in the present generation is cancer epidemiology. Substantial evidence relating mutagenesis to carcinogenesis encourages us to accept the induction of cancer as reasonable evidence of increased risk of mutation. In spite of the shortage of epidemiologists, there are people knowledgeable in cancer epidemiology, and many excellent studies are being conducted. These studies should be continued, expanded in some cases, and modified to be more sensitive to human exposure to chemical mutagens. Because the latent period between exposure and the appearance of malignant tumors is long, epidemiologic studies can never provide immediate answers to questions on the risk of current chemical exposure. However, as a measure of exposure, cancer probably does give useful information on cumulative risk and cumulative genetic risk.

REPRODUCTION

SPERM MORPHOLOGY

Sperm are available from half the adult population, and their morphologic characteristics can be evaluated rather simply by microscopic examination. Many agents are known to influence human sperm morphology (reviewed in Wyrobek and Bruce[509]). Most agents known to be mutagens in other test systems also cause an increase in morphologically abnormal sperm,[462] although the mechanism by which this occurs is unknown. Furthermore, the dose-response relationship and the sensitivity of the response to various agents are unknown. It has nevertheless been suggested that monitoring of sperm is a simple and valuable way to become aware of potential exposure to mutagens. Its greatest value may be in monitoring persons exposed occupationally.

FERTILITY

A commonly used test in experimental animals is the dominant-lethal test, generally assumed to monitor the induction of chromosomally abnormal sperm. There are reports of loss of fertility of human males exposed to various chemicals. It is difficult to attribute such effects to genetic events, rather than to cellular effects. An increase in genetically defective sperm, detected by a decrease in fertility, would require a very large and carefully controlled study. The use of birth control and the changing social patterns of family size virtually rule out evidence on fertility as useful in monitoring mutagenesis.

PHENOTYPIC EFFECTS IN CHILDREN OF EXPOSED PARENTS

Much thought has been directed to the possibility of selecting sentinel phenotypes that result, at least in part, from mutation and that can be used to measure increases in mutation rate. Only a small number of single-gene traits that would be especially useful for this purpose have been identified. However, because the frequency of mutation is so low, a very large population is necessary to estimate or detect a change in the frequency of new mutants. This problem could be solved in part if there were complete and readily accessible health records for large political units. Newcombe[320] has studied the problem of computer linkage with public records.

The Centers for Disease Control (CDC) has a Birth Defects Surveillance Program. Approximately one-third of the births in the United States each year are monitored for defects. Any significant increase in specific defects or any geographic or temporal cluster of defects would be detected rapidly. Such an effect would be followed up by an intensive investigation into the causal agents. The CDC surveillance data reported between 1977 and 1979 showed no increase in birth defects across the nation. That is mildly reassuring, in view of the known introduction of many new chemicals into the environment during that period. One should be cautious, however, about feeling reassured by these negative data.

One shortcoming of this approach is that the time between mutation and conception might be very long, making it difficult to relate an increase in inherited defect to the responsible agent. On the positive side is the fact that clinical defects are part of the concern with chemical mutagens, and the relevance to human risk and health load is direct.

MONITORING TECHNIQUES OF GREATEST POTENTIAL

CHROMOSOMAL ANALYSIS OF PERIPHERAL LYMPHOCYTES

Many mutagens break chromosomes, and there is substantial experience in the measurement of the effects of such agents as ionizing radiation on the chromosomes of peripheral lymphocytes. Many technical problems have been identified and solved. Analysis of chromosomes is relatively expensive and time-consuming and must be done by or under the direct supervision of experienced cytogeneticists. Thus, it is impractical to use chromosome monitoring except for special populations, such as those of industrial workers with known or suspected exposure to mutagens. In these situations, it is recommended that analysis of chromosomes in peripheral lymphocytes be a routine part of health surveillance. One must be cautious in the interpretation, however. Whereas people who have been exposed to mutagenic chemicals and exhibit increased chromosomal abnormalities are thought to be at greater risk of mutation and cancer, there is no direct evidence that they are at a higher risk than others in the population who have been exposed. Chromosomes tell us about populations, but not about individuals. We also do not know how to extrapolate chromosomal damage into risk estimation. The data are more useful as indicators of exposure than of genetic damage. Additional research may reveal other information.

BODY-FLUID ANALYSIS

The various microbial systems used to test blood and urine are useful measures of mutagenic exposure. Positive results cannot be interpreted in terms of health risk, but negative results can be reassuring. These tests are especially useful in monitoring occupational exposure, because such exposure is discovered promptly. Analysis of body fluids should be used in all situations in which positive results are interpreted as indexes of exposure.

SISTER CHROMATID EXCHANGE

It is premature to recommend SCE for routine testing of mutagenic exposure, but the results are sufficiently encouraging to urge its widespread use to learn more about the variables that influence the results. In the case of x-ray exposure, SCE is a sensitive indicator of genetic effects, but this may not be true for some or all chemical mutagens. There is little basis for translating SCE results into health risk. Nevertheless, to test its validity, measures of SCE should be incorporated into studies of special exposure groups.

9

A MUTAGEN ASSESSMENT PROGRAM

Before a program to assess mutagenic chemicals can be devised, a set of critical factors should be considered. These include the potential risks of mutation, the strengths and weaknesses of short-term tests, the difficulties of extrapolating from screening tests and tests with small mammals to a statement of possible human genetic damage, and the even more difficult problem of relating human genetic damage to effects on welfare of future generations. These factors have been discussed in previous chapters. In particular, we have emphasized the contrast between the enormous technical advances in short-term tests and the inability to assess human impact adequately.

In devising a mutagen assessment program, we acknowledge that the attempt is tentative. Certainly, progress will demand continued modification of any scheme of this nature. Completion of the GENE-TOX Program of the Environmental Protection Agency may provide useful information for revision. Thus, our recommendation should be regarded as an interim one.

The recommended program has five levels:

1. Screening of a large number of chemicals with short-term tests.
2. Classification of chemicals by mutagenic potency in individual test systems.
3. Consideration of available animal carcinogenicity data.
4. Further testing of chemicals that are of special importance.
5. Risk estimation, if a risk-benefit analysis is required.

203

AN OVERVIEW OF THE MUTAGEN ASSESSMENT PROGRAM

Figure 9-1 is a flowchart of the testing program. To emphasize that there is no means to determine directly whether a substance causes human germinal mutations, we use the expression "mammalian mutagen" for a substance that is mutagenic in the mouse or other mammal. The

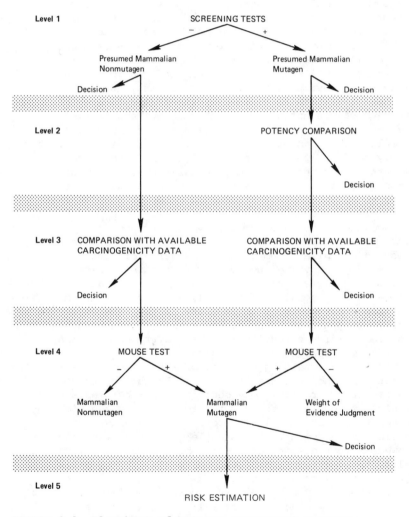

FIGURE 9-1 Flowchart of mutagen assessment program.

determination that a substance is a mammalian mutagen constitutes a strong presumption that the substance is mutagenic in man as well, but we reserve the expression "human mutagen" for the time when direct human germ-cell assessments become possible.

Screening tests are a set of short-term tests chosen to detect different kinds of genetic end points and to represent phylogenetically different organisms (Table 9-1). A positive result in a single properly conducted and duplicated test defines an agent as a mutagen. The results of screening tests designate the compound as a "presumed mammalian mutagen" or a "presumed mammalian nonmutagen." It is a presumed mammalian mutagen only if results are positive in two or more screening tests that involve different end points or divergent test systems.

Classification as a presumed mammalian mutagen or nonmutagen may itself be sufficient information for a risk-benefit evaluation. If the screening test results are negative, this is ordinarily taken as evidence that the chemical is not a mammalian mutagen, because the short-term tests are very sensitive and encompass a number of relevant end points. However, if the chemical is to be widely used or if people are likely to be exposed to large amounts, additional tests may be desirable. Likewise, a compound that produces positive results in one or more tests may have benefits that could outweigh a small risk and therefore necessitate further tests.

Knowledge of mutagenic potency is not required to classify a substance as a presumed mammalian mutagen or presumed mammalian nonmutagen. However, relative potency may be of great value in deciding to continue testing (Level 2). For example, if the substance is weakly mutagenic and socially beneficial, additional tests may be justified that would be unnecessary if the substance were highly mutagenic or of no great benefit. We suggest later a scale by which to assign mutagens to groups according to relative mutagenic potency in a test system.

For the overwhelming majority of tested chemicals, we expect that the screening tests will be sufficient for a manufacturing or regulatory decision. Further tests can consist of supplementary short-term tests. These might be chosen to confirm or clarify results pertaining to a particular end point. For example, if the screening tests showed an increase in chromosomal breaks in mammalian cells, this pattern could be confirmed in a Drosophila chromosomal-rearrangement test.

For especially difficult or important decisions, rodent tests are recommended (Figure 9-1). If the result is clearly positive, the substance is a mammalian mutagen,

TABLE 9-1 Mutagen Test Systems

Principal Short-Term Tests

A. Gene mutation
   1. Microbial test with and without metabolic activation:
      Salmonella reversion tests
   2. Mammalian cell-culture test with and without metabolic activation:
      HGPRT or TK
   3. Drosophila X-linked lethal test

B. Chromosomal mutation
   In vitro mammalian cell test with and without metabolic activation

C. Genomic mutation
   No short-term test has been adequately developed and validated;
   when this has been done, such a test should be included

Mouse Tests for Confirmation or Risk Estimation

A. For confirmation
   1. Specific-locus test (perhaps preceded by spot test)
   2. Dominant-lethal test

B. For risk estimation
   1. Dominant-mutation tests (skeletal and cataract)
   2. Heritable-translocation test

Supplementary Tests

A. DNA damage
   1. Direct assays of DNA damage
   2. Unscheduled DNA synthesis
   3. Sister chromatid exchange
   4. Yeast mitotic crossing-over and gene conversion

B. Alternatives to S-9 metabolic activation
   1. Mammalian cell homogenate
   2. Host-mediated assay

C. Acquisition of tumor-like traits by cultured mammalian cells
   ("neoplastic transformation")

D. Additional mutation tests
   1. Tests using E. coli and other bacteria
   2. Fungal tests
   3. Drosophila chromosome tests
   4. Mouse spot test
   5. Other mouse tests (aneuploidy and micronucleus)

regardless of the outcome of short-term tests. However, if the result is negative, the decision depends on the short-term test results. If these are negative, then a negative result in a mouse test confirms that the compound is a mammalian nonmutagen. If the short-term test results are positive, a negative result in a mouse test creates an ambiguous situation (discussed later).

Most potentially mutagenic compounds are likely to be tested for carcinogenicity (Level 3). The results of such testing, perhaps with the results from short-term mutagenicity tests, may be sufficient for a decision. In that case, a mouse test for mutagenicity is not needed, and limited mammalian mutation-testing resources can be conserved.

If carcinogenicity data are unavailable or inconclusive, the next step (Level 4) is to test for mutagenicity in the mouse. In many cases, the presence or absence of mutagenicity in the short-term tests and in the mouse may be sufficient evidence for a decision. In the most difficult cases, a quantitative risk estimate may be needed.

SCREENING SYSTEMS

The success of a mutagen assessment program depends strongly on the efficacy of the screening system, for most of the decisions regarding individual chemicals must be made on the basis of short-term screening tests. The criteria for choosing test systems are discussed in Chapter 6. On the basis of these criteria, the Committee has selected a set of tests, listed as "principal short-term tests" in Table 9-1. Confirmatory rodent tests and supplementary tests are also listed.

There are three end points to be tested: gene mutations, chromosomal mutations, and genomic mutations. Excellent short-term tests are available for gene mutations. The most thoroughly examined and widely used is the Salmonella/-microsome system developed by Ames and his associates. Coupled with appropriate activation systems, this is the principal test among microbial systems. Among mammalian systems, the hypoxanthine-guanine phosphoribosyl transferase (HGPRT) system in Chinese hamster cells (V79 or CHO) and the thymidine kinase (TK) system in mouse lymphoma cells are well developed. The third gene-mutation test selects for recessive-lethal mutations in Drosophila; the Muller-5 system is most popular for detecting X-linked recessive lethal mutations.

To detect chromosomal mutations, mammalian cell-culture

systems can be used with and without metabolic activation. In vitro cytogenetic tests are well validated and widely used. In addition, there are Drosophila tests for detecting chromosomal rearrangements, but they are more expensive than cell-culture tests. The most widely used Drosophila test monitors translocations on the basis of altered linkage associations of marker genes. As far as is known, substances that induce chromosomal rearrangements in Drosophila also induce recessive lethal mutations; this is as expected, inasmuch as some chromosomal changes produce recessive lethal effects. Thus, the Drosophila germinal test encompasses two mutational events. There is little point in doing a chromosomal-rearrangement test with an X-linked-lethal test, except to confirm the result of an in vitro mammalian cytogenetic assay or for more detailed analysis of mechanisms.

No short-term genomic mutation tests have been validated sufficiently to warrant recommendation as routine short-term screening tests. Tests for detection of aneuploidy are being developed in fungi, field vole, and Drosophila. As such tests become standardized and validated, they should be added to the assessment system. It is likely that chemicals that induce aneuploidy will not be detectable in other systems, because they may react with a proteinaceous target, rather than act on DNA directly.

Table 9-1 lists a group of mouse tests that can be used for confirmation if, for any reason, mammalian germinal tests are deemed necessary. It may sometimes be desirable, before a germinal test, to do a somatic spot test, which is more sensitive and less expensive than germinal tests. It may help to provide guidance as to appropriate concentrations and other experimental conditions.

Our suggested test program uses two tiers of short-term tests, as listed in Table 9-2. Tier I consists of a Salmonella reversion test, a mammalian cell-culture gene-mutation test (using either HGPRT or TK), and a mammalian cell chromosomal-breakage test. All tests should be conducted with and without metabolic activation. If all three tests are negative, the chemical is classified as a presumed mammalian nonmutagen. If two or all three of the three tests are clearly positive, the chemical is classified as a presumed mammalian mutagen. The combination of a positive result in one test and negative results in two tests is ambiguous, and the system moves to Tier II--the Drosophila X-linked-lethal test. If this test is positive, the substance is classified as a presumed mammalian mutagen; if it is negative, the substance is considered to be a presumed mammalian nonmutagen. If both mammalian in vitro

TABLE 9-2 A Decision Function for Short-Term Tests

Tier I	Tier II
1. Salmonella/microsome gene mutation 2. Mammalian cell gene mutation (HGPRT or TK) 3. Mammalian cell chromosomal breakage	4. Drosophila X-linked lethal mutation

Decision Function
MM - Presumed mammalian mutagen
MN - Presumed mammalian nonmutagen
M - Mutagen
? - Go to Tier II

Outcome in Test				Decision
1	2	3	4	
+	+	+		MM
+	+	−		MM
+	−	+		MM
−	+	+		MM
+	−	−		M?
−	+	−		M?
−	−	+		M?
−	−	−		MN
			+	MM
			−	MN

gene-mutation tests (HGPRT and TK) are done and the result of either is positive, we recommend that the outcome in this test system be regarded as positive.

We do not intend to imply that this is the only possible decision function. For example, a chemical may already have undergone several tests not included in this system. In such circumstances, a weight-of-evidence approach is appropriate, as described in the EPA proposed guidelines for mutagenicity risk assessment.[475]

Many of the tests listed as supplementary in Table 9-1 have very desirable properties. With further research and validation, we can expect the set of useful tests to increase further. It may often be possible to resolve ambiguous, inconsistent, or doubtful cases by further tests and perhaps in this way avoid using mouse tests. Supplementary tests are also useful when the primary tests are inappropriate. For example, Drosophila is not suitable for testing insecticides.

EVALUATION OF THE ASSESSMENT PROGRAM

To evaluate the assessment program empirically, we obtained data on 3,251 chemicals that had been reviewed at the Environmental Mutagen Information Center for 23 tests. From this group, we selected information on nine tests included among either the principal or supplementary tests in our program; five of these are in our two screening tiers. Thirty-six chemicals had been tested thoroughly enough in these five tests for conclusions to be reached through our decision function (Table 9-2). These are listed as Groups A and B in Table 9-3. Group C includes some special cases that are discussed later.

The data in these tables have been critically reviewed by peer committees and represent the consensus of these committees. We have learned of later information that would change some of the items, but because not all the data could be reviewed, we have left the table intact in the interest of consistency.

It is apparent that the chemicals have been tested haphazardly; that is not surprising, inasmuch as there is no agreed-on testing system. It is also clear that this sample of chemicals constitutes a set most of which would be classified as presumed mammalian mutagens by our assessment program. Unfortunately, negative results often go unpublished. People doing research are reluctant to present negative results, and journals are reluctant to publish them. Yet, such results are important for the evaluation of test systems and for regulatory decisions. We suggest that there be a central repository for negative results; it could issue periodic lists of chemicals that yielded such results, and interested parties could obtain the details from the repository.

Group A in Table 9-3 consists of 33 chemicals that would have been classified as presumed mammalian mutagens on the basis of Tier I testing. The internal consistency of Tier I tests in this group is high; for example, only three of the 33 chemicals had negative results in the Salmonella/microsome test. Of the 33 chemicals, 20 were subjected to the Drosophila X-linked recessive lethal test, and 19 had positive results. Note that there are only two cases of a discrepancy between L51 and V79. Benzo[a]pyrene probably does not represent a real inconsistency; although it is listed as negative for V79 by the Environmental Mutagen Information Center, it has

TABLE 9-3 Results of Mutagenicity Tests[a] of Various Widely Tested Chemicals[b]

Chemical	Tier I Tests				Tier II Test	Supplementary Tests			
	Sal	L51	V79	CYC	SRL	UDS	SCE	DLT	SLT
Group A--Classified as presumed mammalian mutagen on the basis of Tier I tests:									
Mitomycin C	-	+		+	+	+	+	+	+
Cyclophosphamide	+	+		+	+		+	+	+
DDT	-		+	+	-			+	
Dibenz[a,h]anthracene	+		+		+	-			
Diethylnitrosamine	+	+	+	+	+	+		-	-
3-Methylcholanthrene	+		+	-	+	+	+		
Benz[a]anthracene	+		+			-			
Quinoline	+			+	+	+	+		
2-Oxetanone	+	+				+	+		
Dimethylbenzanthracene	+		+			+	+		
Amethopterine	-	+		+		-	+	+	+
Ethyl methanesulfonate	+	+	+		+	+/-	+	+	
Dimethylnitrosamine	+	+	+	+	+	+/-	+	+	
Methyl methanesulfonate	+	+	+		+	+	+	+	+
N-Methyl-N'-nitro-N-nitrosoguanidine	+	+	+		+	+	+	+	
Epoxystyrene	+		+		+	+		-	
2-Amino-4-nitroaniline	+			+	+		+	+	
ICR 70	+		+		+			-	
Benzo[b]triphenylene	+		+			-			

Compound							
Methylnitrosourea	+	+	+	+	+	+	−
Aflatoxin B1	+	+	+	+	+	+	−
Furylfuramide	+	+	+	+	+		
N-Ethyl-N-nitroso-N'-nitroguanidine	+	+	+	+	+	+	−
Nitro-p-phenylenediamine	+	+		+	+	+	−
N-Acetoxy-2-acetylaminofluorene	+	+	+	+	+	+	+
Sodium nitrite	+	+	+	+	+		−
Benz[a]anthracene^c	+	+	+	+	+		
Daunomycin	+	+	+	+	+	+	
Hycanthone methanesulfonate	+	+		+	+	+	−
Sodium azide	+	+	+	−	+	+	
4-Acetylaminofluorene	+	−	−	−			
Benzo[a]pyrene	+	−	+	+	+		
2-Acetylaminofluorene	+	+	+/−	+	+		−

Group B--Classified as presumed mammalian mutagen on the basis of Tier II test:

Compound							
Caffeine	−	−	+	+	+		−
Styrene	+/−	−	−	+	+		+
Procarbazine hydrochloride	−	+	+	+	+	+	
Methylazoxymethanol acetate	+	+	+	+			

TABLE 9-3 continued

Chemical	Tier I Tests				Tier II Test	Supplementary Tests			
	Sal	L51	V79	CYC	SRL	UDS	SCE	DLT	SLT
Group C--Special cases:									
Ethanol	-			-			-	+	
Fluothane	-		-		+				
Captan	+/-		+		-	-		+	
TPA	-	-					+		

a. Sal = Salmonella/microsome.
    L51 = L5178Y/TK$^+$/- mouse lymphoma cell line.
    V79 = Chinese hamster lund cell-line specific locus.
    CYC = Mammalian cell-culture cytogenetic.
    SRL = Drosophila recessive lethal.
    UDS = Unscheduled DNA synthesis.
    SCE = Sister chromatid exchange.
    DLT = Mouse dominant-lethal mutation.
    SLT = Mouse specific locus.
  b. This information represents the consensus evaluation of EMIC, which is accurate for data published through December 1981. Results for individual chemicals may not reflect recent experimental evidence.
  c. 7-(Bromomethyl)-12-methylbenzanthracene.

been reported as a mutagen in the review of Bradley et al.[37] (see Table 9-4).

Group B consists of four chemicals whose classification might not have been possible on the basis of Tier I tests, but that would be considered presumed mammalian mutagens because of their positive response in the Tier II test. Some of these might have been classified as presumed mammalian mutagens on the basis of Tier I tests alone, if all four Tier I tests had been used.

Examination of Groups A and B shows that in the over-whelming majority of these cases a decision would have been reached on the basis of Tier I tests alone. The more expensive Drosophila tests would not be needed most of the time. Note, however, that the collection of chemicals in Table 9-3 is biased in favor of definite and strong mutagens, because these are more fully represented in the literature. A group of chemicals containing weak mutagens might have led to less consistent decisions. For example, 2-acetyl-aminofluorene gave inconsistent outcomes of the two gene-mutation tests that used mammalian cell lines. In our scheme, it should also be tested for mammalian cytogenetic effects; if the results are negative, Tier II testing would be required. The failure to find mutagenesis in CHO cells might have been due to insufficient concentration or time of metabolic activation.

The dominant-lethal test is recommended as one of the mouse tests. The deaths are thought to be caused by chromosomal breakage--a conclusion supported by the correlation between this and direct tests of translocations in the mouse. The dominant-lethal test has been found positive for several chemicals that are negative or very weakly positive in direct mouse tests of heritable translocations.[135] Therefore, it appears to be more sensitive than mouse germinal translocation tests, although from the table it appears less sensitive than short-term tests. As mentioned before, the dominant-lethal test may in some cases be detecting effects that are nongenetic or that effect embryos so young as to have little human impact.

Nine chemicals are shown for the specific-locus test. Five are positive. The negatives, as discussed elsewhere in this report, may be due to insufficient numbers or to differences in such things as repair systems, tissue distribution, cell selection, and metabolic activation or inactivation.

Another observation from Table 9-3 is the sensitivity of the sister chromatid exchange (SCE) test and its general agreement with the tier tests. Every tested chemical that produced positive results in the tier system also gave positive results for SCEs. The Committee seriously considered adding SCE tests to the Tier I test battery.

However, in Chapter 6 we state that the test system should detect actual mutations. SCEs are not the same as mutations, and their effect on future generations is not clear. Mainly for this reason, a majority of the Committee prefer not to include SCEs in the tier system.

In Chapter 6, we also say that a system measuring some other end point could be validated by showing that it predicts mutation. The data in Table 9-3 show that mutagens detected by the test systems also produce SCEs. If the trend continues--substances negative by mutation criteria being negative also for SCEs--then the simplicity and low cost of the test would argue for its inclusion in the battery of recommended tests. A demonstration of a causal connection between SCE and mutation would also justify inclusion.

In vivo SCE tests can be especially useful in measuring the tissue distribution of a mutagen. Finding SCEs in a cell demonstrates that the substance or a derivative did indeed reach and affect the chromosomes. This can help in assessing the likely human damage of a chemical demonstrated to be mutagenic in short-term tests. It can also be useful in carcinogenicity testing.

Results of tests for unscheduled DNA synthesis are less consistent with the other results. This suggests that these tests are not yet ready for routine use in a test battery. As data on unscheduled DNA synthesis in mouse spermatids accumulate, this test may become more useful.

Group C of Table 9-3 consists of some special cases that had inconsistent, ambiguous, or puzzling results. Ethanol has been negative in all tests except the mouse dominant-lethal test. It should be tested further. More dose-response data and supplemental tests might be especially helpful.

Fluothane was negative in two Tier I tests (and not subjected to the third), but was positive in the Drosophila test. If fluothane had also had a negative result in the mammalian cytogenetic test, it would be the only example in this series of a substance that was mutagenic according to the Tier II test but was not detected in Tier I.

Captan had one ambiguous result and one positive result in the two Tier I tests used. It was also positive in the mouse dominant-lethal test. Because results in the Drosophila test were negative, captan is a doubtful mutagen that requires more testing.

TPA is an example of a substance with a possible false-positive result in the SCE test, but again the data are too fragmentary to permit any conclusion.

We conclude that the assessment program in this chapter is effective for detection of mutagens. Among the results on chemicals that have been fully tested in our tier system, there are no false-negatives by the criterion of being negative in the short-term tests and positive in the mouse test. Ethanol and TPA might have false-negative results, but neither has been tested fully. However, we have no way of knowing whether our system would produce false-positives--substances that are deemed mutagens by our criteria, but are not mutagenic in man. There are no human data to provide definitive information.

CLASSIFYING MUTAGENS BY STRENGTH OF MUTAGENICITY

Classifying chemicals into those which produce a significant increase in mutation in test systems and those which do not is usually sufficient for a decision regarding mutagenic risk. The potency of the mutagen then is not a factor. In more complex cases, a quantitative classification is required. As mentioned earlier, there are usually inconsistencies in the potency of a chemical among different tests. Yet, if chemicals are put into 5-10 potency groups, the rank order is roughly preserved.

It seems simple and reasonable to divide potency values into geometrically equal intervals for a given test system. This is preferable to simple percentile ranking, because to some extent it takes potency ratios into account. A logarithmic scale provides a broader range than an arithmetic scale. It also takes advantage of the typical pharmacologic finding that the distribution of susceptibility has a log-normal, rather than a normal distribution. That this scaling is suitable is shown by the roughly symmetrical frequency distribution in Table 9-6. The scale we are suggesting provides scores that are independent of the units in which concentration is measured.

The Committee also considered a scheme in which the range of mutagenic potencies, arranged from lowest to highest, was divided into a small, fixed number of geometrically equal intervals. The idea behind this is that, if the ranges differ greatly from one test system to another, we might make the scale easier to interpret by normalizing the values to fit a fixed number of intervals.

Essentially this principle was used by Clive.[66] This would be especially advantageous if the scores from different tests were to be averaged.

However, the alternative of dividing the scale logarithmically seemed likely to be simpler and more easily interpreted by most users. We expect that most decision-makers would prefer to have separate data from each of the tests, rather than some sort of average, and this preference removes one of the strongest reasons for normalizing.

Therefore, we proceed as follows: Suppose that the least potent chemical subjected to a given test produces a potency value of X, which falls in the range 10^k - 10^{k+1} units. Then each chemical examined with this test would be assigned to one of the following potency groups:

Group 1: potency value between 10^k and 10^{k+1},
Group 2: potency value between 10^{k+1} and 10^{k+2},
Group 3: potency value between 10^{k+2} and 10^{k+3},

and so on, until the highest observed value is categorized. Chemicals that produce no significant mutagenic effect are assigned to Group 0.

Although the range of potencies for different test systems is expected to vary, it is unlikely that any system would have more than 10 potency groups. For the various chemicals tested in V79 Chinese hamster cells and in the Salmonella/microsome tests, which are listed in Tables 9-4 and 9-5, eight potency groups were generated for each assay. The numbers of chemicals per potency range are given in Table 9-6.

As mentioned earlier, if the number of potency groups were to differ markedly among a set of test systems, an investigator might elect to standardize the grouping to a common number of potency groups--for example, by using logarithms to a different base for each group. However, there is some satisfaction in knowing that for the unstandardized grouping the difference between two chemicals in adjacent groups is approximately an order of magnitude.

The data in Tables 9-4 and 9-5 include 23 chemicals that have been tested in both systems. The values for these are given in Table 9-7 and plotted in Figure 9-2. It is clear that, when the data are plotted as logarithms, there is a rough linear relationship. The correlation coefficient is 0.74. (When the two outliers at the lower right are omitted, the correlation becomes 0.89.)

The high correlation is not surprising, inasmuch as the two tests are intended to detect the same end point, gene mutations. The graph shows that a rough classification of

TABLE 9-4 Arrangement of Data of Chemical Mutagenic Potency in V79
Chinese Hamster Cells[a]

Chemical	Potency[b]
Group 1	Range 10^{-5}–10^{-4}
1-Nitrosopyrolidine	1.0×10^{-5}
N-Nitrosomorpholine	1.5×10^{-5}
Dipropylnitrosamine	2.4×10^{-5}
Diethylnitrosamine	4.8×10^{-5}
1-Methyl-4-nitrosopiperazine	7.7×10^{-5}
3-β-D-Glucopyranosyl-1-methyl-1-nitrosourea	9.0×10^{-5}
Group 2	Range 10^{-4}–10^{-3}
Dimethylnitrosamine	1.3×10^{-4}
Methylpropylnitrosamine	1.4×10^{-4}
Methylazoxymethanol acetate	4.5×10^{-4}
Ethyl methanesulfonate	7.1×10^{-4}
Dipentylnitrosamine	7.7×10^{-4}
Group 3	Range 10^{-3}–10^{-2}
N'-(Trichloromethylthio)-4-cyclohexane	1.0×10^{-3}
Dibutylnitrosamine	1.0×10^{-3}
2-Deoxy-2-(3-methyl-3-nitrosoureido-)-D- glucopyranose	1.3×10^{-3}
Methyl methanesulfonate	1.5×10^{-3}
Furylfuramide	3.1×10^{-3}
cis-Benzo[a]pyrene-4,5-dihydrodiol	5.8×10^{-3}
p,p'-DDE	6.0×10^{-3}
cis-3-Methylcholanthrene-11,12-dihydrodiol	8.2×10^{-3}
Methylnitrosourea	8.4×10^{-3}
Benz[a]anthracene-8,9-diol-10,11-epoxide	9.3×10^{-3}
Group 4	Range 10^{-2}–10^{-1}
Streptozotocin tetraacetate	1.5×10^{-2}
7-Methylbenz[a]anthracene	1.5×10^{-2}
5-Hydroxydibenz[a,h]anthracene	1.6×10^{-2}
1-Hydroxybenzo[a]pyrene	1.6×10^{-2}
Benzo[a]pyrene-3,6-quinone	2.0×10^{-2}
6-Hydroxybenzo[a]pyrene	2.2×10^{-2}
3-Hydroxybenzo[a]pyrene	2.4×10^{-2}
Benzo[a]pyrene-11,12-epoxide	2.6×10^{-2}
1-Hydroxy-3-methylcholanthrene	2.8×10^{-2}

TABLE 9-4   continued

Chemical	Potency[b]
p,p'-DDT	3.0×10^{-2}
Benz[a]anthracene-10,11-diol-8,9-epoxide	4.0×10^{-2}
trans-Benzo[a]pyrene-11,12-dihydrodiol	4.2×10^{-2}
Benzo[a]pyrene-4,5-epoxide	4.7×10^{-2}
5'-Bromodeoxyuridine	5.6×10^{-2}
Benz[a]anthracene-5,6-dihydroepoxide	6.5×10^{-2}
5-Hydroxydibenz[a,h]anthracene	7.4×10^{-2}
Group 5	Range 10^{-1}-10^0
Dibenz[a,c]anthracene	1.0×10^{-1}
3-Methylcholanthrene-11,12-epoxide	2.2×10^{-1}
MNNG	2.9×10^{-1}
N-Acetoxy-2-acetylaminofluorene	5.9×10^{-1}
Cytosine arabinoside	7.7×10^{-1}
Group 6	Range 10^0-10^1
7,12-Dimethylbenz[a]anthracene	1.6×10^0
3-Methylcholanthrene	2.2×10^0
7-8-Dihydrobenzo[a]pyrene-7,8-epoxide	2.5×10^0
7-Bromomethylbenz[a]anthracene	3.4×10^0
ICR-170	3.8×10^0
(±)-trans-Benzo[a]pyrene-7,8-dihydrodiol-9,10-epoxide	5.0×10^0
7-Methylbenz[a]anthracene-5,6-epoxide	5.0×10^0
1,2-Epoxy-1,2,3,4-tetrahydrobenz[a]anthracene	6.9×10^0
Group 7	Range 10^1-10^2
Adriamycin	1.0×10^1
Tetrahydrobenzo[a]pyrene	1.0×10^1
Benzo[a]pyrene	1.4×10^1
Daunorubicin	3.3×10^1
Group 8	Range 10^2-10^3
7,8-dihydrodiol-9,10-epoxide	2.0×10^2

_____

a. Data from Bradley et al.[37]

b. Mutagenic potency was defined by Bradley et al. as the concentration (μM) that increases mutation frequency 10-fold above spontaneous background, calculated over a certain dose range and assuming a linear dose-response relationship.

These data are expressed as reciprocals to give an ascending scale, in accordance with model groupings.

TABLE 9-5 Arrangement of Data of Chemical Mutagenic
Potency in the Salmonella/microsome Test[a]

Chemical	Potency[b]
Group 1	Range $10^{-3}-10^{-2}$
Ethyl p-toluenesulfonate	5.0×10^{-3}
1,2-Epoxybutane	6.0×10^{-3}
Group 2	Range $10^{-2}-10^{-1}$
Diethylnitrosamine	1.0×10^{-2}
Benzyl chloride	2.0×10^{-2}
N-Nitrosopyrrolidine	2.0×10^{-2}
Dimethylnitrosamine	2.0×10^{-2}
Dimethylcarbamyl chloride	4.0×10^{-2}
N-Nitrosomorpholine	6.0×10^{-2}
Di-n-propylnitrosamine	8.0×10^{-2}
Group 3	Range $10^{-1}-10^{0}$
1,2,7,8-Diepoxyoctane	1.0×10^{-1}
1,2,3,4-Diepoxybutane	1.2×10^{-1}
N-Methyl-4-aminoazobenzene	1.4×10^{-1}
Di-n-butylnitrosamine	1.5×10^{-1}
2-Nitrosonaphthalene	1.6×10^{-1}
Ethyl methanesulfonate	1.6×10^{-1}
5-Nitro-2-furoic acid	2.6×10^{-1}
Isophosphamide	2.6×10^{-1}
4-Aminoazobenzene	2.9×10^{-1}
Melphalan	2.9×10^{-1}
4-Acetylaminofluorene	3.0×10^{-1}
N-Hydroxy-4-aminoazobenzene	3.5×10^{-1}
Styrene oxide	3.7×10^{-1}
Uracil mustard	4.0×10^{-1}
α-Naphthylamine	4.2×10^{-1}
2,4-Diaminotoluene	4.3×10^{-1}
2,3-Epoxy-1-propanol (glycidol)	5.8×10^{-1}
Benzo[e]pyrene	6.0×10^{-1}
Methyl methanesulfonate	6.3×10^{-1}
Group 4	Range $10^{0}-10^{1}$
1-(2-Hydroxyethyl)-2-methyl-5-nitro-imidazole (metronidazole)	1.1×10^{0}
N-Nitrosoethylurea	1.1×10^{0}
Methylbis(2-chloroethyl)amine	1.3×10^{0}
Cyclophosphamide	1.4×10^{0}
Benzidine	1.4×10^{0}
Azobenzene	1.4×10^{0}
p-Dimethylaminobenzenediazo sodium sulfonate	1.8×10^{0}
Propyleneimine	2.0×10^{0}
Ethyleneimine	2.0×10^{0}
Aflatoxin B2	2.1×10^{0}
Chrysene-5,6-oxide	2.2×10^{0}
1'-Acetoxysafrole	2.4×10^{0}

TABLE 9-5 continued

Chemical	Potency[b]
Hycanthone methanesulfonate	2.5×10^0
4,4'-methylenebis-2-chloroaniline	2.7×10^0
1,1-Diphenyl-2-propynyl-$\underline{N}$-cyclohexyl carbamate	2.8×10^0
1,2-Dimethyl-5-nitroimidazole	3.5×10^0
β-Propiolactone	4.1×10^0
$\underline{N}$-Nitrosomethylurea	4.4×10^0
10-Chloromethyl-9-methylanthracene	4.6×10^0
Dibenz[a,h]anthracene-5,6-oxide	5.3×10^0
5-Nitro-2-furamidoxime	5.3×10^0
Chlornaphazin	5.6×10^0
1,3-Propane sulfone	6.6×10^0
1-Phenyl-1-(3,4-xylyl)-2-propynyl-$\underline{N}$-cyclohexyl carbamate	7.5×10^0
Diazoacetylglycine hydrazide	7.9×10^0
β-Naphthylamine	8.5×10^0
2-Nitrobiphenyl	8.7×10^0
7,9-Dimethylbenz[c]acridine	9.4×10^0
2,7-Bisacetylaminofluorene	9.5×10^0
Group 5	Range 10^1-10^2
9-Aminoacridine	1.0×10^1
Benz[a]anthracene	1.1×10^1
Dibenz[a,h]anthracene	1.1×10^1
4-Nitrobiphenyl	1.1×10^1
o-Aminoazotoluene	1.5×10^1
7-10-Dimethylbenz[c]acridine	1.5×10^1
Diazoacetylglycine ethyl ester	1.7×10^1
2-Nitrofluorene	1.8×10^1
Dibenzo[a,j]acridine	1.8×10^1
4-Amino-$\underline{trans}$-stilbene	1.9×10^1
7,12-Dimethylbenz[a]anthracene	1.9×10^1
2,3-Epoxypropionaldehyde (glycidaldehyde)	1.9×10^1
Dibenzo[a,i]pyrene	2.0×10^1
7,8-Dihydrobenzo[a]pyrene	2.0×10^1
7-Bromomethyl-12-methylbenz[a]anthracene	2.0×10^1
β-Naphthylhydroxylamine	2.1×10^1
2,7-Diaminofluorene	2.2×10^1
1-Aminoanthracene	2.2×10^1
4-Dimethylamino-$\underline{trans}$-stilbene	2.2×10^1
7-Methylbenz[a]anthracene	2.2×10^1
1-Aminopyrene	2.3×10^1
Captan	2.5×10^1
Diazoacetylglycine amide	2.8×10^1
7-Hydroxymethyl-12-methylbenz[a]anthracene	3.0×10^1
4-Aminobiphenyl	3.1×10^1
10-Bromomethylanthracene	3.5×10^1
Chrysene	3.8×10^1
Proflavin	3.8×10^1
PNNG	4.0×10^1
$\underline{N}$-Hydroxy-2-acetylaminofluorene	4.8×10^1
BNNG	4.9×10^1
$\underline{N}$-Acetoxy-2-acetylaminofluorene	5.0×10^1
10-Chloromethyl-9-chloroanthracene	5.5×10^1
3-Methylcholanthrene	5.8×10^1

Chemical	Potency[b]
Folpet	6.4×10^1
Acridine orange	6.6×10^1
2',3-Dimethyl-4-aminobiphenyl	7.5×10^1
4-Hydroxyaminoquinoline-1-oxide	7.6×10^1
7-Chloromethyl-12-methylbenz[a]anthracene	8.0×10^1
Ethidium bromide	8.0×10^1
9,10-Dichloromethylanthracene	8.8×10^1
ICR-10	9.0×10^1

Group 6	Range 10^2-10^3
2-Acetylaminofluorene	1.08×10^2
Adriamycin	1.08×10^2
3-Hydroxybenzo[a]pyrene	1.11×10^2
Aflatoxin M1	1.12×10^2
Aflatoxin G1	1.16×10^2
Benzo[a]pyrene	1.21×10^2
7-Chloromethylbenz[a]anthracene	1.21×10^2
Sodium azide	1.50×10^2
6-Aminochrysene	1.55×10^2
Dibenz[a,c]anthracene	1.75×10^2
2-Aminofluorene	2.05×10^2
α-Naphthylhydroxylamine	2.29×10^2
1-[(5-Nitrofurfurylidene)-amino]hydantoin	2.30×10^2
ICR-170	2.60×10^2
6-Hydroxymethylbenzo[a]pyrene	2.70×10^2
Benzo[a]pyrene-4,5-oxide	2.95×10^2
ENNG	3.50×10^2
Daunorubicin	3.56×10^2
2-Aminoanthracene	5.10×10^2
ICR-191	5.11×10^2
N-Hydroxy-2-aminofluorene	5.83×10^2
3-Methoxy-4-aminoazobenzene	7.47×10^2

Group 7	Range 10^3-10^4
2-Nitrosofluorene	1.04×10^3
MNNG	1.375×10^3
1-(5-Nitro-2-thiazolyl)-2-imidazolidinone	1.752×10^3
Streptozotocin	1.949×10^3
Aflatoxicol	2.2×10^3
4-Nitroquinoline-1-oxide	2.906×10^3
Aflatoxin B1	7.057×10^3

Group 8	Range 10^4-10^5
Azaserine	12.0×10^4
N-[4-(5-Nitro-2-furyl)-thiazolyl]formamide	16.5×10^4
Cigarette-smoke condensate	18.2×10^4
2-(2-Furyl)-3-(5-nitro-2-furyl)-acrylamide	20.8×10^4

a. Data from McCann et al.[276]
b. Mutagenic potency was defined by McCann et al. as the number of revertants per nanomole.

TABLE 9-6 Frequency of Chemicals in Various Potency Groups in the Salmonella/microsome and V79 Chinese Hamster Systems[a]

Potency Group[b]	Salmonella/microsome		V79 Chinese Hamster	
	Potency Range	Frequency	Potency Range	Frequency
1	$10^{-3}-10^{-2}$	2	$10^{-5}-10^{-4}$	6
2	$10^{-2}-10^{-1}$	7	$10^{-4}-10^{-3}$	5
3	$10^{-1}-10^{0}$	20	$10^{-3}-10^{-2}$	10
4	$10^{0}-10^{1}$	30	$10^{-2}-10^{-1}$	16
5	$10^{1}-10^{2}$	42	$10^{-1}-10^{0}$	5
6	$10^{2}-10^{3}$	22	$10^{0}-10^{1}$	8
7	$10^{3}-10^{4}$	7	$10^{1}-10^{2}$	4
8	$10^{4}-10^{5}$	4	$10^{2}-10^{3}$	1

a. Data from Bradley et al.[37] and McCann et al.[276]
b. For the Salmonella system, the potency is the number of revertants per nanomole. For the V79 system, it is the concentration (μM) that increases mutation frequency to 10 times the spontaneous value.

mutagens by potency would give reasonably consistent results across the two tests.

A plot of this sort is useful for qualitative analysis, especially of outliers. A study of the test conditions (e.g., the activating systems used) the particular strain of test organisms (e.g., its sensitivity to frame shifts vs. base substitutions), or the chemical nature of the mutagen may reveal the basis for the discrepancy and ultimately yield deeper insights. For example, the discrepancy in the two tests for furylfuramide (the extreme outlier in Figure 9-2) could be due to different nitroreductase activities in the two systems, which would lead to differences in capacity to convert the chemical into an active form.

It is important to be aware of the criteria used by the authors of the studies cited in selecting their data, because similar requirements should apply to schemes to which uniform standards will be applied. Test protocols, test strains or cell lines, genetic loci, metabolic-activation requirements, mutant-selection protocols, and many other factors were evaluated before data were acceptable for publication. This kind of evaluation is absolutely necessary in constructing a relative-potency scale like the one we propose. Although not all GENE-TOX evaluations are complete, the Committee views the current GENE-TOX effort as a good source of protocol and data evaluation and recommends that GENE-TOX criteria be considered in selecting data from well-known test systems.

The Committee considered ways in which scores from various test systems might be combined into a single number that could be used for decision-making. We rejected this approach on two grounds. First, there is inconsistency from test to test for some chemicals, and a useful overall score would require some measure of statistical reliability. Second, we believe that the individual scores from the tests in our scheme would be more useful than their average, which would necessarily lose some information. Qualitative differences that might not

TABLE 9-7 Comparison of Mutagenic Potency of 23 Chemicals Tested in Salmonella/microsome and V79 Chinese Hamster Systems

| | Potency | | | |
| | Salmonella | | V79 Chinese Hamster | |
Chemical	P^a	log P	P'^b	-log P'
Diethylnitrosamine	1.0×10^{-2}	-2.00	2.1×10^4	-4.32
1-Nitrosopyrolidine	2.0×10^{-2}	-1.70	9.6×10^4	-4.98
Dimethylnitrosamine	2.0×10^{-2}	-1.70	8.0×10^3	-3.90
N-Nitrosomorpholine	6.0×10^{-2}	-1.22	6.7×10^4	-4.83
Dipropylnitrosamine	8.0×10^{-2}	-1.10	4.2×10^4	-4.62
Ethyl methanesulfonate	1.6×10^{-1}	-0.80	1.4×10^3	-3.15
Methyl methanesulfonate	6.3×10^{-1}	-0.20	6.65×10^2	-2.82
Methylnitrosourea	4.4×10^0	0.64	1.18×10^2	-2.07
Benz[a]anthracene-5,6-dihydroepoxide	5.3×10^0	0.72	1.54×10^1	-1.19
7,12-Dimethylbenz[a]anthracene	1.9×10^1	1.28	6.0×10^{-1}	0.22
7-Methylbenz[a]anthracene	2.2×10^1	1.34	6.6×10^1	-1.82
N-Acetoxy-2-acetylamino-fluorene	5.0×10^1	1.70	1.7×10^0	-0.23
3-Methylcholanthrene	5.8×10^1	1.76	4.6×10^{-1}	0.34
Adriamycin	1.08×10^2	2.03	1.0×10^{-1}	1.00
3-Hydroxybenzo[a]pyrene	1.11×10^2	2.05	4.1×10^1	-1.61
Benzo[a]pyrene	1.21×10^2	2.08	7.0×10^{-2}	1.15
Dibenz[a,c]anthracene	1.75×10^2	2.24	1.0×10^1	-1.00
ICR-170	2.60×10^2	2.41	2.7×10^{-1}	0.57
Benzo[a]pyrene-4,5-epoxide	2.95×10^2	2.47	2.1×10^1	-1.32
Daunorubicin	3.56×10^2	2.55	3.0×10^{-2}	1.52
MNNG	1.38×10^3	3.14	3.5×10^0	-0.54
Streptozotocin tetraacetate	1.95×10^3	3.29	6.67×10^1	-1.82
Furylfuramide	2.08×10^4	4.32	3.18×10^2	-2.50

a. Number of revertants per nanomole.
b. Concentration (µM) that increases mutation frequency 10-fold above the spontaneous frequency.

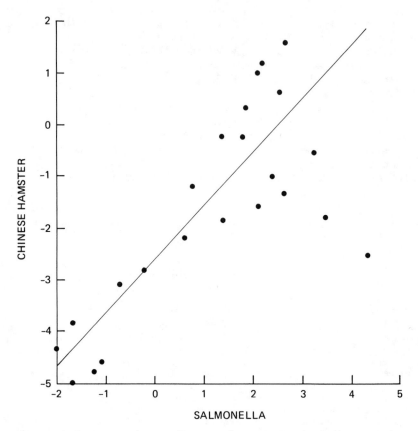

FIGURE 9-2 Comparison of potencies of chemicals tested in Salmonella/microsome and V79 Chinese hamster systems. Ordinate: -log P', Chinese hamster. Abscissa: log P, Salmonella/microsome. Correlation, R = 0.74.

appear in an average could be brought out with our scheme. We therefore believe that it is premature to suggest any composite index of mutagenicity and recommend that all the scores of a given chemical be used.

CARCINOGENICITY TESTING

Many of the chemicals tested in a mutagenicity program will also be independently tested for carcinogenicity. Indeed, the Salmonella/microsome test is widely used as an initial screen for carcinogenicity. A decision regarding

the use of a chemical often involves both mutagenesis and
carcinogenesis. A substance that is weakly mutagenic
might be controlled on the grounds of carcinogenicity,
even though it would not be on the grounds of mutagenicity
alone.

Carcinogenic risk may be sufficient for a decision to
control the use of a chemical; in this case, a mouse
mutation test is not needed. The combination of carcinogenicity information and results from short-term mutagenicity
tests may be sufficient for a decision. In some cases, if
the risk-benefit calculation based on cancer is equivocal,
even an uncertain mutational increment may be enough to
tip the balance.

FURTHER TESTING WITH MICE

If the previous tests do not suffice for a decision,
further testing in mammals is indicated. If the purpose
is to get mammalian germinal data on whether a substance
produces mutations, the specific-locus test is suitable
because of its low background rate and the extent to which
the test has been performed. It should be recognized,
however, that chemicals that yield inconclusive results in
short-term tests are likely to yield negative or inconclusive
results in mouse tests. The dominant-lethal test may be
used if the expected effect is chromosomal.

As shown in Figure 9-1, a clearly positive result in a
germinal mouse test is sufficient to classify a chemical
as a mammalian mutagen, regardless of the results in other
tests. Such mouse tests are the specific-locus, dominant-
skeletal, cataract, and heritable-translocation tests.
The dominant-lethal test does not permit genetic validation,
so it is not included. Additional evidence of mutability
is required. In practice, positive results in the mouse
have been preceded by positive tests in short-term tests,
so we expect this situation to occur rarely, if ever.

The most difficult situation in our assessment program
arises when a chemical that had positive results in
screening tests has a negative result in a mouse test.
Several chemicals that are mutagenic in diverse submammalian systems have been claimed to be nonmutagenic in
the mouse specific-locus system. Several explanations
have been offered to explain this contradiction.

One is that the mouse is inherently resistant to many
mutagens. When a highly reactive chemical, one that binds
tightly to serum or tissue components immediately on
administration, or one that is subject to rapid enzymatic
destruction is administered, it is possible that only an

insignificant fraction of the dose administered will reach
the germ cells. In other cases, a particular strain
derived from highly inbred mice might lack some mutagen-
activating capacity that is common in wild mice or in
humans. The mouse is not universally resistant to
mutagens; for example, it responds strongly to ENU. Its
resistance to other chemical mutagens is difficult to
prove or disprove with the limited data now available.
Chapter 4 cites examples of differences in enzymatic
activation and detoxification between various mammals and
between strains of the same species. In this connection,
it has recently been reported[311] that, whereas 48 rat
strains were all positive for the Ah phenotype (which
regulates many drug-metabolizing enzyme activities), 24 of
68 mouse strains were negative. This suggests that one
may well find differences in chemical mutagenesis between
different mouse strains, and it further complicates
extrapolation from mice to humans. All mice used in the
specific-locus tests have been Ah-positive.

Another factor is that the mouse may have an active
repair system in the testes. The nonlinear response and
dose-fractionation effect offer some evidence of this,[383]
but other explanations are possible. There is direct
evidence that the chemical reaches the testes. This kind
of information is available on a large scale only for ENU,
and information on other chemicals is needed. Although
these studies suggest that similar phenomena apply in man,
this remains uncertain.

The second explanation is that the numbers of progeny
examined in the tests were too small to permit detection
of modest mutagenic responses. The historical spontaneous-
mutation frequency in male mice is about 0.000058 per
seven loci, so a test that examined 10,000 progeny from
treated males and revealed no mutants would be unable to
exclude, at the 95% confidence level, a total mutation
rate less than 5 times the spontaneous rate. For an
explanation of this calculation, see the appendix to
Chapter 6.

For these reasons and others given earlier, the Committee
is reluctant to recommend that a chemical be regarded as
nonmutagenic in humans because of negative evidence in the
mouse when other tests have been positive. Such decisions
must be made case by case, with all the relevant evidence
taken into account. Such evidence might, for example, be
that the mouse and human are known to metabolize the
chemical in the same way or to have similar repair systems
or that there is consistency in these factors in the mouse
and another mammal. The Committee feels that it is prudent
to regard the chemical as a potential human mutagen unless

there is evidence that the mouse is a good human surrogate with respect to this chemical.

If a chemical is mutagenic by the consensus of short-term tests, a decision to continue with mouse tests will usually mean that it has important benefits. It might, for example, be an effective drug with limited use whose benefit outweighs a substantial genetic risk. It might be a chemical of great social benefit and one on which the evidence from short-term tests (perhaps including others that are not parts of the minimal battery) is that it is a weak or doubtful mutagen.

The Committee recognizes that there may be valuable chemicals that are acceptable, despite entailing a genetic risk. The drug hycanthone, which has been used in the treatment of schistosomiasis, could be an example. The proper procedure is to show that the risk is acceptable with respect to risk-benefit considerations. It is manifestly impossible to prove that a chemical is not a weak human mutagen. It is reasonable to argue on the basis of confidence limits in the mouse and other relevant evidence that the risk is small enough to be outweighed by the benefits of the drug.

Screening tests can usually determine whether the expected risk is gene or chromosomal mutation or both. For estimating the risk from dominant phenotypes, the Committee favors a dominant-mutation test in mice as most relevant to the human situation. If the risk is primarily chromosomal breakage, the heritable-translocation test is preferred.

The only estimate of dominant effects in humans comes from mouse data. BEIR III and UNSCEAR both used skeletal anomalies and cataracts as a basis for human radiation-risk estimates. With chemicals, there are greater uncertainties in extrapolating from mouse to man. The skeletal and cataract systems have not been used widely enough for their validity to be assessed, but at present there is little choice but to use these if an estimate must be made. We suggest that the human impact in the first 5-10 generations be estimated as 4 times the first-generation estimate, as explained in Chapter 7. As is also discussed in Chapter 7, there is no feasible way to estimate the total genetic impact.

The estimation of effects of chromosomal breakage can be based on cytologic examination of chromosomes during meiosis or on the presence of partial sterility in the offspring of treated parents. In either case, the impact on successive generations can be estimated from knowledge of the transmission and clinical impact of human chromo-somal rearrangements.

228

The dominant-skeletal-mutation test requires considerable anatomic knowledge and experience to distinguish true genetic changes in the absence of breeding tests. It is also time-consuming. The cataract test has a more specific phenotype and requires a shorter time per mouse, but it screens for a considerably smaller number of loci. Neither of the tests has been validated by use in several laboratories with a variety of strains and many chemicals. It would be highly desirable to make comparisons with other small mammals. Without such information, an assessment of the human dominant-mutation risk is very uncertain. In view of this, we recommend that in any risk-benefit decision the risk component take into account all relevant test and pharmacologic information.

10

SOME ADDITIONAL ISSUES AND RESEARCH SUGGESTIONS

Several issues, both scientific and judgmental, are
outside the specific responsibility of the Committee or do
not fit into the existing framework of mutation-risk
assessment, yet are not totally irrelevant. These issues
are discussed in this chapter with some suggestions for
research.

TRANSPOSABLE GENETIC ELEMENTS

High mutation rates produced by elements (transposons,
insertion sequences, etc.) capable of inserting themselves
into DNA and of moving from one place to another in the
genome are mentioned in Chapter 3. These have been
recognized in bacteria for several years. Similar elements
in maize have been studied for three decades or more. If
such an element inserts into a gene, it is likely to
disrupt the gene's function in some way that leads to its
recognition as a mutant gene.

Although the subject is in its infancy, it is already
clear that a substantial fraction, possibly a majority, of
spontaneous mutations in Drosophila have such a cause. If
that turns out to be true and generalizable to mammals
(there is reason to believe that such elements are present
in mice and humans), it will require a revision in our
thinking about mutation and mutagens, and it would mean
that the kinds of mutagenic mechanisms discussed in this
report account for only a part of the spontaneous-mutation
rate. On the one hand, we can conclude optimistically
that classical mutagens are relatively less important. On
the other hand, we can assume pessimistically that chemicals
not detectable with existing test systems increase the
rate of transposon-induced mutations.

It is possible that the kinds of chemicals that affect the transposition process differ from those causing nucleotide changes and chromosomal breakage. The mechanisms may be more similar to those of crossing-over than to those of mutation, and the target might be a protein, rather than DNA. Very little is known about which chemicals increase and which decrease the rate of transposition.

The enzyme reverse transcriptase makes DNA from an RNA model--the reverse of the usual process. In this way, RNA viruses (retroviruses) can be incorporated into the chromosome as DNA copies. There is now evidence that DNA can be moved from one place to another in the genome by this method: the DNA is transcribed to RNA, which in turn is transcribed to chromosomal DNA. Roughly, the consequences are the same as those of a transposon.

Little can usefully be said today as to how this information bears on mutagen testing systems. But chemicals that affect transposition may be as important as those which affect base changes or chromosomal breakage. If so, it will be necessary to design test systems for finding and assessing the importance of such chemicals.

ANTIMUTAGENS

It was emphasized in Chapters 3 and 9 that the net effect of mutation on the human population is harmful. That is true of spontaneous, as well as induced, mutation. The current spontaneous-mutation rate may or may not be too high from the standpoint of evolution (thousands or more generations), but there is no doubt that for several generations in the future we would be better off if our spontaneous-mutation rate (and induced-mutation rate) were lower.

Perhaps it will be possible to counter the effects of an increase in environmental mutagens by lowering the spontaneous-mutation rate (which must be due in part to chemical influences) with exogenous chemicals. It is not likely that a pill that reduces the mutation rate and possibly reduces carcinogenesis as a byproduct and that has no adverse side effects will suddenly appear. But new research has led to much greater knowledge of what controls the rates of mutation.

Reducing the mutation rate can be approached in two ways. The first is to identify substances that counteract known mutagens. Such chemicals have been found, but they might have an opposite effect elsewhere--e.g., converting nonmutagens into mutagens. Intermediate metabolism (especially toxification and detoxification) is so complicated that it is difficult to be sure that one understands all the effects of an added chemical. The second approach involves direct chemical intervention in the mutation process itself. A number of processes are known to affect mutation and premutational damage, but it is also possible that the bulk of mutation is caused by errors in repair. It may be possible to interfere with error-prone systems while keeping repair error-free. However, such treatment may well increase cell death, which itself may cause harm that offsets a reduction in mutation.

There is obviously no way of knowing what will develop in this field. That ways of reducing mutation rates can be found seems likely, but whether they will be safe enough for practical application is problematic.

GENETIC HETEROGENEITY

Several genetically determined conditions predispose to a high mutation rate, and some are known to increase the susceptibility to environmental mutagens in particular. For example, persons with xeroderma pigmentosum are deficient in enzymes that repair DNA damage done by ultraviolet radiation, and they develop skin tumors on areas of the body exposed to sunlight. For their own protection, they should not be farmers, cowboys, or lifeguards on sunny beaches. Some chemicals mimic ultraviolet radiation in their effects on DNA, and such persons are expected to be especially susceptible to them.

Modern genetics is revealing genotypes with special sensitivity to various drugs and special susceptibility to the effects of chemical mutagens. Research is advancing very rapidly, and we can expect more and more such genotypes to be discovered. Individual genotypes of high susceptibility are very rare, but it is important that persons with those genotypes be identified so that they can be protected. The protection is likely to benefit both the persons in question and their descendants, because of the high correlation between mutagenicity and carcinogenicity.

It is clearly not feasible to set protection standards so rigidly that even the most susceptible persons are suitably protected. If a small fraction of the population has 100 times as high a mutation rate associated with a particular chemical as the population average, setting exposure standards for this chemical at one-hundredth of what they would otherwise be may deprive the population at large of the benefits of the chemical. More lives might be saved by identifying susceptible persons and protecting them individually from the chemical. The issue is especially acute, for example, for workers in a factory where they may be exposed to mutagenic chemicals. If persons of special susceptibility to mutagens were prevented from working in areas close to a suspected chemical or were transferred to other work, this would very likely improve the average health now and in future generations. Although this may have the appearance of job discrimination, there are precedents, such as the practice of transferring pregnant women to safer jobs with the understanding that they will not lose pay or seniority because of the transfer.

We believe that society will eventually have to recognize genetic heterogeneity in a practical way. Individual differences are likely to become more important as more is learned about them. Our social and legal systems will have to acknowledge that treating everyone equally is in fact treating some unfairly.

There is a more elementary consideration: The genetic risk associated with mutagenic chemicals is zero after reproduction ceases and in persons who are not going to reproduce. Hence, a policy that assigns mutagenically risky jobs to older persons would protect future genera-tions. Such a practice has been followed in some industries and laboratories where specific jobs, often involving only a few minutes of exposure above normal limits, were assigned to persons past reproductive age.

The Committee does not condone unnecessary exposure of anyone to mutagens, but there will always be some situations of greater risk than others and some situations in which a social benefit is associated with a risky process. A policy of assigning nonreproductive or postreproductive persons to such risky positions would be a step toward better genetic health in the future. Such a policy might have a dividend in protecting against the effects of carcinogens, in that most mutagens are also carcinogenic. Because of the long latent period--20-40 yr for most cancers--an older person may not live to develop cancer, and, if cancer does develop, the number of years of life lost is less than it would be for a younger person.

LONG-RANGE COST-BENEFIT ANALYSIS AND INTERGENERATION EQUITY

Mutational risk-benefit analysis is quite different from most risk-benefit analyses. It is not unusual for

the benefits and risks to go to different persons;
ideally, there is some form of compensation. However, it
is unusual for the benefits and risks to be many generations
apart. In the case of chemical mutagens, most of the
beneficiaries are living now, whereas most of those at
risk have not yet been born and perhaps will not be born
for many centuries. How can our generation objectively
weigh benefits to itself against risks to future generations? In only a few instances--such as soil and water
conservation, preservation of native vegetation and
wilderness areas, and treatment of endangered species--do
we give much thought to future generations.

Each generation hands benefits to its descendants. We
profit by the scientific and technologic advances made by
our forefathers, and the higher living and health standards
that we enjoy are parts of this benefit. To the extent
that a beneficial chemical increases the knowledge,
technology, and wealth that our generation passes to the
future, we can say that we are offsetting mutagenic
effects. That is not intended to argue against all
efforts to protect the genetic health of our descendants,
but it does argue against a policy so overprotective as to
stultify the development of chemicals that benefit us and
may benefit future generations as well.

SOME SUGGESTIONS FOR RESEARCH

A recurring theme throughout this report is the
uncertainty of much of our knowledge. The lack of understanding ranges from factors that influence the mutation
process itself to the effects of mutation on future human
populations. Yet, within the last two decades there have
been enormous advances in fundamental genetics, and their
application has permitted informed decisions about the use
of genotoxic chemicals. We can expect continuing rapid
advances, with consequent narrowing of uncertainty.

The following brief discussion outlines some research
that the Committee believes can considerably increase our
knowledge of chemical mutagenesis and of its effects on
our descendants. The list that follows is not intended to
be exhaustive or detailed; specific research methods are
in the province of the researchers themselves. Nor have
we tried to be original or imaginative; most of the
suggestions have been made before, and some of the
programs have already begun. The list represents our
judgment of some of the fields of greatest need and
promise.

BASIC RESEARCH IN GENETICS AND MUTAGENESIS

We list this first, because we believe that it is by
far the most important. The great developments in short-
term test systems, such as the Salmonella/microsome
system, are direct outgrowths of molecular and cellular
genetics. These highly effective tests could not have
been developed without basic knowledge. Furthermore,
individual research workers, not advisory committees,
recognized the need for and developed these tests. In our
opinion, the most innovative and ultimately the most
important advances are likely to come from basic research.

DEVELOPMENT AND VALIDATION OF TESTS FOR GENOMIC MUTATION

There are no quick, inexpensive, sensitive, and validated
tests for aneuploidy. Fungal tests are being developed,
and Drosophila tests are being validated. X-chromosome
aneuploidy can be detected in the mouse, but the test is
too expensive for general use. The detection of XX, XY,
and YY spermatids in the vole appears promising, but a
test system has not been developed for routine use.

MOLECULAR DOSIMETRY

Various methods for molecular dosimetry have been
proposed and developed, but they are not practical for
routine use and have not been validated. A dosimetric
method that could be applied directly to humans would be
particularly valuable.

NEW METHODS FOR MEASURING MUTATION IN MAMMALS

We have stressed the disadvantages of large-scale
testing of possible mutagens in mammals. In vivo
mammalian tests are expensive and sample only a small
fraction of the genome. New methods are needed that
screen a substantial fraction of the genome and that
provide detailed information on the nature of mutation.
Methods analogous to those used to measure X-linked lethal
mutations in Drosophila are being developed. There is
also a need for molecular approaches.

METABOLISM OF MUTAGENS AND PROMUTAGENS

The recent recognition that there are numerous activating and detoxification systems and that they differ in
different species and in different strains of a given
species calls for continued comparative studies in various
mammals to provide a broader basis for induction and for
predicting human effects.

VALIDATION AND EXTENSION OF SKELETAL AND CATARACT TESTS IN MAMMALS

The dominant skeletal and cataract mutation tests are
potentially valuable tools for mutagenicity evaluation,
but require validation before they can be used confidently
for chemical-mutagen risk estimates. Small mammals other
than mice should be used to test the generality of the
mouse results. Fortunately, such studies do not require
special genetic strains that are difficult to develop and
that are now available only in the mouse. It would be
useful to have a better understanding of the relationship
between human disease and skeletal effects in mice. For
example, it might be desirable for those versed in human
skeletal anomalies to study skeletal mutation in mice with
a view to strengthening the bridge between skeletal
changes in mice and the total dominant-mutation rate in
man. Such studies could possibly be extended to other
organ systems.

METABOLIC ACTIVATION SYSTEMS

The metabolic activation of chemicals varies substantially within and among species, including man.
Theoretically, a human activation system would be more
suitable than a rat system for estimating human risk.
However, that is not practical, and more research is
needed to find a system that leads to the best human
predictions.

TRANSPOSABLE ELEMENTS

The influence of transposons and insertion elements in
basic mutagenesis is just beginning to be understood, and
it is not known how pervasive or important transposition
is in mammals. This is a very active field, and we expect
that important results will be available soon.

STRUCTURE-FUNCTION RELATIONSHIPS OF VARIOUS CHEMICALS

Knowledge of chemical structure is only a rough indicator of chemical mutagenicity. The rapidity of the growth of knowledge of the molecular basis of mutation implies that further research will lead to much better prediction of mutagenic potential on the basis of chemical structure.

EXPERIMENTS WITH SMALL MAMMALS

Results of attempts to measure effects on vital statistics of the descendants of irradiated mice have been equivocal. In particular, Spalding et al.[429] irradiated mice with large doses for many generations, with no measurable effects. With potent chemical mutagens (such as ENU), better mating systems, and more accurate measures of phenotypic change, better experiments could be done today; and they should not be confined to mice. Although crude, such studies would give information (sorely lacking today) on the effect of an increase in mutation rate on vital statistics.

NORMAL INCIDENCE AND SOCIAL COST OF GENETIC DISEASE

There have been only two large attempts to ascertain all cases of genetic disease in a large defined population, and these had discrepant results. With proper attention to epidemiologic details, computerized data recording, and record linkage, a great deal of the uncertainty about the present burden of genetic disease could be removed. Correlations among relatives would permit estimates of the mutational component.

INDIVIDUAL DIFFERENCES IN MUTATION RATE AND MUTAGEN SUSCEPTIBILITY

It is increasingly evident that there are large varia-tions in human susceptibility to chemicals, some of which are mutagenic. It is possible that a small fraction of the population produces most of the mutations. It is important to understand such variability, and in particular to find ways to identify and protect those who are especially susceptible. Those who are susceptible to mutagens are also likely to be susceptible to carcinogens, so there is an additional reason for such studies.

GLOSSARY

ABCW RELATIONSHIP The relationship noted by Abrahamson, Bender, Conger, and Wolff wherein the per-gene rate of radiation-induced mutation is directly proportional to the haploid amount of an organism's DNA.

ADDITIVE FACTOR One of a group of nonallelic genes that affect the same phenotypic characteristic and have a cumulative effect on the phenotype. (See also QUANTITATIVE INHERITANCE)

ADDUCT A chemical addition product. For example, when the mutagenic alkylating agent ethyl methanesulfonate reacts with DNA, any of the normal bases in DNA (i.e., adenine, thymine, guanine, and cytosine) may be converted into adducts, such as N7-ethylguanine and N3-ethylcytosine.

ALKALINE SUCROSE CENTRIFUGATION A centrifugation procedure that can be used to measure the occurrence of single-strand breaks in DNA.

ALKYLATING AGENT A substance that causes the addition of an alkyl group to an organic compound; according to the number of reactive groups they contain, alkylating agents are classified as monofunctional, bifunctional, or polyfunctional; many chemical mutagens are alkylating agents.

ALKYLATION The addition of alkyl groups, such as methyl or ethyl groups, to a chemical; for example, the mutagen ethyl methanesulfonate (EMS) adds ethyl groups to DNA, forming adducts, such as N7-ethylguanine; EMS is said to be an alkylating agent and to alkylate DNA.

ALLELE One member of a pair or series of homologous genes that can occur at a particular locus on a homologous chromosome; one of two or more alternative forms of a gene, including inactive forms.

237

ANEUPLOID   An organism or cell whose somatic nuclei do not contain an exact multiple of the haploid number of chromosomes, one or more chromosomes being represented more (or fewer) times than the rest.   (See also MONO-SOMIC and TRISOMIC)

ASCUS   The saclike structure (a meiosporangium) in which ascospores (the products of meiosis) are produced in Ascomycete fungi.

AUTOSOME   A chromosome other than a sex chromosome; a chromosome not associated with the sex of the organism and therefore possessed in matching pairs by diploid members of both sexes.

AUXOTROPH   An organism or cell that is unable to carry out some particular synthesis and hence requires the product of that synthesis to be present in the growth media.   (See also PROTOTROPH)

8-AZAGUANINE   An analogue of the normal DNA and RNA purine base guanine; selection for resistance to the toxic effects of 8-azaguanine is the basis of several mutation-detection systems.

BACK MUTATION   Mutation of a mutated gene to its former condition.   (See also REVERSION and SUPPRESSION)

BASE-PAIR SUBSTITUTION   A point mutation in which one base pair in DNA is replaced by another, such as adenine:thymine → guanine:cytosine or adenine:thymine → thymine:adenine.   (See also TRANSITION MUTATION and TRANSVERSION MUTATION)

CENTROMERE   A specialized part of a chromosome that attaches to a spindle fiber in mitosis or meiosis.

CHROMATID   One of the identical longitudinal halves of a chromosome, sharing a common centromere with a sister chromatid; produced by the replication of a chromosome during interphase.

CHROMATID GAP   A small achromatic region of a (stained) chromatid, detected in cytogenetic analysis; "gap" is used, rather than "break," if the achromatic region is smaller than the width of the chromatid.

CHROMOSOME   A nucleoprotein structure, generally more or less rodlike during nuclear division; a physical structure that bears genes; each species has a character-istic number of chromosomes.

CHROMOSOMAL MUTATION   A mutational change that simul-taneously affects many genes, in that it involves segments of chromosomes, rather than a single genetic locus.   (See also GENE MUTATION, POINT MUTATION, and GENOMIC MUTATION)

CODING SEQUENCE   The region of a gene (DNA) that encodes the amino acid sequence of a protein.   (See also INTRON and EXON)

CODOMINANT Pertaining to a pair of alleles in which both members of the pair are expressed in a heterozygote.

CODON Three contiguous nucleotides in mRNA that specify the amino acid to be inserted at a specific position in a polypeptide during translation; of the 64 possible codons that are formed by the four types of nucleotides in RNA (nucleotides of adenine, guanine, cytosine, and uracil), 61 specify an amino acid and three (nonsense codons) specify no amino acid, but rather serve as termination signals in protein synthesis.

COLCEMID A chemical that inhibits the formation of the mitotic spindle that is involved in the division of eukaryotic cell nuclei; colcemid (or the related substance colchicine) is used in some procedures to facilitate cytogenetic analysis.

COMPLEMENTATION The ability of recessive mutations in two different segments of DNA that are involved in determining the same phenotype to interact in such a way that, when both are present, a nonmutant phenotype results.

CONJUGATION In toxicology: A detoxification reaction (e.g., by acylation, alkylation, or esterification) in which a toxicant is metabolically joined to another substance (e.g., a glucuronide, riboside, glutathione, or sulfate), generally increasing the water solubility of the toxicant and thereby facilitating its excretion. In genetics: A process by which two organisms of a unicellular or filamentous species come into contact and exchange genetic material; the genetic exchange may be unidirectional (e.g., in bacteria) or reciprocal (e.g., in Paramecium).

CROSSING-OVER A process whereby genes are exchanged by breakage and rejoining of homologous chromatids; crossing-over typically is reciprocal and occurs as a regular part of meiosis; it also occurs, but at a lower frequency, in mitosis. (See also MITOTIC CROSSING-OVER)

CYTOCHROME P-450 A family of heme-containing isozymes involved in the metabolic processing of thousands of substances, notably the toxification and detoxification of xenobiotics. (See also MONOOXYGENASES)

DAMAGE In the context of this report, the amount of mutational change produced in germ cells. (See also IMPACT)

DEFICIENCY A deletion.

DELETION The loss of a part of a chromosome, often involving several genes, sometimes only a portion of one gene.

DETOXIFICATION The metabolic conversion of a substance
into another substance of lower toxicity; the mammalian
liver is an important site of detoxification processes,
among which are monooxygenase reactions and conjugations.
(See also METABOLIC ACTIVATION and TOXIFICATION)

DIPLOID An organism or cell having two complete sets of
chromosomes, with each set typically of a different
parental origin; the chromosome number twice that
typically present in gametes. (See also HAPLOID and
POLYPLOID)

DISOMIC Having two of a given chromosome in an otherwise
haploid cell or organism.

DNA CROSS-LINKS Chemical linkages between the two strands
of DNA, for instance by bifunctional adducts.

DNA DAMAGE Any modification of DNA that alters its coding
properties or its normal function in replication or
transcription.

DNA POLYMERASE Any of several enzymes that catalyze the
formation of DNA from deoxyribonucleoside triphosphates,
using one strand of DNA as a template.

DOMINANT Pertaining to the member of a pair of alleles
that expresses itself in heterozygotes to the exclusion
of the other member of the pair; the trait produced by
a dominant allele. (See also RECESSIVE)

DOSE Amount of material reaching the target, such as the
number of adducts per nucleotide. Used loosely as
equivalent to "exposure."

DUPLICATION A chromosomal aberration in which a segment
of the chromosome is repeated.

ELECTROMORPH A mutant allele of a gene that is distinguished from other alleles by a change in the electrophoretic mobility of the protein encoded by that gene.

ELECTROPHILE An agent that, having affinity for a pair of
electrons, reacts with a substance that offers a pair
of electrons in bond formation (i.e., with a nucleophile);
because there are many nucleophilic sites in DNA,
electrophiles can react with DNA to produce a variety
of adducts; many mutagens and carcinogens react with
DNA as electrophiles.

ELECTROPHORETIC MOBILITY The movement of charged particles
or molecules (e.g., proteins) when they are placed in
an electric field in electrophoresis; electrophoresis
can be used to separate molecules on the basis of
slight differences in charge and is therefore used in
the identification and characterization of mutant
proteins.

ENDONUCLEASE An enzyme that cleaves internal phosphodiester bonds that connect adjacent nucleotides in a

nucleic acid molecule; DNA endonucleases thus introduce strand breaks into DNA molecules. (See also EXONUCLEASE)

EUKARYOTIC Pertaining to cells or organisms that have membrane-bound, structurally discrete cell nuclei and cell organelles; the cell type of animals, plants, and all other cellular organisms except bacteria and blue-green algae. (See also PROKARYOTIC)

EXCISION REPAIR The enzymatic removal from DNA of a polynucleotide segment that includes DNA damage (such as single-strand breaks and damaged bases) followed by resynthesis and rejoining of the DNA.

EXON The portion of a gene that contains the amino acid coding sequences and that remains represented in mature mRNA after mRNA precursors have been spliced to remove internal noncoding regions (i.e., introns).

EXONUCLEASE An enzyme that digests a nucleic acid (e.g., DNA) by removing nucleotides from the ends of strands or internal strand breaks (i.e., it does not cleave internal phosphodiester bonds). (See also ENDONUCLEASE)

EXPOSURE Amount of material ingested, inhaled, or otherwise received by an organism. (See also DOSE)

FIDELITY The biochemical concept that describes the accuracy of the enzymatic copying of DNA or RNA.

FORWARD MUTATION Mutation at any site in a nonmutant gene giving rise to a mutant allele of that gene.

FRAMESHIFT MUTATION A gene mutation that occurs by the addition or deletion of one or a few base pairs and causes a shift in the reading frame of the genetic code, thereby altering the message encoded by all DNA base pairs that are read after the point of the mutation.

G_1, G_2 Parts of the interphase of the eukaryotic cell cycle when DNA is not being replicated; G_1 precedes DNA replication, and G_2 follows replication.

GAMETE A mature germ cell (i.e., a sperm or an egg) possessing a haploid chromosome set and capable of initiating formation of a new organism by fusion with another gamete.

GENE CONVERSION An unequal exchange of genetic markers during recombination that results in limited homozygosity in chromosomal regions that were previously heteroallelic. (See also MITOTIC GENE CONVERSION)

GENE MUTATION Mutation due to a molecular change in a gene, as opposed to a large chromosomal mutation; includes point mutations and intragenic deletions. (See also GENOMIC MUTATION)

GENOME A complete set of chromosomes or of chromosomal genes.

GENOMIC MUTATION A change in the number of chromosomes in the genome that does not alter the structure or arrangement of genes in the chromosomes. (See also ANEUPLOIDY, POLYPLOIDY, CHROMOSOMAL MUTATION, GENE MUTATION, and POINT MUTATION)

GENOTOXICITY The capacity to cause an adverse effect on a genetic system, including mutagenesis and other indicators of genetic damage.

GENOTYPE The genetic constitution of an organism; the specific genes possessed by an organism. (See also PHENOTYPE)

HAPLOID An organism or cell having a single complete set of chromosomes; the chromosome number of typical gametes; monoploid. (See also DIPLOID and POLYPLOID)

HEMIZYGOTE An organism in which a given gene (such as a sex-linked gene in the heterogametic sex, e.g., XY mammalian males) is present in single dose.

HERITABILITY A concept that quantifies the proportional contributions of genotype and environment to some trait; broadly, the proportion of the phenotypic variance in a population that is attributable to genetic differences among individuals in the population; narrowly, the proportion of the phenotypic variance that is attributable to additive genetic variability (i.e., the proportion of phenotypic deviation from the population mean that is transmitted to the next generation).

HERITABLE TRANSLOCATION A stable rearrangement of the position of chromosomal segments that leads to successful chromosomal replication.

HETEROALLELIC DIPLOID A diploid that contains two different mutant alleles of a gene; because the mutations are at different sites, a functional (wild-type) allele can be produced from the heteroallelic pair by intragenic (generally nonreciprocal) recombination.

HETEROKARYON A cell or fungal hypha that contains nuclei of more than one genetic origin; nuclei in heterokaryons generally do not fuse, but can divide individually and simultaneously to form new multinucleate (or binucleate) cells or hyphae.

HETEROTHALLIC Having two or more genetically incompatible but morphologically similar haploid phases which function as separate sexes or strains (as in some algae and fungi).

HETEROZYGOTE An organism whose chromosomes bear unlike alleles of a given gene; heterozygotes produce gametes of more than one kind with respect to a particular locus. (See also HOMOZYGOTE)

HGPRT Hypoxanthine-guanine phosphoribosyl transferase (also called HPRT); an enzyme involved in the utiliza-

tion of the purine bases hypoxanthine and guanine in
mammalian cells (there are related enzymes in submammalian species); mutants that lack HGPRT are
resistant to the toxic effects of the guanine analogues
8-azaguanine and 6-thioguanine, which can therefore be
used to select HGPRT mutants and form the basis of
several mutation-detection systems.

HISTOCOMPATIBILITY COMPLEX The set of histocompatibility
genes that are important in the acceptance or rejection
of tissue grafts.

HOMOLOGOUS CHROMOSOMES Chromosomes occurring in pairs,
one derived from each of two parents, normally (except
for sex chromosomes) morphologically alike and bearing
the same gene loci; each member of such a pair is the
homologue of the other.

HOMOZYGOTE An organism whose chromosomes bear identical
alleles of a given allelic pair or series; homozygotes
produce gametes of only one kind with respect to the
given locus. (See also HETEROZYGOTE)

IMPACT Medical and social effects on future generations
of genetic damage in the current generation. (See also
DAMAGE)

INSERTION SEQUENCE One of several short (e.g., IS1 in E.
coli is about 800 base pairs long) segments of DNA that
are able to insert into a variety of places in a chromosome; best characterized in bacteria, insertion sequences
are involved in several types of genetic instability.
(See also TRANSPOSON)

INTERVENING SEQUENCE See INTRON.

INTRON A region of a gene (i.e., DNA) that is transcribed
in the synthesis of RNA, but enzymatically removed (by
"splicing") from the final mRNA before its translation
into an amino acid sequence in protein; introns are
characteristic of gene structure in eukaryotic, but not
prokaryotic, cells. (See also EXON and CODING SEQUENCE)

INVERSION Reversal of the order of a segment of DNA in a
given chromosome.

ISOZYME One of several forms of an enzyme that have
similar catalytic activities, but differ in kinetic
properties and often in electrophoretic mobility.

LOCUS The position that a particular gene occupies in a
chromosome.

MEIOSIS The process by which a eukaryotic cell nucleus
(in which the DNA has been replicated only once)
undergoes two coordinated divisions that yield four
cells, each having ploidy half that of the original
cell; in higher animals, meiosis provides for the
production of haploid sperms or eggs from diploid
spermatocytes or oocytes. (See also MITOSIS)

MENDELIAN Pertaining to the principles of dominance, segregation of alleles, and independent assortment of alleles, as initially discovered by Gregor Mendel.

MERISTEMATIC Pertaining to undifferentiated plant tissues (e.g., root tips) that are characterized by regular, frequent cell division.

METABOLIC ACTIVATION The metabolic conversion of a promutagen into a mutagen--an aspect of toxification; the possibility that a chemical may undergo toxification in vivo provides the rationale for using S-9 mixtures or other metabolic activation systems with many in vitro genetic-toxicity tests. (See also DETOXIFICATION)

METAPHASE The stage of nuclear division in which the chromosomes are highly condensed and in the equatorial plane of the spindle before centromere separation; the stage of mitosis at which chromosomal morphology is optimal for cytogenetic analysis.

MICRONUCLEUS A nucleus, separate from and additional to the main nucleus of a cell, produced during telophase of mitosis or meiosis by lagging chromosomes or chromosomal fragments derived from spontaneous or experimentally induced chromosomal structural changes; the smaller of the two nuclei that occur in the cells of ciliate protozoans.

MICROSOME A phospholipid-nucleoprotein complex derived from the ribosomes and endoplasmic reticulum of eukaryotic cells; site of diverse enzymatic reactions important in the metabolism of toxicants and other chemicals.

MISSENSE MUTATION A mutation that changes one codon into another, leading to incorporation of a different amino acid in protein synthesis and sometimes resulting in an inactive protein. (See also NONSENSE MUTATION)

MITOCHONDRION A membrane-bound organelle of eukaryotic organisms that replicates independently of the cell nucleus and contains its own DNA and its own protein-synthesizing apparatus; its function is to provide energy to the cell in the form of adenosine triphosphate by oxidative phosphorylation.

MITOSIS The process by which the nucleus of a eukaryotic cell (in which the DNA has been replicated) divides, providing for the exact division of the cell to produce two daughter cells of the same ploidy as the original cell. (See also MEIOSIS)

MITOTIC CROSSING-OVER Somatic crossing-over; crossing-over during mitosis of somatic cells or other cells (e.g., yeasts) with a ploidy higher than haploid, leading to the segregation of heterozygous alleles.

MITOTIC GENE CONVERSION Nonreciprocal recombination
occurring in mitosis.

MITOTIC RECOMBINATION Mitotic crossing-over and mitotic
gene conversion.

MONOOXYGENASE An enzyme system that inserts one atom of
oxygen into its substrate; the various forms of cytochrome P-450 are a subset of monooxygenases. (See also
DETOXIFICATION)

MONOSOMIC Pertaining to an organism that lacks one
chromosome of a diploid set.

MUTAGEN An agent that causes mutation.

MUTANT An organism that possesses an alteration in its
DNA that makes its genetic function or structure
different from that of a corresponding wild-type
organism.

MUTATION A permanent change in genotype other than one
brought about by genetic recombination.

MUTATIONAL COMPONENT The fraction of the incidence of a
disease or disability that increases in proportion to
the mutation rate; more broadly, the mutational
component of a condition is the proportion of the total
impact of that condition that is attributable to
recurrent mutation; the "impact" of a disease or
disability encompasses the total deleterious effect or
burden imposed on human welfare by the condition.

MUTATION LOAD The decrease in fitness of the average
genotype due to the accumulation of deleterious mutation.

NADP Nicotinamide adenine dinucleotide phosphate; NADP
and the related NAD (the reduced forms are $NADPH_2$ and
$NADH_2$) are coenzymes that are involved in diverse
oxidation-reduction reactions in biologic systems;
among the processes that require $NADPH_2$ is the metabolism of many toxicants by microsomal enzymes in the
mammalian liver.

NONDISJUNCTION The failure of homologous chromosomes to
separate at anaphase I of meiosis; the failure of
chromatids to separate at anaphase of mitosis or at
anaphase II of meiosis.

NONRECIPROCAL RECOMBINATION See GENE CONVERSION.

NONSENSE CODON A codon that does not specify any amino
acid in protein synthesis, but instead specifies
termination of a polypeptide chain; the nonsense codons
are UAA, UAG, and UGA.

NONSENSE MUTATION A mutation that changes a codon for a
particular amino acid into a nonsense codon. (See also
MISSENSE MUTATION)

NUCLEOTIDE The monomeric unit of polynucleotide polymers
known as nucleic acids; consists of three components--a
ribose or a 2-deoxyribose sugar, a pyrimidine or purine

base, and a phosphate group--each of which exists as a phosphate ester of the N-glycoside of the nitrogenous base.

OPERON   A tightly linked (i.e., contiguous) set of related genes and regulatory sites, by which a given genetically controlled metabolic activity is regulated.

OUABAIN   A chemical of botanic origin that inhibits sodium-potassium-activated ATPase in cell membranes, thereby being toxic to the cell; the selection of mutants that are resistant to the toxic effects of ouabain provides the basis of a mutation-detection system in mammalian cells.

PALINDROME   A length of DNA containing inverted repeat sequences capable of buckling to form a base-paired loop with either strand or both strands of previously linear, helical DNA.

PENETRANCE   The frequency with which a gene or gene combination manifests itself in the phenotype of the carriers; penetrance depends on genotype and environment.

PHASE I METABOLISM   Oxidations, reductions, and hydrolyses catalyzed by monooxygenases.

PHASE II METABOLISM   Conjugations, most commonly with glucuronide, sulfate, or glutathione.

PHENOCOPY   A phenotypic variation due to environmental influences that mimics the expression of a genotype other than its own.

PHENOTYPE   The detectable expression of the interaction of genotype and environment; the characteristics of an organism.   (See also GENOTYPE)

PHENOTYPIC EXPRESSION TIME   The time required for the manifestation (expression) of a new mutation, presumably including the time required for the fixation of a premutational lesion in DNA as a mutation and for the dilution of the wild-type gene product in the cell.

PHOTOREACTIVATION   Direct reversal of ultraviolet-light-induced injury to cells, accomplished by postirradiation exposure to visible light; involves the cleavage of pyrimidine dimers by photoreactivating enzymes.

PLASMID   A self-replicating, extrachromosomal DNA molecule in the cytoplasm of some cells; characterized most extensively in bacteria.

PLOIDY   Refers to the number of sets of chromosomes in a cell or organism--1 set in monoploids (haploids), 2 in diploids, 3 in triploids, 4 in tetraploids, etc.

POINT MUTATION   A mutation affecting only one or a few DNA base pairs in a gene.   (See also CHROMOSOMAL MUTATION, GENE MUTATION, and GENOMIC MUTATION)

POLYPEPTIDE A compound containing amino acid residues joined by peptide bonds; a protein consists of one or more specific polypeptide chains.

POLYPLOID An organism or cell having more than two complete sets of chromosomes, e.g., triploid, tetraploid. (See also DIPLOID and HAPLOID)

POSTREPLICATION REPAIR A type of repair of DNA damage that acts not on primary DNA lesions, but on secondary lesions arising as a consequence of unrepaired primary lesions in replicating DNA; the primary lesions lead to discontinuities in the daughter strand produced during replication; in bacteria, the repair of daughterstrand gaps involves a recombinational process (recombinational repair), which operates independently of excision repair; after replication of damaged DNA, postreplication repair reconstructs at least one undamaged copy of the genome of each cell by recombinational filling-in of the gaps; in mammalian cells, post-replication repair may involve a process similar to normal replication, rather than recombination.

PROKARYOTIC Pertaining to cells or organisms (i.e., bacteria and blue-green algae) that do not have membrane-bound cell nuclei and cell organelles. (See also EUKARYOTIC)

PROMOTER In carcinogenesis: A chemical that increases the carcinogenic activity of other agents that initiate carcinogenesis. In genetics: A region of DNA that is the initial binding site for the enzyme (RNA polymerase) that will transcribe a gene into RNA.

PROMUTAGEN A chemical that is not mutagenic itself, but can be metabolically converted into a mutagen.

PROTOTROPH An organism able to carry out a given chemical synthesis; a wild-type organism able to grow on minimal medium. (See also AUXOTROPH)

PSEUDOGENE An inactive, closely situated copy of an active gene; a duplicate gene that has undergone mutation that has rendered it incapable of being properly transcribed or translated.

QUANTITATIVE INHERITANCE Inheritance of a characteristic (e.g., height in man and milk production in cattle) that depends on the cumulative action of many genes, each of which produces a small effect. (See also ADDITIVE FACTOR)

REC Rem-equivalent chemical; a unit used in the Environmental Mutagen Society Committee 17 report (Drake, 1975) for the estimation of genetic risk; the dose (or product of concentration and time) that produces an amount of genetic damage equal to that produced by 1 rem of chronic irradiation.

RECESSIVE Pertaining to the member of a pair of genes
that fails to express itself in heterozygotes in the
presence of its dominant allele; pertaining to the
trait produced by a recessive gene; recessive genes
ordinarily express themselves only in the homozygous
state. (See also DOMINANT)

RECIPROCAL TRANSLOCATION An exchange of segments between
two non-homologous chromosomes.

RECOMBINATION Formation of a new association of genes (or
DNA sequences) of different parental origins; recombination
in eukaryotes typically occurs by the independent
assortment of genes on different chromosomes in meiosis
and by crossing-over or gene conversion; in modern
usage, "recombination" is sometimes restricted to
situations in which new linkage relationships are
established in chromosomes (i.e., to crossing-over and
gene conversion), rather than including independent
assortment; in recombinant-DNA technology, different
isolated DNA sequences are joined in the laboratory
under experimental conditions. (See also MITOTIC
RECOMBINATION)

RECOMBINATIONAL REPAIR Repair by recombination between
sister DNA molecules that fills the gaps opposite
unrepaired lesions left in the daughter DNA strands
after replication of damaged DNA. (See also POST-
REPLICATION REPAIR)

REPLICATION The formation of replicas from a model or
template; applies to the synthesis of new DNA from
preexisting DNA; the process by which genes (hereditary
material; DNA) duplicate themselves.

REVERSE MUTATION Mutation that restores the wild-type
phenotype or gene function in a mutant; may occur
either by restoration of the original DNA sequence
(back mutation) or by indirect compensation for the
original mutation (suppression).

S The part of interphase of the eukaryotic cell cycle
when DNA is replicated.

S-9 A metabolic activation mixture that is used with many
in vitro genetic-toxicity tests to provide for the
conversion of promutagens into mutagens; the enzymatic
activities of an S-9 mixture are those of a postmitochondrial supernatant (i.e., microsomal and
cytosolic enzymes) derived from a mammalian liver
homogenate; the expression "S-9" originally referred to
supernatant from centrifugation at 9,000 rpm.

SENSITIVITY The proportion of human mutagens that are
positive in the system being evaluated. In this report,
because there is no way to measure human mutagenesis,

"sensitivity" means the capacity of the test to detect small increases in the mutation rate.

SEX CHROMOSOME One of a pair of chromosomes that are morphologically dissimilar in one of the two sexes and that are involved in the determination of sex; in mammals, the sex chromosomes are designated the X and Y chromosomes, and females have two X chromosomes and males have one X and one Y chromosome. (See also AUTOSOME)

SEX-LINKED Pertaining to a genetic trait that exhibits a pattern of inheritance indicating that it is determined by a sex chromosome, particularly the X chromosome; pertaining to a gene that is on the X chromosome.

SISTER CHROMATID EXCHANGE The exchange of segments between the two chromatids of a chromosome.

SOMATIC CELL One of the two cell types (the other being a germ cell) of a multicellular diploid organism; it contains a diploid number of chromosomes and is involved in all functions of the organism except fertilization.

SOMATIC CROSSING-OVER See MITOTIC CROSSING-OVER.

S.O.S. REPAIR A repair process that is error-prone, in that it generates mutations; best characterized in the bacterium E. coli, S.O.S. repair depends on recA$^+$ and lexA$^+$ gene functions and is inducible by DNA damage caused by ultraviolet light and some chemical mutagens.

SUPPRESSION The restoration of lost genetic function in a mutant by a second mutation in a different gene (intergenic suppression) or at a second site in the same gene (intragenic suppression). (See also BACK MUTATION and REVERSE MUTATION)

SUPPRESSOR A mutation whose detectable effect is to prevent (suppress) the expression of another mutation when both are present; a suppressor mutation reverses the effect of another mutation, although not occurring at the same position.

6-THIOGUANINE An analogue of the purine base guanine, which is a normal component of DNA and RNA; selection for resistance to the toxic effects of 6-thioguanine is the basis of several mutation-detection systems.

THYMIDINE KINASE (TK) An enzyme involved in the utilization of the nucleoside thymidine (which ultimately becomes part of the structure of DNA); catalyzes the phosphorylation of thymidine to thymidine monophosphate; mutants that lack TK are resistant to the toxic effects of several thymidine analogues, including bromodeoxyuridine and trifluorothymidine; selection of these drug-resistant mutants provides the basis of several mutation-detection systems, most notably in mammalian cells.

TOXICANT   Any substance that, through its chemical action, causes adverse effects in living organisms.

TOXIFICATION   The metabolic conversion of a substance into another substance that has greater toxicity; sometimes occurs as a consequence of processes that are usually associated with detoxification.   (See also METABOLIC ACTIVATION)

TRANSCRIPTION   The synthesis of RNA on a DNA template in such a way that the sequence of nucleotides in the RNA is determined by the sequence of nucleotides in DNA. (See also TRANSLATION)

TRANSITION MUTATION   A base-pair substitution mutation in which the purine:pyrimidine base-pair orientation is preserved, as in adenine:thymine → guanine:cytosine.

TRANSLATION   The process by which a particular messenger RNA (mRNA) nucleotide sequence determines a specific amino acid sequence of a polypeptide chain; occurs as the polypeptide is synthesized and is therefore the second step in the readout of the information in the genetic code (the first is transcription).

TRANSLOCATION   The shift of a portion of a chromosome to another part of the same chromosome or to a different chromosome.   (See also RECIPROCAL TRANSLOCATION)

TRANSPOSITION   Relocation of a DNA sequence within a chromosome.

TRANSPOSON   A genetic element that can transfer itself from one location to another in the genetic material of a cell; best characterized in bacteria, transposons can carry typical bacterial genes and be inserted in chromosomes by means of insertion sequences.

TRANSVERSION MUTATION   A base-pair substitution mutation in which the purine:pyrimidine base-pair orientation is reversed, as in adenine:thymine → thymine:adenine.

TRISOMIC   Pertaining to the presence of one extra chromosome in an otherwise diploid organism.

UNSCHEDULED DNA SYNTHESIS (UDS)   DNA synthesis that occurs at a stage in the cell cycle other than S; incorporation of precursors (e.g., tritiated thymidine) into DNA in the absence of semiconservative replication; a manifestation of genetic repair, whose occurrence has been used as an indicator of induced DNA damage.

VALIDATION   The process by which the consistency of a particular test is determined; the concordance of results of a test in question and previously established tests for a representative sample of chemicals is evaluated.

WILD-TYPE The most frequently encountered phenotype in natural breeding populations; the "normal" phenotype, in contrast which an atypical mutant phenotype; "wild-type" is a somewhat arbitrary designation, in that "wild" populations are composed of genetically highly distinct individuals.

X CHROMOSOME See SEX CHROMOSOME.

XENOBIOTIC Pertaining to a substance that is foreign to the normal constitution of an organism.

X-LINKED See SEX-LINKED.

Y BODY A fluorescent body observed by fluorescence microscopy in sperm and thought to represent a Y chromosome; double Y bodies are thought to arise by sex-chromosome nondisjunction.

Y CHROMOSOME See SEX CHROMOSOME.

ZYGOTE A diploid cell formed by the fusion of two haploid gametes from eukaryotic organisms with sexual reproduction.

REFERENCES

1. Aaron, C.S. Molecular dosimetry of chemical mutagens: selection of appropriate target molecules for determining molecular dose to the germ line. Mutat. Res. 38:303-310, 1976.

2. Aaron, C.S., and W.R. Lee. Molecular dosimetry of the mutagen ethyl methanesulfonate in Drosophila melanogaster spermatozoa: linear relation of DNA alkylation per sperm cell (dose) to sex-linked recessive lethals. Mutat. Res. 49:27-44, 1978.

3. Aaron, C.S., A.A. Van Zeeland, G.R. Mohn, A.T. Natarajan, A.G.A.C. Knaap, A.D. Tates, and B.W. Glickman. Molecular dosimetry of the chemical mutagen ethyl methanesulfonate: quantitative comparison of mutation induction in Escherichia coli, V79 Chinese hamster cells and L5178Y mouse lymphoma cells, and some cytological results in vitro and in vivo. Mutat. Res. 69:201-216, 1980.

4. Abrahamson, S., M.A. Bender, A.D. Conger, and S. Wolff. Uniformity of radiation-induced mutation rates among different species. Nature 245:460-462, 1973.

5. Abrahamson, S., and E.B. Lewis. The detection of mutations in Drosophila melanogaster, pp. 461-487. In A. Hollaender, Ed. Chemical Mutagens: Principles and Methods for Their Detection. Vol. 2. New York: Plenum Press, 1971.

6. Abrahamson, S., F.E. Würgler, C. DeJongh, and H.U. Meyer. How many loci on the X-chromosome of Drosophila melanogaster can mutate to recessive lethals? Environ. Mutagenesis 2:447-453, 1980.

7. Adler, I-D. New approaches to mutagenicity studies in animals for carcinogenic and mutagenic agents. I. Modification of the heritable translocation test. Teratog. Carcin. Mutagen. 1:75-86, 1980.

8. Allen, J.R., D.A. Barsotti, L.K. Lambrecht, and J.P. Van Miller. Reproductive effects of halogenated aromatic hydrocarbons on nonhuman primates. Ann. N.Y. Acad. Sci. 320:419-425, 1979.

9. Amano, E. Genetic and biochemical characterization of waxy mutants in cereals. Environ. Health. Perspect. 37:35-41, 1981.

10. Ames, B.N. A bacterial system for detecting mutagens and carcinogens, pp. 57-66. In H.E. Sutton and M.I. Harris, Eds. Mutagenic Effects of Environmental Contaminants. New York: Academic Press, 1972.

11. Ames, B.N. Identifying environmental chemicals causing mutations and cancer. Science 204:587-593, 1979.

12. Ames, B.N., W.E. Durston, E. Yamasaki, and F.D. Lee. Carcinogens are mutagens: a simple test system combining liver homogenates for activation and bacteria for detection. Proc. Natl. Acad. Sci. U.S.A. 70:2281-2285, 1973.

13. Ames, B.N., F.D. Lee, and W.E. Durston. An improved bacterial test system for the detection and classification of mutagens and carcinogens. Proc. Natl. Acad. Sci. U.S.A. 70:782-786, 1973.

14. Ames, B.N., J. McCann, and E. Yamasaki. Methods for detecting carcinogens and mutagens with the Salmonella/mammalian-microsome mutagenicity test. Mutat. Res. 31:347-364, 1975.

15. Ansari, A.A., M.A. Baig, and H.V. Malling. In vivo germinal mutation detection with "monospecific" antibody against lactate dehydrogenase-X. Proc. Natl. Acad. Sci. U.S.A. 77:7352-7356, 1980.

16. Arenaz, P., and B.K. Vig. Somatic crossing-over in Glycine max (L.) merrill: Activation of dimethyl nitrosoamine by plant seed and comparison with methyl nitrosourea in inducing somatic mosaicism. Mutat. Res. 52:367-380, 1978.

17. Arlett, C.F., D. Turnbull, S.A. Harcourt, A.R. Lehmann, and C.M. Colella. A comparison of the 8-azaguanine and ouabain-resistance systems for the selection of induced mutant Chinese hamster cells. Mutat. Res. 33:261-278, 1975.

18. Auerbach, C. Mutation Research: Problems, Results and Perspectives. London: Halsted Press, 1976. 504 pp.

19. Auerbach, C., and J.M. Robson. Production of mutations by allyl isothiocyanate. Nature 154:81, 1944.

20. Aurias, A., M. Prieur, B. Dutrillaux, and J. Lejeune. Systematic analysis of 95 reciprocal translocations of autosomes. Hum. Genet. 45:259-282, 1978.

21. Awa, A.A., S. Neriishi, T. Honda, M.C. Yoshida, T. Sofuni, and T. Matsui. Chromosome-aberration frequency in cultured blood-cells in relation to radiation dose of A-bomb survivors. Lancet 2:903-905, 1971.

22. Axtel, J.D., and R.A. Brink. Chemically induced paramutation at the R locus in maize. Proc. Natl. Acad. Sci. U.S.A. 58:181-187, 1967.

23. Baden, J.M., M. Kelley, R.S. Wharton, B.A. Hitt, V.F. Simmon, and R.I. Mazze. Mutagenicity of halogenated ether anesthetics. Anesthesiology 46:346-350, 1977.

24. Baker, R.M., D.M. Brunette, R. Mankovitz, L.H. Thompson, G.F. Whitmore, L. Siminovitch, and J.E. Till. Ouabain-resistant mutants of mouse and hamster cells in culture. Cell 1:9-21, 1974.

25. Barrett, J.C., and P.O.P. Ts'o. Relationship between somatic mutation and neoplastic transformation. Proc. Natl. Acad. Sci. U.S.A. 75:3297-3301, 1978.

26. Barrett, J.C., A. Wong, and J.A. McLachlan. Diethylstilbestrol induces neoplastic transformation without measurable gene mutation at two loci. Science 212:1402-1404, 1981.

27. Bartsch, H., C. Malaveille, A.-M. Camus, G. Martel-Planche, G. Brun, A. Hautefeuille, N. Sabadie, A. Barbin, T. Kuroki, C. Drevon, C. Piccoli, and R. Montesano. Validation and comparative studies on 180 chemicals with S. typhimurium strains and V79 Chinese hamster cells in the presence of various metabolizing systems. Mutat. Res. 76:1-50, 1980.

28. Benditt, E.P., and J.M. Benditt. Evidence for a monoclonal origin of human atherosclerotic plaques. Proc. Natl. Acad. Sci. U.S.A. 70:1753-1756, 1973.

29. Bergsma, D., Ed. Birth Defects Compendium. 2nd Edition. New York: Alan R. Liss, 1979. 1222 pp.

30. Berry, M.N., and D.S. Friend. High-yield preparation of isolated rat liver parenchymal cells: A biochemical and fine structural study. J. Cell Biol 43:506-520, 1969.

31. Bhan, A.K., and M.L.H. Kaul. Frequency and spectrum of chlorophyll-deficient mutations in rice after treatment with radiation and alkylating agents. Mutat. Res. 36:311-318, 1976.

32. Bigger, C.A., J.E. Tomaszewski, and A. Dipple. Differences between products of binding of 7,12-dimethylbenz(a)anthracene to DNA in mouse skin and in a rat liver microsomal system. Biochem. Biophys. Res. Commun. 80:229-235, 1978.

33. Bingham, E., R. Niemeier, and W. Dalbey. Metabolism of environmental pollutants by the isolated perfused lung. Fed. Proc. 35:81-84, 1976.

34. Bishop, J.B., and R.L. Kodell. The heritable trans-
    location assay: Its relationship to assessment of
    genetic risk for future generations. Teratog.
    Carcinog. and Mutag. 1:305-332, 1980.
35. Bissell, D.M., and P.S. Guzelian. Microsomal functions
    and phenotypic change in adult rat hepatocytes in
    primary monolayer culture, pp. 119-136. In L.E.
    Gerschenson and E.B. Thompson, Eds. Gene Expression
    and Carcinogenesis in Cultured Liver. New York:
    Academic Press, 1975.
36. Bonati-Pellié, C., and C. Smith. Risk tables for
    genetic counseling in some common congenital
    malformations. J. Med. Genet. 11:374-377, 1974.
37. Bradley, M.O., B. Bhuyon, M.O. Francis, R. Langenbach,
    A. Peterson, and E. Huberman. Mutagenesis by chemical
    agents in V79 Chinese hamster cells: A review and
    analysis of the literature. A report of the GENE-TOX
    Program. Mutat. Res. 87:81-142, 1981.
38. Brandom, W.F., G. Saccomanno, V.E. Archer, P.G.
    Archer, and A.D. Bloom. Chromosome aberrations as a
    biological dose-response indicator of radiation
    exposure in uranium miners. Radiat. Res. 76:159-171,
    1978.
39. Brewen, G.J., R.J. Preston, and N. Gengozian. Analysis
    of x-ray induced chromosomal translocations in human
    and marmoset stem cells. Nature 253:468-470, 1975.
40. Bridges, B.A. Some general principles of mutagenicity
    screening and a possible framework for testing
    procedures. Environ. Health Perspect. 6:221-227,
    1973.
41. Bridges, B.A., J. Clemmesen, and T. Sugimura.
    Cigarette smoking--does it carry a genetic risk?
    Mutat. Res. 65:71-81, 1979.
42. Brockman, H.E., D. De Marini, F.J. de Serres, A.
    Katz, T-M. Ong, A.J.F. Griffiths, and R.S. Stafford.
    Mutation tests in Neurospora crassa. A report for
    the U.S. EPA GENE-TOX Program. Mutat. Res. (in
    press)
43. Brown, M.S., and J.L. Goldstein. Receptor-mediated
    endocytosis: Insights from the lipoprotein receptor
    system. Proc. Natl. Acad. Sci. U.S.A. 76:3330-3337,
    1979.
44. Brusick, D.J. Principles of Genetic Toxicology. New
    York: Plenum Press, 1980. 279 pp.
45. Brusick, D.J., V.F. Simmon, H.S. Rosenkranz, V.A.
    Ray, and R.S. Stafford. An evaluation of the
    Escherichia coli WP$_2$ and WP$_2$uvrA reverse mutation
    assay. Mutat. Res. 76:169-190, 1980.

46. Buckton, K.E., G.E. Hamilton, L. Paton, and A.O. Langlands. Chromosome aberrations in irradiated ankylosing spondylitis patients, pp. 142-150. In H.J. Evans and D.C. Lloyd, Eds. Mutagen-induced Chromosome Damage in Man. New Haven: Yale Univ. Press, 1978.

47. Buening, M.K., P.G. Wislocki, W. Levin, H. Yagi, D.R. Thakker, H. Akagi, M. Koreeda, D.M. Jerina, and A.H. Conney. Tumorigenicity of the optical enantiomers of the diastereomeric benzo(a)pyrene 7,8-diol-9,10-epoxides in newborn mice: Exceptional activity of (+)-7β,8α-dihydroxy-9α,10α-epoxy-7,8,9,10-tetra-hydrobenzo(a)pyrene. Proc. Natl. Acad. Sci. U.S.A. 75:5358-5361, 1978.

48. Cairns, J. The origin of human cancers. Nature 289:353-357, 1981.

49. Campbell, T.C. Chemical carcinogens and human risk assessment. Fed. Proc. 39:2467-2484, 1980.

50. Carpenter, D.A., and G.A. Sega. Unscheduled DNA synthesis induced in mouse spermatids after combined treatment with methyl methanesulfonate and x-rays. Mutat. Res. 50:219-228, 1978.

51. Carper, D., T. Shinohara, J. Piatigorsky, and J.H. Kinoshita. Deficiency of functional messenger RNA for a developmentally regulated β-crystallin poly-peptide in a hereditary cataract. Science 217:463-464, 1982.

52. Carrano, A.V., L.H. Thompson, P.A. Lindl, and J.L. Minkler. Sister chromatid exchange as an indicator of mutagenesis. Nature 271:551-553, 1978.

53. Carter, C.O. Genetics of common single malforma-tions. Brit. Med. Bull. 32:21-26, 1976.

54. Caskey, C.T., and G.D. Kruh. The HPRT locus. Cell 16:1-9, 1979.

55. Cattanach, B.M. Induction of paternal sex-chromosome losses and deletions and of autosomal gene mutations by the treatment of mouse post-meiotic germ cells with triethylenemelamine. Mutat. Res. 4:73-82, 1967.

56. Černá, M., P. Rössner, K. Angelis, J. Nováková, and R.J. Srám. Mutagenicity studies with nitro-furans. III. Mutagenicity testing of nitrofurylacrylic acid in human blood and urine. Mutat. Res. 77:13-20, 1980.

57. Cerniglia, C.E., and D.T. Gibson. Oxidation of benzo[a]pyrene by the filamentous fungus Cunninghamella elegans. J. Biol. Chem. 254: 12174-12180, 1979.

58. Chakrabarty, A.M. Plasmids in Pseudomonas. Ann. Rev. Genet. 10:7-30, 1976.

59. Chapuis-Cellier, C., and P. Arnaud. Preferential transmission of the Z deficient allele of α_1-antitrypsin. Science 205:407-408, 1979.

60. Chasin, L.A. The effect of ploidy on chemical mutagenesis in cultured Chinese hamster cells. J. Cell Physiol. 82:299-307, 1973.

61. Chengelis, C.P., and R.A. Neal. Studies of carbonyl sulfide toxicity: Metabolism by carbonic anhydrase. Toxicol. Appl. Pharmacol. 55:198-202, 1980.

62. Chu, E.H.Y., and H.V. Malling. Mammalian cell genetics. II. Chemical induction of specific locus mutations in Chinese hamster cells in vitro. Proc. Natl. Acad. Sci. U.S.A. 61:1306-1312, 1968.

63. Chung, C.S., O.W. Robison, and N.E. Morton. A note on deaf mutism. Hum. Genet. 23:357-366, 1959.

64. Cleaver, J.E. Methods for studying excision repair of DNA damaged by physical and chemical mutagens, pp. 19-48. In B.J. Kilbey, M. Legator, W. Nichols, and C. Ramel, Eds. Handbook of Mutagenicity Test Procedures. Amsterdam: Elsevier/North Holland, 1977.

65. Cleaver, J.E. Methods for studying repair of DNA damaged by physical and chemical carcinogens. Methods Cancer Res. 11:123-165, 1975.

66. Clive, D. Comparative chemical mutagenicity: Can we make risk estimates?, pp. 1039-1066. In F.J. de Serres and M.D. Shelby, Eds. Comparative Chemical Mutagenesis. New York: Plenum Press, 1981.

67. Clive, D., K.O. Johnson, J.F.S. Spector, A.G. Batson, and M.M.M. Brown. Validation and characterization of the L5178Y/TK[+/-] mouse lymphoma mutagen assay system. Mutat. Res. 59:61-108, 1979.

68. Cohen, G.M., and B.P. Moore. Metabolism of [^{3}H]-benzo(a)pyrene by different portions of the respiratory tract. Biochem. Pharmacol. 25:1623-1629, 1976.

69. Conger, B.V., and J.V. Carabia. Mutagenic effectiveness and efficiency of sodium azide versus ethyl methane-sultonate in maize: Induction of somatic mutations at the yg$_2$ locus by treatment of seeds differing in metabolic state and cell population. Mutat. Res. 46:285-296, 1977.

70. Constantin, M.J. Utility of specific locus systems in higher plants to monitor for mutagens. Environ. Health Perspect. 27:69-75, 1978.

71. Constantin, M.J., F.J. de Serres, R.A. Nilan, S. Sandhu, and M.D. Shelby. Proceedings of the Conference on Pollen Systems to Detect Biological Activity of Environmental Pollutants. Environ. Health Perspect. 37:1-168, 1981.

72. Cornfield, J. Carcinogenic risk assessment. Science 198:693-699, 1977.

73. Countryman, P.I., and J.A. Heddle. The production of micronuclei from chromosome aberrations in irradiated cultures of human lymphocytes. Mutat. Res. 41:321-332, 1976.

74. Cox, R., I. Damjanov, S.E. Abanobi, and D.S. Sarma. A method for measuring DNA damage and repair in the liver in vivo. Cancer Res. 33:2114-2121, 1973.

75. Craymer, L. A new genetic testing procedure for potential mutagens. Drosophila Information Service 51:62, 1974.

76. Crouch, E., and R. Wilson. Interspecies comparison of carcinogenic potency. J. Toxicol. Environ. Health 5:1095-1118, 1979.

77. Crow, J.F. Chemical risk to future generations. Scientist and Citizen, pp. 113-117, June-July 1968.

78. Crow, J.F. Human population monitoring, pp. 591-605. In A. Hollaender, Ed. Chemical Mutagens: Principles and Methods for Their Detection. Vol. 2. New York: Plenum Press, 1971.

79. Crow, J.F. Minor viability mutants in Drosophila. Genetics 92:s165-s172, 1979.

80. Crow, J.F. The evaluation of chemical mutagenicity data in relation to population risk: Impact of various types of genetic damage and risk assessment. Environ. Health Perspect. 6:1-5, 1973.

81. Crow, J.F., and C. Denniston. The mutation component of genetic damage. Science 212:888-893, 1981.

82. Crump, K.S., D.G. Hoel, C.H. Langley, and R. Peto. Fundamental carcinogenic processes and their implications for low dose risk assessment. Cancer Res. 36:2973-2979, 1976.

83. Czygan, P., H. Greim, A.J. Garro, F. Hutterer, F. Schaffner, H. Popper, O. Rosenthal, and D.Y. Cooper. Microsomal metabolism of dimethylnitrosamine and the cytochrome P-450 dependency of its activation to a mutagen. Cancer Res. 33:2983-2986, 1973.

84. Damjanov, I., R. Cox, D.S. Sarma, and E. Farber. Patterns of damage and repair of liver DNA induced by carcinogenic methylating agents in vivo. Cancer Res. 33:2122-2128, 1973.

85. Davies, P.J., W.E. Evans, and J.M. Parry. Mitotic recombination induced by chemical and physical agents in the yeast Saccharomyces cerevisiae. Mutat. Res. 29:301-314, 1975.

86. Decad, G.M., D.P. Hsieh, and J.L. Byard. Maintenance of cytochrome P-450 and metabolism of aflatoxin B_1 in primary hepatocyte cultures. Biochem. Biophys. Res. Commun. 78:279-287, 1977.

87. DeJongh, L.F. A Study of Chromosomal Inversions and Translocations Induced by X-Rays in Premeiotic and Postmeiotic Germ Cells of Drosophila melanogaster Males. Ph.D. Thesis. Madison: Univ. of Wisconsin, 1975. 117 pp.

88. Demars, R., and K.R. Held. The spontaneous azaguanine-resistant mutants of diploid human fibroblasts. Humangenetik 16:87-110, 1972.

89. Den Engelse, L., and E.J. Philippus. In vivo repair of rat liver DNA damaged by dimethylnitrosamine or diethylnitrosamine. Chem.-Biol. Interactions 19:111-124, 1977.

90. de Serres, F.J., and J. Ashby, Eds. Evaluation of Short-Term Tests for Carcinogens: Report of the International Collaborative Program. New York: Elsevier/North Holland, 1981. 827 pp.

91. de Serres, F.J., and G.R. Hoffmann. Summary report in the performance of yeast assays, pp. 68-76. In F.J. de Serres and J. Ashby, Eds. Evaluation of Short-Term Tests for Carcinogens. New York: Elsevier/North Holland, 1981.

92. de Serres, F.J., and A. Hollaender, Eds. Chemical Mutagens: Principles and Methods for Their Detection. Vol. 6. New York: Plenum Press, 1980. 485 pp.

93. de Serres, F.J., and H.V. Malling. Measurement of recessive lethal damage over the entire genome and at two specific loci in the ad-3 region of a two-component heterokaryon of Neurospora crassa, pp. 311-342. In A. Hollaender, Ed. Chemical Mutagens: Principles and Methods for Their Detection. Vol. 2. New York: Plenum Press, 1971.

94. de Serres, F.J., and M.D. Shelby, Eds. Higher plant systems as monitors of environmental mutagens. Proceedings of the NIEHS-sponsored workshop. Environ. Health Perspect. 27:1-206, 1978.

95. de Serres, F.J., and M.D. Shelby. Recommendations on data production and analysis using the Salmonella/-microsome mutagenicity assay. Environ. Mutagenesis 1:87-92, 1979.

96. Dixon, R.L., and I.P. Lee. Metabolism of benzo(a)pyrene by isolated perfused testis and testicular homogenate. Life Sci. 27:2439-2444, 1980.

97. Dixon, R.L., I.P. Lee, and R.J. Sherins. Methods to assess reproductive effects of environmental chemicals: Studies of cadmium and boron administered orally. Environ. Health Perspect. 13:59-67, 1976.

98. Drake, J.W. Environmental mutagenic hazards. Report of Committee-17, Environmental Mutagen Society. Science 187:503-514, 1975.

99. Drake, J.W. The Molecular Basis of Mutation. San Francisco: Holden-Day, 1970. 273 pp.

100. Drake, J.W., and R.H. Baltz. The biochemistry of mutagenesis. Ann. Rev. Biochem. 45:11-37, 1976.

101. Drake, J.W., and R.E. Koch. Mutagenesis. Stroudsburg: Dowden, Hutchinson & Ross, 1976. 363 pp.

102. Duker, N.J., and G.W. Teebor. Detection of different types of damage in alkylated DNA by means of human corrective endonuclease (correndo-nuclease). Proc. Natl. Acad. Sci. U.S.A. 73:2629-2633, 1976.

103. Dunkel, V.C. Collaborative studies on the Salmonella/-microsome mutagenicity assay. J. Assoc. Anal. Chem. 62:874-882, 1979.

104. Ehling, U.H. Comparison of radiation- and chemically-induced dominant lethal mutations in male mice. Mutat. Res. 11:35-44, 1971.

105. Ehling, U.H. Dominant mutations affecting the skeleton in offspring of x-irradiated male mice. Genetics 54:1381-1389, 1966.

106. Ehling, U.H. Induction of gene mutations in germ cells of the mouse. Arch. Toxicol 46:123-138, 1980.

107. Ehling, U.H. Specific-locus mutations in mice, pp. 233-256. In A. Hollaender and F.J. de Serres, Eds. Chemical Mutagens: Principles and Methods for Their Detection. Vol. 5. New York: Plenum Press, 1978.

108. Ehling, U.H., J. Favor, J. Kratochvilova, and A. Neuhäuser-Klaus. Dominant cataract mutations and specific-locus mutations in mice induced by radiation or ethylnitrosourea. Mutat. Res. 92:181-192, 1982.

109. Ehrenberg, L. Higher plants, pp. 365-386. In A. Hollaender, Ed. Chemical Mutagens: Principles and Methods for Their Detection. Vol. 2. New York: Plenum Press, 1971.

110. Ehrenberg, L., and B. Holmberg. Extrapolation of carcinogenic risk from animal experiments to man. Environ. Health Perspect. 22:33-35, 1978.

111. Ehrenberg, L., S. Osterman-Golkar, D. Segerbäck, K. Svensson, and C.J. Calleman. Evaluation of genetic risks of alkylating agents. III. Alkylation of haemoglobin after metabolic conversion of ethene to ethene oxide in vivo. Mutat. Res. 45:175-184, 1977.

112. Elespuru, R.K., and M.B. Yarmolinsky. A colorimetric assay of lysogenic induction designed for screening potential carcinogenic and carcinostatic agents. Environ. Mutagenesis 1:65-78, 1979.

113. Emmerling-Thompson, M., and M.M. Nawrocky. Genetic basis for using Tradescantia clone 4430 as an environmental monitor of mutagens. J. of Heredity 71:261-265, 1980.

114. Essigmann, J.M., R.G. Croy, A.M. Nadzan, W.F. Bushby, Jr., V.N. Reinhold, G. Büchi, and G.N. Wogan. Structural identification of the major DNA adduct formed by aflatoxin B$_1$ in vitro. Proc. Natl. Acad. Sci. U.S.A. 74:1870-1874, 1977.

115. Evans, H.J. Cytological methods for detecting chemical mutagens, pp. 1-29. In A. Hollaender, Ed. Chemical Mutagens: Principles and Methods for Their Detection. Vol. 4. New York: Plenum Press, 1976.

116. Evans, H.J., K.E. Buckton, G.E. Hamilton, and A. Carothers. Radiation-induced chromosome aberrations in nuclear-dockyard workers. Nature 277:531-534, 1979.

117. Evans, H.J., and M.L. O'Riordan. Human peripheral blood lymphocytes for the analysis of chromosome aberrations in mutagen tests. Mutat. Res. 31:135-148, 1975.

118. Evans, H.J., and Vijayalaxmi. Induction of 8-azaguanine resistance and sister chromatid exchange in human lymphocytes exposed to mitomycin C and X rays in vitro. Nature 292:601-605, 1981.

119. Fahl, W.E., G. Michalopoulos, G.L. Sattler, C.R. Jefcoate, and H.C. Pitot. Chatacteristics of microsomal enzyme controls in primary cultures of rat hepatocytes. Arch. Biochem. Biophys. 192:61-72, 1979.

120. Falconer, D.S. The inheritance of liability to certain diseases, estimated from the incidence among relatives. Ann. Hum. Genet. 29:51-76, 1965.

121. Festing, M. Mouse strain identification. Nature 238:351-352, 1972.

122. Fishbein, L. Potential industrial carcinogenic and mutagenic alkylating agents, pp. 329-363. In D.B. Walters, Ed. Safe Handling of Chemical Carcinogens, Mutagens, Teratogens, and Highly Toxic Substances. Vol. I. Ann Arbor, Michigan: Ann Arbor Science, 1980.

123. Fisher, R.A. The Genetical Theory of Natural Selection. Oxford: Clarendon Press, 1930. 291 pp.

124. Food Safety Council. Proposed system for food safety assessment. Fd. Cosmet. Toxicol. 16(Suppl. 12), 1978.

125. Foureman, P.A. A translocation X;Y system for detecting meiotic nondisjunction and chromosome breakage in males of Drosophila melanogaster. Environ. Health Perspect. 31:53-58, 1979.

126. Fredrickson, D.S., and R.I. Levy. Familial hyperlipoproteinemia, pp. 545-614. In J.B. Stanbury, J.B. Wyngoarden, and D.S. Fredrickson, Eds. The Metabolic

Basis of Inherited Disease. New York: McGraw-Hill, 1972.

127. Freeling, M. Toward monitoring specific DNA lesions in the gene by using pollen systems. Environ. Health Perspect. 37:13-17, 1981.

128. Funes-Cravioto, F., C. Zapata-Gayon, B. Kolmodin-Hedman, B. Lambert, J. Lindsten, E. Norberg, M. Nordenskjöld, R. Olin, and A. Swensson. Chromosome aberrations and sister-chromatid exchange in workers in chemical laboratories and a rotoprinting factory and in children of women laboratory workers. Lancet 2:322-325, 1977.

129. Gabridge, M.D., A. Denunzio, and M.S. Legator. Microbial mutagenicity of streptozotocin in animal-mediated assays. Nature 221:68-70, 1969.

130. Galloway, S.M., P.E. Perry, J. Meneses, D.W. Nebert, and R.A. Pedersen. Cultured mouse embryos metabolize benzo[a]pyrene during early gestation: Genetic differences detectable by sister chromatid exchange. Proc. Natl. Acad. Sci. U.S.A. 77:3524-3528, 1980.

131. Garry, V.F., J. Hozier, D. Jacobs, R.L. Wade, and D.G. Grey. Ethylene oxide: evidence of human chromosomal effects. Environ. Mutagenesis 1:375-382, 1979.

132. Gaylor, D.W. The ED_{01} study: summary and conclusions. J. Environ. Pathol. Toxicol. 3:179-183, 1980.

133. Gellert, R.J., and W.L. Heinrichs. Effects of DDT homologs administered to female rats during the perinatal period. Biol. Neonate 26:283-290, 1975.

134. Generoso, W.M., J.B. Bishop, D.G. Gosslee, G.W. Newell, C. Sheu, and E. von Halle. Heritable translocation test in mice. Mutat. Res. 76:191-215, 1980.

135. Generoso, W.M., K.T. Cain, C.V. Cornett, E.W. Russell, C.S. Hellwig, and C.Y. Horton. Differences in the ratio of dominant-lethal mutations to heritable translocations produced in mouse spermatids and fully mature sperm after treatment with triethyl-enemelamine (TEM). Genetics 100:633-640, 1982.

136. Generoso, W.M., K.T. Cain, and S.W. Huff. Chemical induction of sex-chromosome loss in female mice, pp. 111-112. In Report of the Oak Ridge National Laboratory, Biology Division, Annual Program. ORNL-4915. June 30, 1973.

137. Generoso, W.M., K.T. Cain, S.W. Huff, and D.G. Gosslee. Heritable-translocation test in mice, pp. 55-78. In A. Hollaender and F.J. de Serres, Eds. Chemical Mutagens: Principles and Methods for Their Detection. Vol. 5. New York: Plenum Press, 1978.

138. Generoso, W.M., K.T. Cain, M. Krishna, and S.W. Huff. Genetic lesions induced by chemicals in

spermatozoa and spermatids of mice are repaired in the egg. Proc. Natl. Acad. Sci. U.S.A. 76:435-437, 1979.

139. Generoso, W.M., S.W. Huff, and K.T. Cain. Relative rates at which dominant-lethal mutations and heritable translocations are induced by alkylating chemicals in postmeiotic male germ cells of mice. Genetics 93:163-171, 1979.

140. Gentile, J.M., E.D. Wagner, and M.J. Plewa. The detection of weak recombinogenic activities in the herbicides alachlor and propachlor using a plant-activation bioassay. Mutat. Res. 48:113-116, 1977.

141. Goldstein, A., L. Aronow, and S.M. Kalman, Eds. Principles of Drug Action: The Basis of Pharmacology. 2nd Edition. New York: John Wiley & Sons, 1974. 854 pp.

142. Grafström, R., P. Moldéus, B. Anderson, and S. Orrenius. Xenobiotic metabolism by isolated rat small intestinal cells. Med. Biol. 57:287-293, 1979.

143. Grant, W.F. Chromosome aberrations in plants as a monitoring system. Environ. Health Perspect. 27:37-43, 1978.

144. Green, M.H.L., and W.J. Muriel. Mutagen testing using Trp[+] reversion in Escherichia coli. Mutat. Res. 38:3-32, 1976.

145. Green, M.H.L., W.J. Muriel, and B.A. Bridges. Use of a simplified fluctuation test to detect low levels of mutagens. Mutat. Res. 38:33-42, 1976.

146. Green, S., A. Auletta, J. Fabricant, R.W. Kapp, Jr., M. Manandhar, C. Sheu, and B.L. Whitfield. Dominant lethal assay, p. 64. In Current Status of Bioassays in Genetic Toxicology (GENE-TOX). Conference held December 3-5, 1980. Washington, D.C.: U.S. Environmental Protection Agency, 1980. (abstract)

147. Griffiths, A.J.F. Neurospora prototroph selection system for studying aneuploid production. Environ. Health Perspect. 31:75-80, 1979.

148. Gupta, R.S., and L. Siminovitch. Genetic markers for quantitative mutagenesis studies in Chinese hamster ovary cells. Characteristics of some recently developed selective systems. Mutat. Res. 69:113-126, 1980.

149. Gustafsson, J-Å., J. Carlstedt-Duke, A. Mode, and J. Rafter, Eds. Biochemistry, Biophysics and Regulation of Cytochrome P-450. New York: Elsevier/North-Holland, 1980. 626 pp.

150. Hällström, I., and R. Grafström. The metabolism of drugs and carcinogens in isolated subcellular fractions of Drosophila melanogaster. II. Enzyme induction and

metabolism of benzo[a]pyrene. Chem.-Biol. Interact. 34:145-159, 1981.

151. Hällström, I., A. Sundvall, U. Rannug, R. Grafström, and C. Ramel. The metabolism of drugs and carcinogens in isolated subcellular fractions of Drosophila melanogaster. I. Activation of vinyl chloride, 2-aminoanthracene and benzo[a]pyrene as measured by mutagenic effects in Salmonella typhimurium. Chem.-Biol. Interact. 34:129-143, 1981.

152. Hanawalt, P.C., P.K. Cooper, A.K. Ganesan, and C.A. Smith. DNA Repair in bacteria and mammalian cells. Ann. Rev. Biochem. 48:783-836, 1979.

153. Harris, C.C., R.H. Yolken, H. Krokan, and I.C. Hsu. Ultrasensitive enzymatic radioimmunoassay: application to detection of cholera toxin and rotavirus. Proc. Natl. Acad. Sci. U.S.A. 76:5336-5339, 1979.

154. Heddle, J.A., and K. Athanasiou. Mutation rate, genome size and their relation to the rec concept. Nature 258:359-361, 1975.

155. Heddle, J.A., R.D. Benz, and P.I. Countryman. Measurement of chromosomal breakage in cultured cells by the micronucleus technique, pp. 191-200. In H.J. Evans and D.C. Lloyd, Eds. Mutagen-Induced Chromosome Damage in Man. New Haven: Yale Univ. Press, 1978.

156. Heddle, J.A., M. Hite, B. Kirkheart, K.H. Larsen, J.T. MacGregor, G.W. Newell, and M.F. Salamone. The induction of micronuclei as a measure of genotoxicity, pp. 50-51. In Current Status of Bioassays in Genetic Toxicology (GENE-TOX). Conference held on December 3-5, 1980. Washington, D.C.: U.S. Environmental Protection Agency, 1980. (abstract)

157. Heidelberger, C. Chemical carcinogenesis. Ann. Rev. Biochem. 44:79-121, 1975.

158. Heinrichs, W.L., and M.R. Juchau. Extrahepatic drug metabolism: The gonads, pp. 319-332. In T. Gram, Ed. Extrahepatic Metabolism of Drugs and Other Foreign Compounds. New York: Spectrum, 1980.

159. Herbst, A.L., M.M. Hubby, R.R. Blough, and F. Azizi. A comparison of pregnancy experience in DES-exposed and DES-unexposed daughters. J. Reprod. Med. 24:62-69, 1980.

160. Hill, A., and S. Wolff. Increased induction of sister chromatid exchange by diethylstilbesterol in lymphocytes from pregnant and premenopausal women. Cancer Res. 42:893-896, 1982.

161. Himelstein-Braw, R., H. Peters, and M. Faber. Morphological study of the ovaries of leukaemic children. Brit. J. Cancer 38:82-87, 1978.

162. Hodgdon, A.L., A.H. Marcus, P. Arenaz, J.L. Rosichan,

T.P. Bogyo, and R.A. Nilan. Ontogeny of the barley plant as related to mutation expression and detection of pollen mutations. Environ. Health Perspect. 37:5-7, 1981.

163. Hoffmann, G.R. Genetic effects of dimethyl sulfate, diethyl sulfate, and related compounds. Mutat. Res. 75:63-129, 1980.

164. Hollaender, A., Ed. Chemical Mutagens: Principles and Methods for Their Detection. Vol. 1. New York: Plenum Press, 1971. 310 pp.

165. Hollaender, A., Ed. Chemical Mutagens: Principles and Methods for Their Detection. Vol. 2. New York: Plenum Press, 1971. 300 pp.

166. Hollaender, A., Ed. Chemical Mutagens: Principles and Methods for Their Detection. Vol. 3. New York: Plenum Press, 1973. 304 pp.

167. Hollaender, A., Ed. Chemical Mutagens: Principles and Methods for Their Detection. Vol. 4. New York: Plenum Press, 1976. 364 pp.

168. Hollaender, A., and F.J. de Serres, Eds. Chemical Mutagens: Principles and Methods for Their Detection. Vol. 5. New York: Plenum Press, 1978. 348 pp.

169. Hollander, D.H., M.S. Tockman, Y.W. Liang, D.S. Borgaonkar. and J.K. Frost. Sister chromatid exchanges in the peripheral blood of cigarette smokers and in lung cancer patients; and the effect of chemotherapy. Human Genet. 44:165-171, 1978.

170. Hollstein, M., J. McCann, F.A. Angelosanto, and W.W. Nichols. Short-term tests for carcinogens and mutagens. Mutat. Res. 65:133-226, 1979.

171. Hook, E.B. Monitoring human mutations and consideration of a dilemma posed by an apparent increase in one type of mutation rate, pp. 483-528. In N.E. Morton and C.S. Chung, Eds. Genetic Epidemiology. New York: Academic Press, 1978.

172. Hsie, A.W., J.P. O'Neill, and V.K. McElheny, Eds. Banbury Report 2. Mammalian Cell Mutagenesis: The Maturation of Test Systems. New York: Cold Spring Harbor Laboratory, 1979. 504 pp.

173. Hsu, I.C., C.C. Harris, M. Yamaguchi, B.F. Trump, and P.W. Schafer. Induction of ouabain-resistant mutation and sister chromatid exchanges in Chinese hamster cells with chemical carcinogens mediated by human pulmonary macrophages. J. Clin. Invest. 64:1245-1252, 1979.

174. Huberman, E. Mutagenesis and cell transformation of mammalian cells in culture by chemical carcinogens. J. Environ. Pathol. Toxicol. 2:29-42, 1978.

175. Huberman, E., L. Aspiras, C. Heidelberger, P. Grover,

and P. Sims. Mutagenicity of mammalian cells of epoxides and other derivatives of polycyclic hydrocarbons. Proc. Natl. Acad. Sci. U.S.A. 68:3195-3199, 1971.

176. Huberman, E., and L. Sachs. Cell-mediated mutagenesis of mammalian cells with chemical carcinogens. Int. J. Cancer 13:326-333, 1974.

177. Huberman, E., and L. Sachs. Mutability of different genetic loci in mammalian cells by metabolically activated carcinogenic polycyclic hydrocarbons. Proc. Natl. Acad. Sci. U.S.A. 73:188-192, 1976.

178. Iatropoulos, M.J., W. Hobson, V. Knauf, and H.P. Adams. Morphological effects of hexachlorobenzene toxicity in female rhesus monkeys. Toxicol. Appl. Pharmacol. 37:433-444, 1976.

179. Ichikawa, S. In situ monitoring with Tradescantia around nuclear power plants. Environ. Health Perspect. 37:145-164, 1981.

180. Inouye, E. Gene-Environmental Interaction in Common Diseases. Baltimore: Univ. Park Press, 1977.

181. International Agency for Research on Cancer. IARC Monographs, Supplement 2. Long-Term and Short-Term Screening Tests for Carcinogens: A Critical Appraisal. Lyons, 1980. 426 pp.

182. International Commission for Protection against Environmental Mutagens and Carcinogens. ICPEMC News No. 1. Mutat. Res. 54:379-381, 1978.

183. Irving, C.C. Interaction of chemical carcinogens with DNA, pp. 189-224. In H. Busch, Ed. Methods in Cancer Research. Vol. 12. New York: Academic Press, 1973.

184. Jackson, L.G., and R.N. Schimke. Clinical Genetics: A Source Book for Physicians. New York: John Wiley, 1979. 652 pp.

185. Jacobs, L., and R. Demars. Quantification of chemical mutagenesis in diploid human fibroblasts: Induction of azaguanine-resistant mutants of N-methyl-N'-nitro-N-nitrosoguanidine. Mutat. Res. 53:29-53, 1978.

186. Jacobs, P.A. Chromosome mutations: frequency at birth in humans. Humangenetik 16:137-140, 1972.

187. Jacobs, P.A. Correlation between euploid structural chromosome rearrangements and mental subnormality in humans. Nature 249:164-165, 1974.

188. Jacobs, P.A. Population surveillance: A cytogenetic approach, pp. 463-481. In N.E. Morton and C.S. Chung, Eds. Genetic Epidemiology. New York: Academic Press, 1978.

189. Jacobs, P.A., M. Melville, S. Ratcliffe, A.J. Keay,

and J. Syme. A cytogenetic survey of 11,680 newborn infants. Ann. Hum. Genet. 37:359-376, 1974.

190. Jagannath, D.R., D.M. Vultaggio, and D.J. Brusick. Genetic activity of 42 coded compounds in the mitotic gene conversion assay using Saccharomyces cerevisiae strain D4, pp. 456-467. In F.J. de Serres and J. Ashby, Eds. Evaluation of Short-Term Tests for Carcinogens. New York: Elsevier/North-Holland, 1981.

191. Jakoby, W.B. The glutathione S-transferases: A group of multifunctional detoxification proteins, pp. 383-414. In A. Meister, Ed. Advances in Enzymology and Related Areas of Molecular Biology. New York: John Wiley and Sons, 1978.

192. Jennette, K.W. Chromate metabolism in liver microsomes. Biol. Trace Element Res. 1:55-62, 1979.

193. Jick, H., J. Porter, and A.S. Morrison. Relation between smoking and age of natural menopause. Lancet 1:1354-1355, 1977.

194. Johnson, F.M. Mutation-rate determinations based on electrophoretic analysis of laboratory mice. Mutat. Res. 82:125-135, 1981.

195. Johnson, F.M., and S.E. Lewis. Electrophoretically detected germinal mutations induced in the mouse by ethylnitrosourea. Proc. Natl. Acad. Sci. U.S.A. 78:3138-3141, 1981.

196. Johnson, F.M., G.T. Roberts, R.K. Sharma, F. Chasalow, R. Zweidinger, A. Morgan, R.W. Hendren, and S.E. Lewis. The detection of mutants in mice by electrophoresis: results of a model induction experiment with procarbazine. Genetics 97:113-124, 1981.

197. Jones, C.A., and E. Huberman. A sensitive hepatocyte-mediated assay for the metabolism of nitrosamines to mutagens for mammalian cells. Cancer Res. 40:406-411, 1980.

198. Kada, T., K. Hirano, and Y. Shirasu. Screening of environmental chemical mutagens by the Rec-assay system with Bacillus subtilis, pp. 149-173. In F.J. de Serres and A. Hollaender, Eds. Chemical Mutagens: Principles and Methods for Their Detection. Vol. 6. New York: Plenum Press, 1980.

199. Käfer, E., B.R. Scott, G.L. Dorn, and R. Stafford. Aspergillus nidulans: Systems and results of tests for chemical induction of mitotic segregation and mutation. I. Diploid and duplication assay systems. A report of the U.S. EPA GENE-TOX Program. Mutat. Res. 98:1-48, 1982.

200. Kahl, G.F., E. Klaus, C. Legraverend, D.W. Nebert, and O. Pelkonen. Formation of benzo(a)pyrene metabolite-

nucleoside adducts in isolated perfused rat and mouse liver and in mouse lung slices. Biochem. Pharmacol. 28:1051-1056, 1979.

201. Kao, F-T., and T.T. Puck. Genetics of somatic mammalian cells. VII. Induction and isolation of nutritional mutants in Chinese hamster cells. Proc. Natl. Acad. Sci. U.S.A. 60:1275-1281, 1968.

202. Kapp, R.W., Jr. Detection of aneuploidy in human sperm. Environ. Health Perspect. 31:27-31, 1979.

203. Kassinova, G.V., S.V. Kovaltsova, S.V. Marfin, and I.A. Zakharov. Activity of 40 coded compounds in differential inhibition and mitotic crossing-over assays in yeast, pp. 434-455. In F.J. de Serres and J. Ashby, Eds. Evaluation of Short-Term Tests for Carcinogens. New York: Elsevier/North-Holland, 1981.

204. Kato, R. Characteristics and differences in the hepatic mixed function oxidases of different species. Pharmacol. Ther. 6:41-98, 1979.

205. Kety, S.S., D. Rosenthal, P.H. Wender, and F. Schulsinger. The types and prevalence of mental illness in the biological and adoptive families of adopted schizophrenics, pp. 345-362. In D. Rosenthal and S.S. Kety, Eds. The Transmission of Schizophrenia. New York: Pergamon Press, 1968.

206. Kihlman, B.A. Root tips for studying the effects of chemicals on chromosomes, pp. 489-514. In A. Hollaender, Ed. Chemical Mutagens: Principles and Methods for Their Detection. Vol. 2. New York: Plenum Press, 1971.

207. Kilbey, B.J., M. Legator, W. Nichols, and C. Ramel, Eds. Handbook of Mutagenicity Test Procedures. Amsterdam: Elsevier Scientific Publishing Company, 1977. 485 pp.

208. Kinoshita, N., and H.V. Gelboin. β-Glucuronidase catalyzed hydrolysis of benzo(a)pyrene-3-glucuronide and binding to DNA. Science 199:307-309, 1978.

209. Klekowski, E.J., Jr. Detection of mutational damage in fern populations: An in situ bioassay for mutagens in aquatic ecosystems, pp. 79-99. In A. Hollaender and F.J. de Serres, Eds. Chemical Mutagens: Principles and Methods for Their Detection. Vol. 5. New York: Plenum Press, 1978.

210. Klekowski, E.J., Jr. Mutational load in a fern population growing in a polluted environment. Amer. J. Bot. 63:1024-1030, 1976.

211. Klekowski, E.J., Jr., and B.B. Berger. Chromosome mutations in a fern population growing in a polluted environment: A bioassay for mutagens in aquatic environments. Amer. J. Bot. 63:239-246, 1976.

212. Klekowski, E., and D.E. Levin. Mutagens in a river heavily polluted with paper recycling wastes: Results of field and laboratory mutagen assays. Environ. Mutagenesis 1:209-219, 1979.

213. Knudson, A.G., Jr. Genetics and etiology of human cancer. Adv. Hum. Genet. 8:1-66, 1977.

214. Knudson, A.G. Germinal and somatic mutation in cancer, pp. 287-310. In N.E. Morton and C.S. Chung. Genetic Epidemiology. New York: Academic Press, 1978.

215. Kohn, K.W., L.C. Erickson, R.A. Ewig, and C.A. Friedman. Fractionation of DNA from mammalian cells by alkaline elution. Biochemistry 15:4629-4637, 1976.

216. Kohn, K.W., C.A. Friedman, R.A. Ewig, and Z.M. Iqbal. DNA chain growth during replication of asynchronous L1210 cells. Alkaline elution of large DNA segments from cells lysed on filters. Biochemistry 13:4134-4139, 1974.

217. Koropatnick, D.J., and H.F. Stich. DNA fragmentation in mouse gastric epithelial cells by precarcinogens, ultimate carcinogens and nitrosation products: an indicator for the determination of organotropy and metabolic activation. Int. J. Cancer 17:765-772, 1976.

218. Kozak, C.A., R.E.K. Fournier, L.A. Leinwald, and F.H. Ruddle. Assignment of the gene governing cellular ouabain resistance to Mus musculus chromosome 3 using human/mouse microcell hybrids. Biochem. Genetics 17:23-34, 1979.

219. Krahn, D.E., and C. Heidelberger. Liver homogenate-mediated mutagenesis in Chinese V79 cells by polycyclic aromatic hydrocarbons and aflatoxins. Mutat. Res. 46:27-44, 1977.

220. Kratochvilova, J. Dominant cataract mutations detected in offspring of gamma-irradiated male mice. J. Heredity 72:302-307, 1981.

221. Kratochvilova, J., and U.H. Ehling. Dominant cataract mutations induced by gamma-irradiation of male mice. Mutat. Res. 63:221-223, 1979.

222. Kuroki, T., C. Drevon, and R. Montesano. Microsome-mediated mutagenesis in V79 Chinese hamster cells by various nitrosamines. Cancer Res. 37:1044-1050, 1977.

223. Kuroki, T., C. Malaveille, C. Drevon, C. Piccoli, M. MacLeod, and J.K. Selkirk. Critical importance of microsome concentration in mutagenesis assay with V79 Chinese hamster cells. Mutat. Res. 63:259-272, 1979.

224. Lambert, B., U. Ringborg, and A. Lindblad. Prolonged increase of sister-chromatid exchanges in lymphocytes of melanoma patients after CCNU treatment. Mutat. Res. 59:295–300, 1979.

225. Langenbach, R., H.J. Freed, D. Raveh, and E. Huberman. Cell specificity in metabolic activation of aflatoxin B$_1$ and benzo(a)pyrene to mutagens for mammalian cells. Nature 276:277–280, 1978.

226. Laqueur, G.L., and M. Spatz. Toxicology of cycasin. Cancer Res. 28:2262–2267, 1968.

227. Larimer, F.W., A.A. Hardigree, W. Lijinsky, and J.L. Epler. Mutagenicity of N-nitrosopiperazine derivatives in Saccharomyces cerevisiae. Mutat. Res. 77:143–148, 1980.

228. Larimer, F.W., D.W. Ramey, W. Lijinsky, and J.L. Epler. Mutagenicity of methylated N-nitrosopiperidines in Saccharomyces cerevisiae. Mutat. Res. 57:155–161, 1978.

229. Latt, S.A. Sister chromatid exchanges, indices of human chromosome damage and repair: Detection by fluorescence and induction by mitomycin C. Proc. Natl. Acad. Sci. U.S.A. 71:3162–3166, 1974.

230. Latt, S.A., J. Allen, S.E. Bloom, A. Carrano, E. Falke, D. Kram, E. Schneider, R. Schreck, R. Tice, R. Whitfield, and S. Wolff. Sister-chromatid exchanges: a report of the GENE-TOX Program. Mutat. Res. 87:17–62, 1981.

231. Latt, S.A., and R.R. Schreck. Sister chromatid exchange analysis. Amer. J. Hum. Genet. 32:297–313, 1980.

232. Lawley, P.D. DNA as a target of alkylating carcinogens. Brit. Med. Bull. 36:19–24, 1980.

233. Leck, I. Descriptive epidemiology of common malformations. Brit. Med. Bull. 32:45–52, 1976.

234. Lederberg, J. Recombination mechanisms in bacteria. J. Cell Comp. Physiol. 45:75–107, 1955.

235. Lee, I.P., and R.L. Dixon. Factors influencing reproductive and genetic toxic effects on male gonads. Environ. Health Perspect. 24:117–127, 1978.

236. Lee, I.P., and J. Nagayama. Metabolism of benzo(a)pyrene by the isolated perfused rat testis. Cancer Res. 40:3297–3303, 1980.

237. Lee, W.R. Dosimetry of alkylating agents, pp. 191–200. In V.K. McElheny and S. Abrahamson, Eds. Banbury Report 1. Assessing Chemical Mutagens: The Risk to Humans. New York: Cold Spring Harbor Laboratory, 1979.

238. Lee, W.R. Dosimetry of chemical mutagens in eukaryote germ cells, pp. 177–202. In A. Hollaender and F.J.

de Serres, Eds. Chemical Mutagens: Principles and Methods for Their Detection. Vol. 5. New York: Plenum Press, 1978.

239. Lee, W.R. Molecular dosimetry of chemical mutagens: Determination of molecular dose to the germ line. Mutat. Res. 38:311-316, 1976.

240. Lee, W.R., S. Abrahamson, R. Valencia, E.S. von Halle, F.E. Würgler, and S. Zimmering. The sex-linked recessive lethal test for mutagenesis in Drosophila melanogaster. Mutat. Res. (in press)

241. Leffler, S., P. Pulkrabek, D. Grunberger, and I.B. Weinstein. Template activity of calf thymus DNA modified by a dihydrodiol epoxide derivative of benzo(a)pyrene. Biochemistry 16:3133-3136, 1977.

242. Legator, M.S., and H.V. Malling. The host-mediated assay, a practical procedure for evaluating potential mutagenic agents in mammals, pp. 569-589. In A. Hollaender, Ed. Chemical Mutagens: Principles and Methods for Their Detection. Vol. 2. New York: Plenum Press, 1971.

243. Legator, M.S., L. Truong, and T.H. Connor. Analysis of body fluids including alkylation of macromolecules for detection of mutagenic agents, pp. 1-23. In A. Hollaender and F.J. de Serres, Eds. Chemical Mutagens: Principles and Methods for Their Detection. Vol. 5. New York: Plenum Press, 1978.

244. Lehmann, A.R., and B.A. Bridges. DNA repair. Essays Biochem. 13:71-119, 1977.

245. Lehmann, H., and R.G. Huntsman. Man's Haemoglobins. 2nd ed. New York: Harper & Row, 1974. 478 pp.

246. Lett, J.T., I. Caldwell, C.J. Dean, and P. Alexander. Rejoining of x-ray induced breaks in the DNA of leukaemia cells. Nature 214:790-792, 1967.

247. Levi, A.J., A.M. Fisher, L. Hughes, and W.F. Hendry. Male infertility due to sulphasalazine. Lancet 2:276-278, 1979.

248. Lewis, E.B. The theory and application of a new method of detecting chromosomal rearrangements in Drosophila melanogaster. Amer. Nat. 88:225-239, 1954.

249. Lilja, H.S., E. Hyde, D.S. Longnecker, and J.D. Yager, Jr. DNA damage and repair in rat tissues following administration of azaserine. Cancer Res. 37:3925-3931, 1977.

250. Lin, W.S., and M. Kapoor. Induction of aryl hydrocarbon hydroxylase in Neurospora crassa by benzo[α]-pyrene. Curr. Microbiol. 3:177-180, 1979.

251. Lind, C., H. Vadi, and L. Ernster. Metabolism of

benzo(a)pyrene-3, 6-quinone and 3-hydroxybenzo(a)-pyrene in liver microsomes from 3-methylcholanthrene-treated rats. A possible role of DT-diaphorase in the formation of glucuronyl conjugates. Arch. Biochem. Biophys. 190:97-108, 1978.

252. Lindgren, D., and K. Lindgren. Investigations of environmental mutagens by the waxy method, p. 22. Newsletter of the Environmental Mutagen Society. No. 6. October 1972.

253. Littlefield, L.G., S.P. Colyer, and R.J. DuFrain. Comparison of sister-chromatid exchanges in human lymphocytes after G_0 exposure to mitomycin in vivo vs in vitro. Mutat. Res. 69:191-197, 1980.

254. Lloyd, D.C. The problems of interpreting aberration yields induced by in vivo irradiation of lymphocytes, pp. 77-88. In H.J. Evans and D.C. Lloyd, Eds. Mutagen-induced Chromosome Damage in Man. New Haven: Yale Univ. Press, 1978.

255. Löfroth, G., S. Osterman-Golkar, and R. Wennerberg. Urinary excretion of methylated purines following inhalation of dimethyl sulphate. Experientia 30:641-642, 1974.

256. Lohman, P.H.M. International Commission for Protection Against Environmental Mutagens and Carcinogens (ICPEMC). Environ. Health Perspect. 28:301-302, 1979.

257. Loprieno, N. Screening of coded carcinogenic/-noncarcinogenic chemicals by a forward-mutation system with the yeast Schizosaccharomyces pombe, pp. 424-433. In F.J. de Serres and J. Ashby, Eds. Evaluation of Short-Term Tests for Carcinogens. New York: Elsevier/North-Holland, 1981.

258. Loprieno, N., R. Barale, E.S. von Halle, and R.C. von Borstel. Report on Schizosaccharomyces pombe. GENE-TOX workshop program. Mutat. Res. (in press)

259. Lu, A.Y.H., and S.B. West. Multiplicity of mammalian microsomal cytochromes P-450. Pharmacol. Rev. 31:277-295, 1979.

260. Luria, S.E., and M. Delbrück. Mutations of bacteria from virus sensitivity to virus resistance. Genetics 28:491-511, 1943.

261. Lutz, W.K. In vivo covalent binding of organic chemicals to DNA as a quantitative indicator in the process of chemical carcinogenesis. Mutat. Res. 65:289-356, 1979.

262. Lyon, E.S., and W.B. Jakoby. The identity of alcohol sulfotransferases with hydroxysteroid sulfotrans-ferases. Arch. Biochem. Biophys. 202:474-481, 1980.

263. Ma, T-H. Micronuclei induced by x-rays and chemical mutagens in meiotic pollen mother cells of Tradescantia. Mutat. Res. 64:307-313, 1979.

264. Ma, T-H. Tradescantia micronucleus bioassay and pollen tube chromatid aberration test for in situ monitoring and mutagen screening. Environ. Health Perspect. 37:85-90, 1981.

265. MacGregor, J.T., and L.E. Sacks. The sporulation system of Bacillus subtilis as the basis of a multi-gene mutagen screening test. Mutat. Res. 38:271-286, 1976.

266. Magee, P.N. Activation and inactivation of chemical carcinogens and mutagens in the mammal. Essays Biochem. 10:105-136, 1974.

267. Maier, P., P. Manser, and G. Zbinden. Granuloma pouch assay. II. Induction of 6-thioguanine resistance by MNNG and benzo(a)pyrene in vivo. Mutat. Res. 77:165-173, 1980.

268. Maier, P., and G. Zbinden. Specific locus mutations induced in somatic cells of rats by orally and parenterally administered procarbazine. Science 209:299-302, 1980.

269. Malling, H.V. Perspectives in mutagenesis. Environ. Mutagen. 3:103-108, 1981.

270. Malling, H.V., and L.R. Valcovic. A biochemical specific locus mutation system in mice. Arch. Toxicol. 38:45-51, 1977.

271. Marquardt, H., U. von Laer, and F.K. Zimmermann. Das spontane, nitrosamid- und nitrit-induzierte Mutationsmuster von 6 Adenin-genloci der Hefe. Z. Vererbungsl. 98:1-9, 1966.

272. Martin, C.N., A.C. McDermid, and R.C. Garner. Testing of known carcinogens and noncarcinogens for their ability to induce unscheduled DNA synthesis in HeLa cells. Cancer Res. 38:2621-2627, 1978.

273. Martin, D. Search for toxic chemicals in environment gets a slow start, is proving difficult and expensive. The Wall Street Journal 191(90):48, May 9, 1978.

274. Maugh, T.H., II. Chemical carcinogens: How dangerous are low doses? Science 202:37-41, 1978.

275. McCann, J., and B.N. Ames. The Salmonella/microsome mutagenicity test: predictive value for animal carcinogenicity, pp. 87-108. In W.G. Flamm and M.A. Mehlman, Eds. Mutagenesis, Advances in Modern Toxicology. Vol. 5. Washington, D.C.: Hemisphere Publishing Company (Wiley), 1978.

276. McCann, J., E. Choi, E. Yamasaki, and B.N. Ames. Detection of carcinogens as mutagens in the Salmonella/-

microsome test: assay of 300 chemicals. Proc. Natl.
Acad. Sci. U.S.A. 72:5135-5139, 1975.

277. McCann, J., N.E. Spingarn, J. Kobori, and B.N. Ames.
Detection of carcinogens as mutagens: bacterial
tester strains with R factor plasmids. Proc. Natl.
Acad. Sci. U.S.A. 72:979-983, 1975.

278. McGrath, R.A., and R.W. Williams. Radiobiology:
reconstruction in vivo of irradiated Escherichia
coli deoxyribonucleic acid; the rejoining of broken
pieces. Nature 212:534-535, 1966.

279. McKusick, V.A. Medelian Inheritance in Man: Catalogs
of autosomal dominant, autosomal recessive, and X-
linked phenotypes. 5th ed. Baltimore: The Johns
Hopkins Univ. Press, 1978. 975 pp.

280. Mehta, R.D., and R.C. von Borstel. Mutagenic activity
of 42 encoded compounds in the haploid yeast reversion
assay, strain XV185-14C, pp. 414-423. In F.J. de
Serres and J. Ashby, Eds. Evaluation of Short-Term
Tests for Carcinogens. New York: Elsevier/North-
Holland, 1981.

281. Miller, E.C. Some current perspectives on chemical
carcinogenesis in humans and experimental animals.
Cancer Res. 38:1479-1496, 1978.

282. Miller, E.C., and J.A. Miller. Mechanisms of chemical
carcinogenesis. Cancer 47:1055-1064, 1981.

283. Miller, J.A. Carcinogenesis by chemicals: An overview.
G.H.A. Clowes Memorial Lecture. Cancer Res. 30:559-
576, 1970.

284. Miller, J.A., and E.C. Miller. Perspectives on the
metabolism of chemical carcinogens, pp. 25-50. In P.
Emmelot and E. Kriek, Eds. Environmental Carcinogenesis: Occurrence, Risk Evaluation and Mechanism.
Amsterdam: Netherlands Cancer Society, 1979.

285. Minnich, V., M.E. Smith, D. Thompson, and S. Kornfeld.
Detection of mutagenic activity in human urine using
mutant strains of Salmonella typhimurium. Cancer
38:1253-1258, 1976.

286. Mohan Rao, P.K. Biological effects of combination
treatments with ionizing radiation (X-rays) and
diethyl sulfate (dES) in barley. Mutat. Res. 16:322-
327, 1972.

287. Mohan Rao, P.K. The relative merits of the three
methods of measuring mutation frequency in barley.
Radiat. Bot. 12:323-329, 1972.

288. Mohn, G.R., and J. Ellenberger. Appreciation of the
value of different bacterial test systems for
detecting and for ranking chemical mutagens. Arch.
Toxicol. 46:45-60, 1980.

289. Mohn, G.R., and J. Ellenberger. The use of Escherichia
     coli K12/343/113(λ) as a multi-purpose indicator
     strain in various mutagenicity testing procedures,
     pp. 95-118. In B.J. Kilbey, M. Legator, W. Nichols,
     and C. Reimel, Eds. Handbook of Mutagenicity Test
     Procedures. Amsterdam: Elsevier/North Holland, 1977.
290. Moreau, P., and R. Devoret. Potential carcinogens
     tested by induction and mutagenesis of prophage λ in
     Escherichia coli K12, pp. 1451-1472. In H.H. Hiatt,
     J.D. Watson, and J.A. Winsten, Eds. Origins of Human
     Cancer. Vol. 4. Book C. New York: Cold Spring Harbor
     Laboratory, 1977.
291. Mrak, E.M. Report of the Secretary's Commission on
     Pesticides and Their Relationship to Environmental
     Health. Washington, D.C.: U.S. Department of Health,
     Education, and Welfare, 1969. 677 pp.
292. Mukhtar, H., R.M. Philpot, and J.R. Bend. The post-
     natal development of microsomal epoxide hydrase,
     cytosolic glutathione S-transferase, and mitochondrial
     and microsomal cytochrome P-450 in adrenals and
     ovaries of female rats. Drug Metab. Dispos. 6:577-
     583, 1978.
293. Muller, H.J. Artificial transmutation of the gene.
     Science (N.Y.) 66:84-87, 1927.
294. Muller, H.J., and I.H. Herskowitz. Concerning the
     healing of chromosome ends produced by breakage in
     Drosophila melanogaster. Am. Naturalist 88:177-208,
     1954.
295. Muller, H.J., and I.I. Oster. Some mutational
     techniques in Drosophila, pp. 249-278. In W.J.
     Burdette, Ed. Methodology in Basic Genetics. San
     Francisco: Holden-Day, Inc., 1963.
296. Müller, R., and M.F. Rajewsky. Sensitive radio-
     immunoassay for detection of O_6-ethyl-deoxyguanosine
     in DNA exposed to the carcinogen ethylnitrosourea in
     vivo or in vitro. Z. Naturforsch. 33:897-901, 1978.
297. Murthy, M.S.S. Induction of gene conversion in
     diploid yeast by chemicals: Correlation with mutagenic
     action and its relevance in genotoxicity screening.
     Mutat. Res. 64:1-17, 1979.
298. Nance, W.E., L.A. Corey, and J.A. Boughman. Monozygote
     twin kinships: A new design for genetic and epidemiologic
     research, pp. 87-132. In N.E. Morton and C.S. Chung,
     Eds. Genetic Epidemiology. New York: Academic Press,
     1978.
299. National Council on Radiation Protection and Measurements.
     Genetic effects, pp. 22-64. In NCRP Report No. 64.
     Influence of Dose and Its Distribution in Time on

Dose-Response Relationships for Low-LET Radiations. Bethesda, Maryland: National Council on Radiation Protection and Measurements, 1980.

300. National Research Council, Advisory Center on Toxicology. Drinking Water and Health. Vol. 1. Washington, D.C.: National Academy of Sciences, 1977. 939 pp.

301. National Research Council, Advisory Committee on the Biological Effects of Ionizing Radiations. Considerations of Health Benefit-Cost Analysis for Activities Involving Ionizing Radiation Exposure and Alternatives. (BEIR II.) Washington, D.C.: National Academy of Sciences, 1977. 440 pp.

302. National Research Council, Advisory Committee on the Biological Effects of Ionizing Radiations. The Effects on Populations of Exposure to Low Levels of Ionizing Radiation. (BEIR I.) Washington, D.C.: National Academy of Sciences, 1972. 217 pp.

303. National Research Council, Advisory Committee on the Biological Effects of Ionizing Radiations. The Effects on Populations of Exposure to Low Levels of Ionizing Radiation: 1980. (BEIR III.) Washington, D.C.: National Academy of Sciences, 1980. 524 pp.

304. National Research Council, Environmental Studies Board. Principles for Evaluating Chemicals in the Environment. Washington, D.C.: National Academy of Sciences, 1975. 454 pp.

305. Nebert, D.W. Clinical pharmacology: Possible clinical importance of genetic differences in drug metabolism. Brit. Med. J. 283:537-542, 1981.

306. Nebert, D.W. Genetic differences in susceptibility to chemically induced myelotoxicity and leukemia. Environ. Health Perspect. 39:11-22, 1981.

307. Nebert, D.W. Multiple forms of inducible drug-metabolizing enzymes: A reasonable mechanism by which any organism can cope with adversity. Mol. Cell. Biochem. 27:27-46, 1979.

308. Nebert, D.W. Pharmacogenetics: An approach to understanding chemical and biologic aspects of cancer. J. Natl. Cancer Inst. 64:1279-1290, 1980.

309. Nebert, D.W., H.J. Eisen, M. Negishi, M.A. Lang, L.M. Hjelmeland, and A.B. Okey. Genetic mechanisms controlling the induction of polysubstrate mono-oxygenase (P-450) activities. Ann. Rev. Pharmacol. Toxicol. 21:431-462, 1981.

310. Nebert, D.W., and J.S. Felton. Importance of genetic factors influencing the metabolism of foreign compounds. Fed. Proc. 35:1133-1141, 1976.

311. Nebert, D.W., N.M. Jensen, H. Shinozuka, H.W. Kunz,

and T.J. Gill. The Ah phenotype: Survey of forty-eight rat strains and twenty inbred mouse strains. Genetics 100:79-87, 1982.

312. Nebert, D.W., M. Negishi, M.A. Lang, L.M. Hjelmeland, and H.J. Eisen. The Ah locus, a multigene family necessary for survival in a chemically adverse environment: Comparison with the immune system. Advanc. Genet. 21:1-52, 1982.

313. Neel, J.V. Evaluation of the effects of chemical mutagens on man: The long road ahead. Proc. Natl. Acad. Sci. U.S.A. 67:908-915, 1970.

314. Neel, J.V. Monitoring for genetic effects in man, pp. 113-129. In National Research Council, Study Group on Environmental Monitoring. Environmental Monitoring. Washington, D.C.: National Academy of Sciences, 1977.

315. Neel, J.V., H.W. Mohrenweiser, and M.H. Meisler. Rate of spontaneous mutation at human loci encoding protein structure. Proc. Natl. Acad. Sci. U.S.A. 77:6037-6041, 1980.

316. Neel, J.V., T.O. Tiffany, and N.G. Anderson. Approaches to monitoring human populations for mutation rates and genetic disease, pp. 105-150. In A. Hollaender, Ed. Chemical Mutagens: Principles and Methods for Their Detection. Vol. 3. New York: Plenum Press, 1973.

317. Negishi, M., D.C. Swan, L.W. Enquist, and D.W. Nebert. Isolation and characterization of a cloned DNA sequence associated with the murine Ah locus and a 3-methylcholanthrene-induced form of cytochrome P-450. Proc. Natl. Acad. Sci. U.S.A. 78:800-804, 1981.

318. Newbold, R.F., C.B. Wigley, M.H. Thompson, and P. Brookes. Cell-mediated mutagenesis in cultured Chinese hamster cells by carcinogenic polycyclic hydrocarbons: Nature and extent of the associated hydrocarbon-DNA reaction. Mutat. Res. 43:101-116, 1977.

319. Newcombe, H.B. Problem of assessing the genetic impact of mutagens on man. Canad. J. Genet. Cytol. 20:459-470, 1978.

320. Newcombe, H.B. Techniques for monitoring and assessing the significance of mutagenesis in human populations, pp. 57-77. In A. Hollaender, Ed. Chemical Mutagens: Principles and Methods for Their Detection. Vol. 3. New York: Plenum Press, 1973.

321. Niculescu-Duväz, I., T. Craescu, M. Tugulea, A. Croisy, and P.C. Jacquignon. A quantitative structure-activity analysis of the mutagenic and carcinogenic

action of 43 structurally related heterocyclic compounds. Carcinogenesis 2:269-275, 1981.

322. Nilan, R.A., J.L. Rosichan, P. Arenaz, A.L. Hodgdon, and A. Kleinhofs. Pollen genetic markers for detection of mutagens in the environment. Environ. Health Perspect. 37:19-25, 1981.

323. Nilan, R.A., and B.K. Vig. Plant test system for detection of chemical mutagens, pp. 143-170. In A. Hollaender, Ed. Chemical Mutagens: Principles and Methods for Their Detection. Vol. 4. New York: Plenum Press, 1976.

324. Nocke-Finck, L., H. Breuer, and D. Reimers. Wirkung von Rifampicin auf den Menstruationszyklus und die Östrogenausscheidung bei Einnahme oraler Kontrazeptiva. Dtsch. Med. Wochenschr. 98:1521-1523, 1973.

325. Nomura, T. Parental exposure to x rays and chemicals induces heritable tumors and anomalies in mice. Nature 296:575-577, 1982.

326. Oakberg, E.F. Effects of radiation on the testis, pp. 233-243. In R.O. Greep and E.B. Astwood, Eds. Handbook of Physiology. Section 7: Endocrinology. Vol. V: Male Reproductive System. Washington, D.C.: American Physiological Society, 1975.

327. Oakberg, E.F. Radiation response of the testis, pp. 1070-1076. Prog. Endocrinol., Proc. Int. Congr. Endocrinol., 3rd ed., Mexico City, 1969.

328. Oehlkers, F. Die Auslösung von Chromosomenmutationen in der Meiosis durch Einwirkung von Chemikalien. Z. Ind. Abst. u. Vererbungsl. 81:313-341, 1943.

329. Okey, A.B., G.P. Bondy, M.E. Mason, G.F. Kahl, H.J. Eisen, T.M. Guenthner, and D.W. Nebert. Regulatory gene product of the Ah locus. Characterization of the cytosolic inducer-receptor complex and evidence for its nuclear translocation. J. Biol. Chem. 254:11636-11648, 1979.

330. Omura, T., and R. Sato. The carbon monoxide-binding pigment of liver microsomes. I. Evidence for its hemoprotein nature. J. Biol. Chem. 239:2370-2378, 1964.

331. O'Neill, J.P., P.A. Brimer, R. Machanoff, G.P. Hirsch, and A.W. Hsie. A quantitative assay of mutation induction at hypoxanthine-guanine phosphoribosyl transferase locus in Chinese hamster ovary cells (CHO/HGPRT system): Development and definition of the system. Mutat. Res. 45:91-101, 1977.

332. Ong, T-M. Use of the spot, plate and suspension test systems for the detection of the mutagenicity of environmental agents and chemical carcinogens in Neurospora crassa. Mutat. Res. 53:297-308, 1978.

333. O'Reilly, R.A. The second reported kindred with hereditary resistance to oral anticoagulant drugs. N. Eng. J. Med. 282:1448-1451, 1970.

334. Ormstad, K., D.P. Jones, and S. Orrenius. Characteristics of glutathione biosynthesis by freshly isolated rat kidney cells. J. Biol. Chem. 225:175-181, 1980.

335. Osterman-Golkar, S., L. Ehrenberg, D. Segerbäck, and I. Hällström. Evaluation of genetic risks of alkylating agents. II. Haemoglobin as a dose monitor. Mutat. Res. 34:1-10, 1976.

336. Owens, I.S., and D.W. Nebert. Aryl hydrocarbon hydroxylase induction in mammalian liver-derived cell cultures. Effects of various metabolic inhibitors on the enzyme activity in hepatoma cells. Biochem. Pharmacol. 25:805-813, 1976.

337. Owens, I.S., and D.W. Nebert. Aryl hydrocarbon hydroxylase induction in mammalian liver-derived cell cultures. Stimulation of "cytochrome $P_1$450-associated" enzyme activity by many inducing compounds. Mol. Pharmacol. 11:94-104, 1975.

338. Paget, G.E., Ed. Mutagenesis in Sub-Mammalian Systems: Status and Significance. Baltimore: Univ. Park Press, 1979. 231 pp.

339. Park, S.D., and J.E. Cleaver. Postreplication repair: Questions of its definicition and possible alteration in xeroderma pigmentosum cell strains. Proc. Natl. Acad. Sci. U.S.A. 76:3927-3931, 1979.

340. Parker, D.R. Radiation-induced exchanges in Drosophila females. Proc. Natl. Acad. Sci. U.S.A. 40:795-800, 1954.

341. Parodi, S., R.A. Mulivor, J.T. Martin, C. Nicolini, D.S.R. Sarma, and E. Farber. Alkaline lysis of mammalian cells for sedimentation analysis of nuclear DNA. Conformation of released DNA as monitored by physical, electron microscopic and enzymological techniques. Biochim. Biophys. Acta 407:174-190, 1975.

342. Parodi, S., M. Taningher, L. Santi, M. Cavanna, L. Sciaba, A. Maura, and G. Brambilla. A practical procedure for testing DNA damage in vivo, proposed for a pre-screening of chemical carcinogens. Mutat. Res. 54:39-46, 1978.

343. Parry, J.M., and D.C. Sharp. Induction of mitotic aneuploidy in the yeast strain D6 by 42 coded compounds, pp. 468-480. In F.J. de Serres and J. Ashby, Eds. Evaluation of Short-Term Tests for Carcinogens. New York: Elsevier/North-Holland, 1981.

344. Parry, J.M., D. Sharp, and E.M. Parry. Detection of

mitotic and meiotic aneuploidy in the yeast <u>Saccharomyces</u> <u>cerevisiae</u>. Environ. Health Perspect. 31:97-111, 1979.

345. Parry, J.M., and F.K. Zimmerman. The detection of monosomic colonies produced by mitotic chromosome non-disjunction in the yeast <u>Saccharomyces</u> <u>cerevisiae</u>. Mutat. Res. 36:49-66, 1976.

346. Patel, J.M., J.C. Wood, and K.C. Leibman. The biotransformation of allyl alcohol and acrolein in rat liver and lung preparations. Drug Metab. Dispos. 8:305-308, 1980.

347. Paterson, M.C. Use of purified lesion-recognizing enzymes to monitor DNA repair <u>in</u> <u>vivo</u>. Advanc. Radiat. Bio. 7:1-53, 1978.

348. Paterson, M.C., and P.J. Smith. Ataxia telangiectasia: an inherited human disorder involving hypersensitivity to ionizing radiation and related DNA-damaging chemicals. Ann. Rev. Genetics 13:291-318, 1979.

349. Pedersen, R.A., and F. Mangia. Ultraviolet-light-induced unscheduled DNA synthesis by resting and growing mouse oocytes. Mutat. Res. 49:425-429, 1978.

350. Pero, R.W., and F. Mitelman. Another approach to <u>in</u> <u>vivo</u> estimation of genetic damage in humans. Proc. Natl. Acad. Sci. U.S.A. 76:462-463, 1979.

351. Petzold, G.L., and J.A. Swenberg. Detection of DNA damage induced <u>in</u> <u>vivo</u> following exposure of rats to carcinogens. Cancer Res. 38:1589-1594, 1978.

352. Plapp, Jr., F.W., and T.C. Wang. Genetic origins of insecticide resistance. In G.P. Georghiou and I. Yamamoto, Eds. Pest Resistance to Pesticides. New York: Academic Press. (in press)

353. Plewa, M.J. Activation of chemicals into mutagens by green plants: A preliminary discussion. Environ. Health Perspect. 27:45-50, 1978.

354. Plewa, M.J., and J.M. Gentile. Mutagenicity of Atrazine: A maize-microbe bioassay. Mutat. Res. 38:287-292, 1976.

355. Plewa, M.J., and E.D. Wagner. Germinal cell mutagenesis in specially designed maize genotypes. Environ. Health Perspect. 37:61-73, 1981.

356. Poirier, M.C., R. Santella, I.B. Weinstein, D. Grunberger, and S.H. Yuspa. Quantitation of benzo(a)-pyrene-deoxyguanosine adducts by radioimmunoassay. Cancer Res. 40:412-416, 1980.

357. Purchase, I.F.H. Inter-species comparisons of carcinogenicity. Br. J. Cancer 41:454-468, 1980.

358. Purchase, I.F.H., E. Longstaff, J. Ashby, J.A. Styles, D. Anderson, P.A. Lefevre, and F.R. Westwood. An evaluation of 6 short-term tests for detecting

organic chemical carcinogens. Br. J. Cancer 37:873-959, 1978.

359. Rall, D.P. Validity of extrapolation of results of animal studies to man. Ann. N.Y. Acad. Sci. 329:85-91, 1979.

360. Rannug, U., A. Johansson, C. Ramel, and C.A. Wachtmeister. The mutagenicity of vinyl chloride after metabolic activation. Ambio 3:194-197, 1974.

361. Rapoport, I.A. The effect of ethylene oxide, glycide, and glycol on genic mutations. Dokl. Akad. Nauk. SSSR 60:467, 1948.

362. Raposa, T. Sister chromatid exchange studies for monitoring DNA damage and repair capacity after cytostatics in vitro and in lymphocytes of leukaemic patients under cytostatic therapy. Mutat. Res. 57:241-251, 1978.

363. Rasmussen, R.E., and P.B. Painter. Evidence for repair of ultra-violet damaged deoxyribonucleic acid in cultured mammalian cells. Nature 203:1360-1362, 1964.

364. Rédei, G.P., M.M. Rédei, W.R. Lower, and S. Sandhu. Identification of carcinogens by mutagenicity for Arabidopsis. Mutat. Res. 74:469-475, 1980.

365. Regan, J.D., and R.B. Setlow. Repair of chemical damage to human DNA, pp. 151-170. In A. Hollaender, Ed. Chemical Mutagens: Principles and Methods for Their Detection. Vol. 3. New York: Plenum Press, 1973.

366. Reimers, T.J., P.M. Sluss, J. Goodwin, and G.E. Seidel. Bigenerational effects of 6-mercaptopurine on reproduction in mice. Biol. Reprod. 22:367-375, 1980.

367. Rethoré, M. Relationships between aneuploidy and development, pp. 101-107. In J.W. Littlefield, J. deGrouchy, and F.J.G. Ebling, Eds. Birth Defects. Proc. of Fifth Internatl. Conference. Excerpta Medica: Amsterdam, 1978.

368. Rice, S.A., and R.E. Talcott. Effects of isoniazid treatment on selected hepatic mixed-function oxidases. Drug Metab. Dispos. 7:260-262, 1979.

369. Rinkus, S.J., and M.S. Legator. Chemical characterization of 465 known or suspected carcinogens and their correlation with mutagenic activity in the Salmonella typhimurium system. Cancer Res. 39:3289-3318, 1979.

370. Rinkus, S.J., and M.S. Legator. The need for both in vitro and in vivo systems in mutagenicity screening, pp. 365-473. In F.J. de Serres and A. Hollaender, Eds. Chemical Mutagens: Principles and Methods for

Their Detection. Vol. 6. New York: Plenum Press, 1980.

371. Ripley, L. S. Model for the participation of quasi-palindromic DNA sequences in frameshift mutation. Proc. Natl. Acad. Sci. U.S.A. 79:4128-4132, 1982.

372. Robbins, A.R., and R.M. Baker. (Na, K)ATPase activity in membrane preparations of ouabain-resistant HeLa cells. Biochemistry 16:5163-5168, 1977.

373. Rosenkranz, H.S., B. Gutter, and W.T. Speck. Mutagenicity and DNA-modifying activity: a comparison of two microbial assays. Mutat. Res. 41:61-70, 1976.

374. Rüdiger, H.W., F. Haenisch, M. Metzler, F. Oesch, and H.R. Glatt. Metabolites of diethylstilboestrol induced sister chromatid exchange in human fibroblasts. Nature 281:392-394, 1979.

375. Russell, L.B. Definition of functional units in a small chromosomal segment of the mouse and its use in interpreting the nature of radiation-induced mutations. Mutat. Res. 11:107-123, 1971.

376. Russell, L.B. Numerical sex-chromosome anomalies in mammals: Their spontaneous occurrence and use in mutagenesis studies, pp. 55-91. In A. Hollaender, Ed. Chemical Mutagens: Principles and Methods for Their Detection. Vol. 4. New York: Plenum Press, 1976.

377. Russell, L.B., P.B. Selby, E. von Halle, W. Sheridan, and L. Valcovic. The mouse specific-locus test with agents other than radiations. Interpretation of data and recommendations for future work. Mutat. Res. 86:329-354, 1981.

378. Russell, L.B., P.B. Selby, E. von Halle, W. Sheridan, and L. Valcovic. Use of the mouse spot test in chemical mutagenesis: Interpretation of past data and recommendations for future work. Mutat. Res. 86:355-379, 1981.

379. Russell, W.L. Comments on mutagenesis risk estimation. Genetics 92:s187-s194, 1979.

380. Russell, W.L. Factors affecting mutagenicity of ethylnitrosourea in the mouse specific-locus test and their bearing on risk estimation, pp. 59-70. In T. Sugimura, S. Kondo, and H. Takebe, Eds. Environmental Mutagens and Carcinogens. New York: Alan R. Liss. (in press)

381. Russell, W.L. Mutation frequencies in female mice and the estimation of genetic hazards of radiation in women. Proc. Natl. Acad. Sci. U.S.A. 74:3523-3527, 1977.

382. Russell, W.L. X-ray-induced mutations in mice. Cold

Spring Harbor Symposium. Quant. Biol. 16:327-336, 1951.

383. Russell, W.L., P.R. Hunsicker, D.A. Carpenter, C.V. Cornett, and G.M. Guinn. Effect of dose fractionation on the ethylnitrosourea induction of specific-locus mutations in mouse spermatogonia. Proc. Natl. Acad. Sci. U.S.A. 79:3592-3593, 1982.

384. Russell, W.L., P.R. Hunsicker, E.M. Kelly, C.M. Vaughan, and G.M. Guinn. Preliminary test of the effect of hycanthone on X-chromosome loss in mice, p. 116. In Oak Ridge National Laboratory. Annual Program. ORNL-4993. June 30, 1974.

385. Russell, W.L., E.M. Kelly, P.R. Hunsicker, J.W. Bangham, S.C. Maddux, and E.L. Phipps. Specific-locus test shows ethylnitrosourea to be the most potent mutagen in the mouse. Proc. Natl. Acad. Sci. U.S.A. 76:5818-5819, 1979.

386. Sankaranarayanan, K., and F. Sobels. Radiation Genetics, pp. 1089-1250. In M. Ashburner and E. Novitski, Eds. The Genetics and Biology of Drosophila. Vol. 1c. New York: Academic Press, 1976.

387. Sarma, D.S.R., S. Rajalakshmi, and E. Farber. Chemical carcinogenesis: interactions of carcinogens with nucleic acids, pp. 235-287. In F.F. Becker, Ed. Cancer: A Comprehensive Treatise. Vol. 1. New York: Plenum Press, 1975.

388. Sato, K., R.S. Slesinski, and J.W. Littlefield. Chemical mutagenesis at the phosphoribosyltrans-ferase locus in cultured human lymphoblasts. Proc. Natl. Acad. Sci. U.S.A. 69:1244-1248, 1972.

389. Sato, R., and T. Omura, Eds. Cytochrome P-450. New York: Academic Press, 1978. 233 pp.

390. Schairer, L.A., J. Van't Hof, C.G. Hayes, R.M. Burton, and F.J. de Serres. Exploratory monitoring of air pollutants for mutagenicity activity with the Tradescantia stamen hair system. Environ. Health Perspect. 27:51-60, 1978.

391. Schalet, A.P., and K. Sankaranarayanan. Evaluation and re-evaluation of genetic radiation hazards in man. I. Interspecific comparison of estimates of mutation rates. Mutat. Res. 35:341-370, 1976.

392. Schmid, W. The micronucleus test. Mutat. Res. 31:9-15, 1975.

393. Schmid, W. The micronucleus test, pp. 235-242. In B.J. Kilbey, M. Legator, W. Nichols, and C. Ramel, Eds. Handbook of Mutagenicity Test Procedures. Amsterdam: Elsevier/North Holland, 1977.

394. Schmid, W. The micronucleus test for cytogenetic analysis, pp. 31-53. In A. Hollaender, Ed. Chemical

Mutagens: Principles and Methods for Their Detection. Vol. 4. New York: Plenum Press, 1976.

395. Schneiderman, M.A., P. Decouflé, and C.C. Brown. Thresholds for environmental cancer: biologic and statistical considerations. Ann. N.Y. Acad. Sci. 329:92-130, 1979.

396. Schull, W.J., M. Otake, and J.V. Neel. Genetic effects of the atomic bombs: A reappraisal. Science 213:1220-1227, 1981.

397. Schwartz, M., K.E. Appel, R. Rickart, and K.W. Kunz. Effect of DMN, phenobarbital and halothane, on the sedimentation characteristics of rat liver DNA. Arch. Toxicol. Suppl. 2:479-482, 1979.

398. Scott, B.R., G.L. Dorn, E. Käfer, and R. Stafford. Aspergillus nidulans: Systems and results of tests for induction of mitotic segregation and mutation. II. Haploid assay systems and overall response of all systems. A report of the U.S. EPA GENE-TOX Program. Mutat. Res. 98:49-94, 1982.

399. Searle, A.G. Mutation induction in mice. Adv. Radiat. Biol. 4:131-207, 1974.

400. Sega, G.A. Molecular dosimetry of chemical mutagens. Measurement of molecular dose and DNA repair in mammalian germ cells. Mutat. Res. 38:317-326, 1976.

401. Sega, G.A. Unscheduled DNA synthesis in the germ cells of male mice exposed in vivo to the chemical mutagen ethyl methanesulfonate. Proc. Natl. Acad. Sci. U.S.A. 71:4955-4959, 1974.

402. Sega, G.A., J.G. Owens, and R.B. Cumming. Studies on DNA repair in early spermatid stages of male mice after in vivo treatment with methyl-, ethyl-, propyl-, and isopropyl methanesulfonate. Mutat. Res. 36:193-212, 1976.

403. Sega, G.A., and R.E. Sotomayor. Unscheduled DNA synthesis in mammalian germ cells. Its potential use in mutagenicity testing, pp. 421-445. In F.J. de Serres and A. Hollaender, Eds. Chemical Mutagens: Principles and Methods for Their Detection. Vol. 7. New York: Plenum Press, 1982.

404. Sega, G.A., R.E. Sotomayor, and J.G. Owens. A study of unscheduled DNA synthesis induced by x-rays in the germ cells of male mice. Mutat. Res. 49:239-257, 1978.

405. Sega, G.A., K.W. Wolfe, and J.G. Owens. A comparison of the molecular action of an S_N1-type methylating agent, methyl nitrosourea and an S_N2-type methylating agent, methyl methanesulfonate, in the germ cells of male mice. Chem.-Biol. Interactions 33:253-269, 1981.

406. Segerbäck, D., C.J. Calleman, L. Ehrenberg, G. Löfroth, and S. Osterman-Golkar. Evaluation of genetic risks of alkylating agents. IV. Quantitative determination of alkylated amino acids in haemo-globin as a measure of the dose after treatment of mice with methyl methanesulfonate. Mutat. Res. 49:71-82, 1978.

407. Selby, P.B. Dominant skeletal mutation: Applications in mutagenicity-testing and risk estimation, pp. 385-406. In J.A. Heddle, Ed. Mutagenicity: New Horizons in Genetic Toxicology. New York: Academic Press, 1982.

408. Selby, P.B. Radiation-induced dominant skeletal mutations in mice: Mutation rate, characteristics, and usefulness in estimating genetic hazard to humans from radiation, pp. 537-544. In S. Okada, M. Imamura, T. Terashima, and H. Yamaguchi, Eds. Radiation Research. Proceedings of the 6th International Congress of Radiation Research. Tokyo: ICRR, 1979.

409. Selby, P.B., and P.R. Selby. Gamma-ray-induced dominant mutations that cause skeletal abnormalities in mice. I. Plan, summary of results, and discussion. Mutat. Res. 43:357-375, 1977.

410. Selby, P.B., and P.R. Selby. Gamma-ray-induced dominant mutations that cause skeletal abnormalities in mice. II. Description of proved mutations. Mutat. Res. 51:199-236, 1978.

411. Selby, P.B., and P.R. Selby. Gamma-ray-induced dominant mutations that cause skeletal abnormalities in mice. III. Description of presumed mutations. Mutat. Res. 50:341-351, 1978.

412. Selkirk, J.K. Benzo(a)pyrene carcinogenesis: A biochemical selection mechanism. J. Toxicol Environ. Health 2:1245-1258, 1977.

413. Selkirk, J.K. Divergence of metabolic activation systems for short-term mutagenesis assays. Nature 270:604-607, 1977.

414. Selkirk, J.K., R.G. Croy, F.J. Wiebel, and H.V. Gelboin. Differences in benzo(a)pyrene metabolism between rodent liver microsomes and embryonic cells. Cancer Res. 36:4476-4479, 1976.

415. Setchell, B.P., and G.M.H. Waites. The blood-testis barrier, pp. 143-172. In R.O. Greep and E.B. Astwood, Eds. Handbook of Physiology. Section 7: Endocrinology. Vol. V: Male Reproductive System. Washington, D.C.: American Physiological Society, 1975.

416. Sharp, D.C., and J.M. Parry. Induction of mitotic gene conversion by 41 coded compounds using the yeast culture JD1, pp. 491-501. In F.J. de Serres

and J. Ashby, Eds. Evaluation of Short-Term Tests for Carcinogens. New York: Elsevier/North-Holland, 1981.

417. Sharp, D.C., and J.M. Parry. Use of repair-deficient strains of yeast to assay the activity of 40 coded compounds, pp. 502-516. In F.J. de Serres and J. Ashby, Eds. Evaluation of Short-Term Tests for Carcinogens. New York: Elsevier/North-Holland, 1981.

418. Shum, S., N.M. Jensen, and D.W. Nebert. The Murine Ah locus: In utero toxicity and teratogenesis associated with genetic differences in benzo(a)pyrene metabolism. Teratology 20:365-376, 1979.

419. Siminovitch, L. On the nature of hereditable variation in cultured somatic cells. Cell 7:1-11, 1976.

420. Simmon, V.F., H.S. Rosenkranz, E. Zeiger, and L.A. Poirier. Mutagenic activity of chemical carcinogens and related compounds in the intraperitoneal host-mediated assay. J. Natl. Cancer Inst. 62:911-918, 1979.

421. Simmons, M.J., and J.F. Crow. Mutations affecting fitness in Drosophila populations. Ann. Rev. Genet. 11:49-78, 1977.

422. Sims, P., P.L. Grover, A. Swaisland, K. Pal, and A. Hewer. Metabolic activation of benzo(a)pyrene proceeds by a diol-epoxide. Nature 252:326-328, 1974.

423. Skopek, T.R., H.L. Liber, D.A. Kaden, and W.G. Thilly. Relative sensitivities of forward and reverse mutation assays in Salmonella typhimurium. Proc. Natl. Acad. Sci. U.S.A. 75:4465-4469, 1978.

424. Soares, E.R. TEM-induced gene mutations at enzyme loci in the mouse. Environ. Mutagenesis 1:19-25, 1979.

425. Sobels, F.H. ICPEMC News No. 2. Mutat. Res. 64:357-361, 1979.

426. Sofuni, T., H. Shimba, K. Ohtaki, and A.A. Awa. G-banding Analysis of Chromosome Aberrations in Hiroshima Atomic Bomb Survivors. Radiation Effects Research Foundation Technical Report #13-77. Hiroshima: Radiation Effects Research Foundation, 1978. 8 pp.

427. Sora, S., L. Panzeri, G. Luchini Bonomini, and M.L. Carbone. Saccharomyces cerevisiae-mitotic gene conversion and mitotic crossing over, pp. 141-168. In G.E. Magni, Ed. Mutagenesi Ambientale. Metodiche di Analisi, Vol. 1. Test in vitro, Centro Nazio nale delle Ricerche, Rome, 1979.

428. Sotomayor, R.E., G.A. Sega, and R.B. Cumming. Unscheduled DNA synthesis in spermatogenic cells of mice treated in vivo with the indirect alkylating

agents cyclophosphamide and mitomen. Mutat. Res. 50:229-240, 1978.

429. Spalding, J.F., M.R. Brooks, and G.L. Tietjen. Lifetime body weights and mortality distributions of mice with 10 to 35 generations of ancestral x-ray exposure. Genetics 63:897-906, 1969.

430. Squire, R.A. Ranking animal carcinogens: A proposed regulatory approach. Science 214:877-880, 1981.

431. Stadler, L.J. Mutations in barley induced by x-rays and radium. Science (N.Y.) 68:186-187, 1928.

432. Staffa, J.A., and M.A. Mehlman, Eds. Innovations in Cancer Risk Assessment (ED_{01} Study). J. Environ. Pathol. Toxicol. 3:1-246, 1980. (Special issue on the proceedings of a symposium sponsored by the National Center for Toxicological Research, U.S. Food and Drug Administration, and the American College of Toxicology.)

433. Stamatoyannopoulos, G. Possibilities for demonstrating point mutations in somatic cells, as illustrated by studies of mutant hemoglobins, pp. 49-62. In K. Berg, Ed. Genetic Damage in Man Caused by Environmental Agents. New York: Academic Press, 1979.

434. Stamatoyannopoulos, G., P.E. Nute, Th. Papayannopoulou, T. McGuire, G. Lim, H.F. Bunn, and D. Rucknagel. Development of a somatic mutation screening system using Hb mutants. IV. Successful detection of red cells containing the human frameshift mutants Hb Wayne and Hb Cranston using monospecific fluorescent antibodies. Am. J. Hum. Genet. 32:484-496, 1980.

435. Steinberger, E. Potential male antifertility agents, pp. 33-49. In F.G. McMahon, Ed. Endocrine-Metabolic Drugs. Vol. VI. New York: Futura, 1974.

436. Stephen, A.M., and J.H. Cummings. Mechanism of action of dietary fibre in the human colon. Nature 284:283-284, 1980.

437. Stevenson, A. The load of hereditary defects in human populations. Rad. Res. 1(Suppl. 1):306-325, 1959.

438. Stewart, B.W., and E. Farber. Strand breakage in rat liver DNA and its repair following administration of cyclic nitrosamines. Cancer Res. 33:3209-3215, 1973.

439. Stich, H.F., R.H.C. San, and Y. Kawazoe. DNA repair synthesis in mammalian cells exposed to a series of oncogenic and non-oncogenic derivatives of 4-nitroquinoline 1-oxide. Nature 229:416-419, 1971.

440. Stich, H.F., R.H.C. San, P. Lam, J. Koropatnick, and L. Lo. Unscheduled DNA synthesis of human cells as a short-term assay for chemical carcinogens, pp. 1499-

1512. In H.H. Hiatt, J.D. Watson, and J.A. Winsten, Eds. Origins of Human Cancer. Book C. New York: Cold Spring Harbor Laboratory, 1977.

441. Straus, D.S. Somatic mutation, cellular differentiation, and cancer causation. J. Natl. Cancer Inst. 67:233-241, 1981.

442. Strauss, G.H., and R.J. Albertini. Enumeration of 6-thioguanine-resistant peripheral blood lymphocytes in man as a potential test for somatic cell mutations arising in vivo. Mutat. Res. 61:353-379, 1979.

443. Sutherland, B.M. Photoreactivating enzyme from human leucocytes. Nature 284:109-112, 1974.

444. Sutherland, B.M., P. Runge, and J.C. Sutherland. DNA photoreactivating enzyme from placental mammals. Origin and characteristics. Biochemistry 13:4710-4715, 1974.

445. Sutton, H.E. An Introduction to Human Genetics. 3rd ed. New York: Holt, Rinehart, and Winston, 1980. 592 pp.

446. Sutton, H.E. Prospects of monitoring environmental mutagenesis through somatic mutations, pp. 237-248. In E.B. Hook, D.T. Janerich, and I.H. Porter, Eds. Monitoring, Birth Defects and Environment: The Problem of Surveillance. New York: Academic Press, 1971.

447. Sutton, H.E. The impact of induced mutations on human populations. Mutat. Res. 33:17-24, 1975.

448. Sutton, H.E., and M.I. Harris, Eds. Mutagenic Effects of Environmental Contaminants. New York: Academic Press, 1972. 195 pp.

449. Swift, M., J. Cohen, and R. Pinkham. A maximum-likelihood method for estimating the disease predisposition of heterozygotes. Am. J. Hum. Genet. 26:304-317, 1974.

450. Swift, M., L. Sholman, M. Perry, and C. Chase. Malignant neoplasms in the families of patients with ataxia-telangiectasia. Cancer Res. 36:209-215, 1976.

451. Szybalski, W., E.H. Szybalska, and G. Ragni. Genetic studies with human cell lines. Natl. Cancer Inst. Monogr. 7:75-89, 1962.

452. Tamura, G., C. Gold, A. Ferro-Luzzi, and B.N. Ames. Fecalase: A model for activation of dietary glycosides to mutagens by intestinal flora. Proc. Natl. Acad. Sci. U.S.A. 77:4961-4965, 1980.

453. Tates, A.D. Microtus oeconomus (Rodentia), a useful mammal for studying the induction of sex-chromosome nondisjunction and diploid gametes in male germ cells. Environ. Health Perspect. 31:151-159, 1979.

454. Taylor, A.M.R., D.G. Harnden, C.F. Arlett, S.A.

Harcourt, A.R. Lehmann, S. Stevens, and B.A. Bridges. Ataxia telangiectasia: a human mutation with abnormal radiation sensitivity. Nature 258:427-429, 1975.

455. Taylor, A.M.R., C.M. Rosney, and J.B. Campbell. Unusual sensitivity of ataxia telangiectasia cells to bleomycin. Cancer Res. 39:1046-1050, 1979.

456. Taylor, L.S. Radiation Protection Standards. Cleveland: CRC Press, 1971. 112 pp.

457. Teramoto, S., R. Saito, H. Aoyama, and Y. Shirasu. Dominant lethal mutation induced in male rats by 1,2-dibromo-3-chloropropane (DBCP). Mutat. Res. 77:71-81, 1980.

458. Therman, E. Human Chromosomes: Structure, Behavior, Effects. New York: Springer-Verlag, 1981. 235 pp.

459. Thor, H., P. Moldéus, N. Danell, and S. Orrenius. Isolated liver cells for the study of drug toxicity, pp. 355-371. In R.W. Estabrook and E. Lindenlaub, Eds. The Induction of Drug Metabolism. New York: Schattauer Verlag, 1979.

460. Tomatis, L. The value of long-term testing for the implementation of primary prevention, pp. 1339-1357. In H.H. Hiatt, J.D. Watson, and J.A. Winsten, Eds. Origins of Human Cancer. Human Risk Assessment. Book C. New York: Cold Spring Harbor Laboratory, 1977.

461. Tomkins, D.J., and W.F. Grant. Monitoring natural vegetation for herbicide-induced chromosomal aberrations. Mutat. Res. 36:73-84, 1976.

462. Topham, J.C. Do induced sperm-head abnormalities in mice specifically identify mammalian mutagens rather than carcinogens? Mutat. Res. 74:379-387, 1980.

463. Traut, H. Aneuploidy patterns in Drosophila melanogaster. Environ. Mutagenesis 3:275-286, 1981.

464. Trimble, B.K., and M.E. Smith. The incidence of genetic disease and the impact on man of an altered mutation rate. Canad. J. Genet. Cytol. 19:375-385, 1977.

465. Tukey, R.H., D.W. Nebert, and M. Negishi. Structural gene product of the [Ah] complex. Evidence for transcriptional control of cytochrome P_1-450 induction by use of a cloned DNA sequence. J. Biol. Chem. 256:6969-6974, 1981.

466. Underbrink, A.G., L.A. Schairer, and A.H. Sparrow. Tradescantia stamen hairs: A radiobiological test system applicable to chemical mutagenesis, pp. 171-207. In A. Hollaender, Ed. Chemical Mutagens: Principles and Methods for Their Detection. Vol. 3. New York: Plenum Press, 1973.

467. United Nations Environment Program (UNEP). The

International Register of Potentially Toxic Chemicals. September 1975.

468. United Nations General Assembly. Report of the United Nations Scientific Committee on the Effects of Atomic Radiation. Official Records of the General Assembly. Thirteenth Session. Supplement No. 17 (A/3838). New York: United Nations, 1958.

469. United Nations General Assembly. Report of the United Nations Scientific Committee on the Effects of Atomic Radiation. Official Records of the General Assembly. Seventeenth Session. Supplement No. 16 (A/5216). New York: United Nations, 1962.

470. United Nations General Assembly. Report of the United Nations Scientific Committee on the Effects of Atomic Radiation. Official Records of the General Assembly. Twenty-first Session. Supplement No. 14 (A/6314). New York: United Nations, 1966.

471. United Nations General Assembly. Report of the United Nations Scientific Committee on the Effects of Atomic Radiation. Official Records of the General Assembly. Twenty-fourth Session. Supplement No. 13 (A/7613). New York: United Nations, 1969.

472. United Nations General Assembly. Report of the United Nations Scientific Committee on the Effects of Atomic Radiation. Ionizing Radiation: Levels and Effects. Vol. II. Official Records of the General Assembly. Twenty-seventh Session. Supplement No. 25 (A/8725). New York: United Nations, 1972.

473. United Nations General Assembly. Report of the United Nations Scientific Committee on the Effects of Atomic Radiation. Official Records of the General Assembly. Thirty-second Session. Supplement No. 40 (A/32/40). New York: United Nations, 1977.

474. U.S. Environmental Protection Agency. Water quality criteria. Fed. Register 44:15926-15981, 1979.

475. U.S. Environmental Protection Agency, Office of Research and Development, Reproductive Effects Assessment Group. Mutagenicity risk assessment: Proposed guidelines. Fed. Register 45(221):74984-74988, November 13, 1980.

476. Vähäkangas, K., D.W. Nebert, and O. Pelkonen. The DNA binding of benzo(a)pyrene metabolites catalysed by rat lung microsomes in vitro and in isolated perfused rat lung. Chem. Biol. Interact. 24:167-176, 1979.

477. Valencia, R., S. Abrahamson, W.R. Lee, E.S. VonHalle, R.C. Woodruff, F.E. Würgler, and S. Zimmering. Chromosome mutation tests for mutagenesis in *Drosophila melanogaster*. Mutat. Res. (in press)

478. Van Thiel, D.H., J.S. Gavaler, C.F. Cobb, R.J. Sherins, and R. Lester. Alcohol-induced testicular atrophy in the adult male rat. Endocrinology 105:888-895, 1979.

479. Van Thiel, D.H., J.S. Gavaler, W.I. Smith, and G. Paul. Hypothalamic-pituitary-gonadal dysfunction in men using cimetidine. N. Eng. J. Med. 300:1012-1015, 1979.

480. van Zeeland, A.A., M.C.E. van Diggelen, and J.W.I.M. Simons. The role of metabolic cooperation in selection of hypoxanthine-guanine-phosphoribosyl-transferase (HG-PRT)-deficient mutants from diploid mammalian cell strains. Mutat. Res. 14:355-363, 1972.

481. Vig, B.K. Soybean (Glycine max): A new test system for study of genetic parameters as affected by environmental mutagens. Mutat. Res. 31:49-56, 1975.

482. Vogel, E. The relation between mutational pattern and concentration by chemical mutagens in Drosophila, pp. 117-132. In R. Montesano, H. Bartsch, and L. Tomatis, Eds. Screening Tests in Chemical Carcinogenesis. IARC Publication No. 12. Lyon: International Agency for Research on Cancer, 1976.

483. Vogel, F., and G. Röhrborn, Eds. Chemical Mutagenesis in Mammals and Man. New York: Springer-Verlag, 1970. 519 pp.

484. von Wettstein, D., A. Kahn, O.F. Nielsen, and S. Gough. Genetic regulation of chlorophyll synthesis analyzed with mutants in barley. Science 184:800-802, 1974.

485. Waldstein, E.A., E-H. Cao, and R.B. Setlow. Adaptive resynthesis of O^6-methylguanine-accepting protein can explain the differences between mammalian cells proficient and deficient in methyl excision repair. Proc. Natl. Acad. Sci. U.S.A. 79:5117-5121, 1982.

486. Waters, M.D. The GENE-TOX program, pp. 449-467. In A.W. Hsie, P.J. O'Neil, and V.K. McElheny, Eds. Mammalian Cell Mutagenesis: The Maturation of Test Systems. Banbury Report 2. New York: Cold Spring Harbor Laboratory, 1979.

487. Weatherall, D.J., and J.B. Clegg. The Thalassaemia Syndromes. 3rd ed. Oxford: Blackwell Scientific Publications, 1981. 875 pp.

488. Weinstein, I.B., A.M. Jeffrey, K.W. Jennette, S.H. Blobstein, R.G. Harvey, C. Harris, H. Autrup, H. Kasai, and K. Nakanishi. Benzo(a)pyrene diol epoxides as intermediates in nucleic acid binding in vitro and in vivo. Science 193:592-595, 1976.

489. Weinstein, I.B., R.A. Mufson, L-S. Lee, P.B. Fisher,

J. Laskin, A.D. Horowitz, and V. Ivanovic. Membrane and other biochemical effects of the phorbol esters and their relevance to tumor promotion, pp. 543-563. In B. Pullman, P.O.P. Ts'o, and H. Gelboin, Eds. Carcinogenesis: Fundamental Mechanisms and Environmental Effects. Boston: Reidel Publishing Co., 1980.

490. Weisburger, J.H., and G.M. Williams. Metabolism of chemical carcinogens, pp. 185-234. In F.F. Becker, Ed. Cancer: A Comprehensive Treatise. New York: Plenum Press, 1975.

491. Williams, G.M. Carcinogen-induced DNA repair in primary rat liver cell cultures; a possible screen for chemical carcinogens. Cancer Lett. 1:231-235, 1976.

492. Williams, G.M. Detection of chemical carcinogens by unscheduled DNA synthesis in rat liver primary cell cultures. Cancer Res. 37:1845-1851, 1977.

493. Williams, G.M. Further improvements in the hepatocyte primary culture DNA repair test for carcinogens: detection of carcinogenic biphenyl derivatives. Cancer Lett. 4:69-75, 1978.

494. Williams, G.M. Review of in vitro test systems using DNA damage and repair for screening of chemical carcinogens. J. Assoc. Official Anal. Chem. 62:857-863, 1979.

495. Williams, G.M., C. Bordet, P.A. Cerutti, R.P. Fuchs, J. Laval, S-H. Lu, S. Parodi, A.E. Pegg, and M.F. Rajewsky. DNA damage and repair in mammalian cells, pp. 201-226. In Long-Term and Short-Term Screening Assays for Carcinogens: A Critical Appraisal. IARC Monographs. Supplement 2. Lyon: International Agency for Research on Cancer, 1980.

496. Williams, G.M., and M.F. Laspia. The detection of various nitrosamines in the hepatocyte primary culture/DNA repair test. Cancer Lett. 6:199-206, 1979.

497. Wills, C. Three kinds of genetic variability in yeast populations. Proc. Natl. Acad. Sci. U.S.A. 61:937-944, 1968.

498. Witkin, E.M. Ultraviolet mutagenesis and inducible DNA repair in Escherichia coli. Bact. Rev. 40:869-907, 1976.

499. Wolff, S. Cytogenetic analyses at chemical disposal sites: Problems and prospects, pp. 61-80. In W.W. Lowrance, Ed. Assessment of Health Effects at Chemical Disposal Sites. New York: Rockefeller Univ. Press, 1981.

500. Wolff, S. Radiation Genetics, pp. 419-475. In M.

Errera and A. Forssberg, Eds. Mechanisms in Radiobiology. Vol. 1: General Principles. New York: Academic Press, 1961.

501. Wolff, S. Sister chromatid exchange. Ann. Rev. Genet. 11:183-201, 1977.

502. Wolff, S. Sister chromatid exchange: The most sensitive mammalian system for determining the effects of mutagenic carcinogens, pp. 229-246. In K. Berg, Ed. Genetic Damage in Man Caused by Environmental Agents. New York: Academic Press, 1979.

503. Wolff, S., and B. Rodin. Saccharin-induced sister chromatid exchanges in Chinese hamster and human cells. Science 200:543-545, 1978.

504. Wong, T-W., and Z. Hruban. Testicular degeneration and necrosis induced by chlorcyclizine. Lab. Invest. 26:278-289, 1972.

505. Wright, A.S. The role of metabolism in chemical mutagenesis and chemical carcinogenesis. ICPEMC Working Paper 2/2. Mutat. Res. 75:215-241, 1980.

506. Wright, S. Evolution in Mendelian populations. Genetics 16:97-159, 1931.

507. Würgler, F.E., and U. Graf. Mutation induction in repair-deficient strains of Drosophila, pp. 223-240. In W.M. Generoso, M.D. Shelby, and F.J. de Serres, Eds. DNA Repair and Mutagenesis in Eukaryotes. New York: Plenum Press, 1980.

508. Würgler, F.E., F.H. Sobels, and E. Vogel. Drosophila as assay system for detecting changes, pp. 335-373. In B.J. Kilbey, M. Legator, W. Nichols, and C. Ramel, Eds. Handbook of Mutagenicity Test Procedures. Amsterdam: Elsevier/North Holland, 1977.

509. Wyrobek, A.J., and W.R. Bruce. The induction of sperm-shape abnormalities in mice and humans, pp. 257-285. In A. Hollaender and F.J. de Serres, Eds. Chemical Mutagens: Principles and Methods for Their Detection. Vol. 5. New York: Plenum Press, 1978.

510. Wyrobek, A.J., J.G. Burkhart, M.C. Francis, L.A. Gordon, R.W. Kapp, G. Letz, H.V. Malling, J.C. Topham, and M.D. Whorton. A review of the mouse-sperm-morphology assay and other animal-sperm assays, pp. 57-58. In Current Status of Bioassays in Genetic Toxicology (GENE-TOX). Conference held December 3-5, 1980. Washington, D.C.: U.S. Environmental Protection Agency, 1980. (abstract)

511. Yahagi, T., M. Nagao, T. Seino, T. Matsushima, T. Sugimura, and M. Okada. Mutagenicities of N-nitrosamines on Salmonella. Mutat. Res. 48:121-130, 1977.

512. Yamaguchi, H., S. Tano, A. Tarasa, S. Hirai, K. Hasegawa, and M. Hiraki. Mutations induced in germinating barley seed by diethylsulphate treatment at the interphase, pp. 393-399. In IAEA. Polyploidy and Induced Mutations in Plant Breeding. Vienna: International Atomic Energy Agency, 1972.

513. Yamasaki, E., and B.N. Ames. Concentration of mutagens from urine by adsorption with the nonpolar resin XAD-2: Cigarette smokers have mutagenic urine. Proc. Natl. Acad. Sci. U.S.A. 74:3555-3559, 1977.

514. Zimmering, S., and K.L. Kammermeyer. Potentiation of chromosome loss induced in the paternal genome by methyl methanesulfonate and procarbazine following matings with repair deficient mei-9^a females of Drosophila melanogaster. Environ. Mutagenesis 2:515-520, 1980.

515. Zimmermann, F.K. A yeast strain for visual screening for the two reciprocal products of mitotic crossing over. Mutat. Res 21:263-269, 1973.

516. Zimmermann, F.K., R. Kern, and H. Rasenberger. A yeast strain for simultaneous detection of induced mitotic crossing over, mitotic gene conversion and reverse mutation. Mutat. Res. 28:381-388, 1975.

517. Zimmermann, F.K., and I. Scheel. Induction of mitotic gene conversion in strain D7 of Saccharomyces cerevisiae by 42 coded chemicals, pp. 481-490. In F.J. de Serres and J. Ashby, Eds. Evaluation of Short-Term Tests for Carcinogens. New York: Elsevier/North-Holland, 1981.

518. Zimmermann, F.K., and R. Schwaier. Induction of mitotic gene conversion with nitrous acid, 1-methyl-3-nitro-1-nitrosoguanidine and other alkylating agents in Saccharomyces cerevisiae. Molec. Gen. Genet. 100:63-76, 1967.

519. Zimmermann, F.K., R. Schwaier, and U. von Laer. Mitotic recombination induced in Saccharomyces cerevisiae with nitrous acid, diethylsulfate and carcinogenic, alkylating nitrosamides. Z. Vererbungsl. 98:230-246, 1966.

520. Zimmermann, F.K., R.C. von Borstel, J.M. Parry, D. Siebert, G. Zetterberg, E.S. von Halle, R. Barale, and N. Loprieno. GENE-TOX workshop program: Report on Saccharomyces cerevisiae. Mutat. Res. (in press)

521. Zubroff, J., and D.S. Sarma. A nonradioactive method for measuring DNA damage and its repair in non-proliferating tissues. Anal. Biochem. 70:387-396, 1976.

A